Conceptual Basis for Rural Nursing

Helen J. Lee, RN, PhD, is an Associate Professor in the Montana State University-Bozeman College of Nursing, Missoula Campus. She teaches undergraduate students in medical surgical nursing and research and graduate students in nursing theory. She obtained her BSN and MN from Montana State University-Bozeman, and a PhD in nursing from The University of Texas at Austin. A native of Montana, she has research interests in rurality, hardiness, perception of health, mobility, and gerontological issues.

Conceptual Basis for Rural Nursing

Helen J. Lee, RN, PhD,
Editor

Springer Publishing Company

Springer Publishing Company, Inc.
536 Broadway
New York, NY 10012-3955

Cover design by Janet Joachim
Acquisitions Editor: Ruth Chasek
Production Editor: Helen Song

00 01 02 / 5 4 3 2

Library of Congress Cataloging-in-Publication Data

Conceptual basis for rural nursing / [edited by] Helen J. Lee.
p. cm.
Includes bibliographical references and index.
1. Rural nursing. I. Lee, Helen J.
[DNLM; 1. Nursing. 2. Rural Health Services—United States.
WY 101 C744 1998]
RT120.R87C66 1998
610.73'43—dc21
DNLM/DLC for Library of Congress 98-18898
CIP

Printed in the United States of America

This book is dedicated to Anna M. Shannon. Her vision, foresight, and commitment provided the structure through which rural nursing theory development had its beginning.

Contents

Contributors

Michelle Bailey, MN, RNCS, FNP, graduated from the rural family nurse practitioner graduate program at Montana State University-Bozeman College of Nursing. She is certified by the ANCC as a Family Nurse Practitioner. She is Adjunct Assistant Professor at the Montana State University-Bozeman College of Nursing and at the Gallatin Community Clinic in Bozeman. During summer 1997 she worked as FNP in the Montana Migrant Council at Fairview and Polson. Previous professional nursing experience includes work with migrant farm workers in northern Colorado and in geriatrics at the Gallatin Rest Home in Bozeman, Montana. Her special interests include transcultural nursing.

Jean Ballantyne,* MN, RN, is an Assistant Professor and Campus Director at Montana State University-Bozeman College of Nursing, Billings Campus. Her specialty area is medical-surgical nursing. She has served as a member and President of the Montana Board of Nursing. Her background includes sixteen years of experience in rural hospital nursing.

Robert J. Boik, PhD, is a Professor of Statistics in the Department of Mathematical Sciences at Montana State University-Bozeman. He teaches in the undergraduate and graduate statistics programs, conducts research, and consults on behavioral science applications. His research interests include linear models and multivariate analysis. He earned a BA degree in Psychology from St. Thomas University, MA and PhD degrees in experimental psychology from Baylor University, and MS and PhD degrees in statistics from Temple University.

*Asterisks indicate members of the editorial board.

Janice A. Buehler,* PhD, RN, is an Associate Professor in the College of Nursing, Montana State University-Bozeman, Billings Campus. She teaches psychiatric-mental health nursing in the undergraduate program and a rural nursing course in the graduate program. She earned her BS in Nursing from Oregon Health Sciences Center, her MS in Psychiatric-mental Nursing from the University of Colorado, and her PhD from University of California, San Francisco.

Catherine D. Caniparoli, MSN, RNCS, ANP, is an Assistant Professor of Nursing in the College of Nursing at Montana State University-Bozeman, Great Falls Campus. She teaches Legal-Ethical Issues in Nursing and Physiological Concepts of Nursing to undergraduates and various courses in the graduate Family Nurse Practitioner's option. She earned her BSN from the University of Portland and certified as an Adult Nurse Practitioner through the American Nurses Association. She has had several faculty primary health care practices and is a member of several professional organizations.

Patricia Carrick, MN, RN, FNP, lives in Dillon, MT where she has worked as a rural hospital nurse for ten years. In that practice she has had opportunities to assist patients in experiences from birth to death and everything between, a spectrum of practice she believes to be unrivaled in any other setting. She loves to travel, struggles with her Spanish language skills, enjoys climbing uphill on skis and lugging heavy loads into remote places. Currently she is obsessed with defining a new practice as a nurse practitioner and applying her communication skills to the business of parenting her beloved teen-aged daughter.

Kathleen Chafey, PhD, RN, is a Professor in the College of Nursing, Montana State University-Bozeman. She holds a BSN from Arizona State University and a MS in Public Health Nursing from the School of Public Health at the University of Minnesota. Her PhD is from the University of Minnesota with an emphasis in developmental psychology, specifically moral development; her dissertation was selected "dissertation of the year" by the Association for Moral Education. Her current research interest includes ethical issues in health care, especially issues of autonomy in aging populations.

Shirley A. Cudney, MA, RNCS, GNP, is a retired Associate Professor from Montana State University-Bozeman College of Nursing where she taught for 18 years. She is certified by the ANA as a Gerontological Nurse Practitioner and was the Principal Investigator of the Nursing Approaches to Quality Care for the Elderly project. In her retirement, she is the nurse monitor for the *Women to Women* outreach project, a telecommunication support group for rural women with chronic illness. She received her BSN from Montana State College and her MA in Nursing Education from Teachers' College, Columbia University, New York.

Barbara A. Derwinski-robinson,* MSN, RNC, is an Associate Professor in the College of Nursing, Montana State University-Bozeman, Billings Campus. She teaches undergraduate and graduate maternity-health care of women nursing and undergraduate research. She earned a diploma from Scranton State General Hospital School of Nursing and a BSN and MSN from the University of Pennsylvania. She is a certified women's health care nurse practitioner, sits on the editorial board of the *Journal of Perinatology* and is a Manuscript reviewer for *Image: The Journal of Nursing Scholarship.* She is a member of Sigma Theta Tau and AWHONN and an educational affiliate of ACOG.

Debra A. Doll, BSN, RN, CPTC, is a regional organ procurement coordinator for LifeCenter Northwest, the federally designated organ procurement agency for Washington, Montana, and Alaska. She earned her BSN from Montana State University-Bozeman and has worked in critical care, home care, and as an LPN clinical educator. She has had more than ten years' experience in organ donation, has completed her certification as a procurement transplant coordinator and is currently pursuing certification as a bereavement specialist in death education. She is a member of the American Association for Death Education and Counseling.

Julia Ann Dybbro, MN, RN, is a 1997 graduate of Montana State University-Bozeman in the Family Nursing Practitioner Master of Nursing program. She has baccalaureate degrees in anthropology and nursing. Currently, she is enrolled in doctoral study at the University of Wisconsin, Milwaukee.

Linda L. Grossman, MN, RN is a 1997 graduate of Montana State University-Bozeman in the Rural Family Nurse Practitioner Master of Nursing program. She earned a BS in nursing from Boise State University and a BS in biology from Southern Utah State College. She has worked in critical care nursing in northwest Montana for six years and plans to continue working as a family nurse practitioner in a rural Montana community.

Doris Henson, MS, MPH, RN, is an Assistant Professor in the College of Nursing at Montana State University-Bozeman. She teaches undergraduate community health nursing and nursing management. She holds a B.S.N. from South Dakota State University, an MS from the University of Colorado, and a MPH from the University of California-Berkeley. She is a member of Sigma Theta Tau, the American Public Health Association, and the National Rural Health Association.

Brett R. Hollis, MN, RN, FNP, is a Faculty Nurse Practitioner in Missoula, Montana. His BSN and MN degrees are from Montana State University-Bozeman. He also holds a Bachelor of Arts in Anthropology/Biology from Kent State University.

Sharon Kiely Howard, MS, RN, CS, is an adjunct Assistant Professor in the College of Nursing at Montana State University-Bozeman, Great Falls Campus. As a native Montanan she received her BSN from Montana State University-Bozeman and her MS from the University of Portland. She is credentialed as a clinical specialist in community health nursing. She teaches undergraduate community health nursing and fosters faculty practice sites and contracts for nursing services. She develops and supervises clinical experiences for nursing students in rural settings distant from the nursing campus. She has been involved in community and professional education about HIV/AIDS and related issues for more than ten years on the local, state and national level. She is a member of MNA, ANA, Sigma Theta Tau, and the American Public Health Association.

Sharon R. Hovey, MN, RNC, is an Associate Professor at Montana State University-Bozeman College of Nursing and is the Great Falls Campus Director. She has practiced in a variety of clinical settings and teaches in the undergraduate curriculum. She is nationally certified in maternal and child health and has conducted research in prenatal care, women's health, and spiritual care. Her specific interests relate to the health and stressors experienced by rural women. She is a member of the American Nurses Association, Sigma Theta Tau International, and the Association of Women's Health, Obstetric and Neonatal Nurses.

Vonna Koehler, PhD, RN, is an Assistant Professor in the Montana State University-Bozeman College of Nursing, Billings Campus. She teaches both undergraduate and graduate students in medical-surgical nursing and primary care. She holds a BSN and MN from Montana State University-Bozeman, and a PhD in physiological nursing from the University of Utah. She was a Robert Wood Johnson Faculty Fellow in Primary Care and is currently preparing for certification as an Adult Nurse Practitioner. She is a member of Sigma Theta Tau International, Phi Kappa Phi, and the American Nurses' Association.

Kathleen Ann Long, PhD, RNCS, FAAN, is Professor and Dean, College of Nursing at the University of Florida. She holds a PhD from Johns Hopkins University, an MSN from Wayne State University, and a BSN from Catholic University. From 1983 through 1995 she was a faculty member and administrator (dean, 1990–95) at Montana State University-Bozeman. Dr. Long has published and spoken extensively on rural nursing theory and practice with particular emphasis on mental health, substance abuse prevention, and the health issues of Native Americans.

Kathleen A. McClain, MN, RNCS, FNP, received her BSN and her MN from Montana State University-Bozeman College of Nursing. She is certified by the American Nurses Association as a family nurse practitioner and is a member of Sigma Theta Tau.

A. Gretchen McNeely, DNSc, RNC, is an Associate Professor and the Dean of the St. Mark's-Westminster School of Nursing at Westminster College of Salt Lake City, Utah. Before her position at Westminster College, Dr. McNeely was Assistant Dean at Montana State University-Bozeman. She earned a BSN from Biola University, an MSN in Family-Child Nursing from Loma Linda University, and a DNSc in Nursing Education Administration at the University of San Diego. Dr. McNeely is certified in pediatric nursing and maintains active membership in many professional organizations including ANA and STTI.

Janis M. Majerus, MN, RN, is the Vice-President of Clinical Services at Northern Rocky Mountain Easter Seal Society, managing adult and child care, Case Management, Home Care and Hospice departments, in Montana, Wyoming, and Idaho. She has worked in acute care in the roles of a staff nurse educator, a quality assurance and process improvement coordinator, and the Project Coordinator for "Strengthen Hospital Nursing," a Robert Wood Johnson & PEW Charitable Trust Grant. She received her BSN and MN from Montana State University-Bozeman. She is a charter member of Zeta Upsilon Chapter of Sigma Theta Tau.

Maureen Malone, MN, RN, is a Public Health Nurse with the Indian Health Service. She earned a BSN from the University of Maryland and MN from Montana State University-Bozeman.

Sarah McNerney, MN, RN, is a 1997 graduate of Montana State University-Bozeman in the Rural Family Nurse Practitioner Master of Nursing program. She also received her BSN from Montana State University-Bozeman. She has worked in acute care nursing for eleven years. She plans to work as a family nurse practitioner in rural Montana.

Deborah D. Myers, MN, RN, is an Assistant Professor in the College of Nursing at Montana State University-Bozeman, Billings Campus. She teaches undergraduate psychosocial and psychiatric nursing courses. She received her BSN and her MN in rural nursing with a clinical focus in psychiatric nursing from Montana State University-Bozeman. She is a member of American Psychiatric Nurses Association and Sigma Theta Tau.

Alice Running, PhD, RN, CS (ANP), is the Orvis Endowed Professor and Coordinator of the Family Nurse Practitioner Program at the Orvis School of Nursing, University of Nevada, Reno. She received her BSN from Minot State College, Minot, ND, her MS from the University of Portland, Portland, OR, and her PhD from the University of Colorado Health Sciences Center-School of Nursing, Denver, CO. Dr. Running was a faculty member at Montana State University from 1992–1995.

Teresa Sadler, MN, RN, CFNP, is a Family Nurse Practitioner in a family practice clinic in rural Arizona. She earned her BS in nursing from Northern Arizona University, and an MN in nursing and nurse practitioner degree from Montana State University-Bozeman. She is a member of Sigma Theta Tau.

Jane Ellis Scharff, MN, RN, CNAA, is a doctoral student at the University of Rochester School of Nursing in Rochester, NY. Her bachelor of science and master of nursing degrees were earned at Montana

State University where she then served as assistant professor of medical-surgical nursing. She earned a nurse practitioner certificate from the University of Colorado and worked in private practice for several years. Most recently a member of the management team at one of Montana's urban hospitals, she is certified in advanced nursing administration. She hopes to return to Montana and build a research program around social policy and its relevance to nursing knowledge and practice.

Anna M. Shannon, DNS, RN, is Dean Emeritus and Professor Emeritus in the College of Nursing at Montana State University-Bozeman. She is a psychiatric nurse and has taught at both the undergraduate and graduate levels. She is a graduate of Missouri Baptist Hospital School of Nursing. She earned a BS in nursing from the University of Missouri, Columbia, an MS in nursing from Washington University, St. Louis, and a DNS from the University of California, San Francisco.

M. Jean Shreffler, PhD, RN, is an Assistant Professor at Montana State University-Bozeman College of Nursing, Missoula Campus. She teaches both graduate and undergraduate nursing management and community health. She earned her BSN and MSN from the University of Cincinnati, College of Nursing and Health, and a PhD in nursing science from the University of Washington. Her scholarly interests are in rural health care, specifically access to care for frontier residents.

Therese Sullivan,* PhD, RN, is an Adjunct Associate Professor in the College of Nursing at Montana State University-Bozeman. She earned her PhD at the University of Washington. Her speciality area is Gerontological Nursing and her interest areas are concept development and nursing history. She is the Archivist for Zeta Upsilon Chapter of Sigma Theta Tau International and is currently engaged in a nursing research study of the Master's Degree Program at the College of Nursing, Montana State University-Bozeman.

Dena J. Sutermaster, MSN, RN, is an Associate Professor in the College of Nursing, Montana State University-Bozeman, Billings Campus. She teaches junior undergraduates medical-surgical and gerontological nursing. She earned her BSN and MSN from the University of Pittsburgh. Her master's speciality was nursing education. Before teaching, she worked in medical-surgical nursing in the roles of a staff nurse, an assistant patient care manager, and an ostomy nurse. She is an active member of several organizations including the Zeta Upsilon Chapter of Sigma Theta Tau, the Montana Nurses' Association, and the Billings Chapter for the Prevention of Elder Abuse.

Teresa S. Turnbull, MN, RN, FNP-C, is a Family Nurse Practitioner in the town of Stevensville in the Bitterroot Valley of Montana. She earned her BSN and MN from Montana State University-Bozeman. She is a member of ANA, Sigma Theta Tau, AANP, and the Montana APRN Association for which she is the state newsletter editor. She supports environmental and humanitarian organizations based in Missoula, MT, where she resides with her husband, Donovan, and daughter, Phoebe.

Sarah Walton, MN, RNCS, FNP, CEN, practices as a Family Nurse Practitioner in Big Timber, Montana. She received her bachelor's and Master's degree in nursing from Montana State University-Bozeman.

Clarann Weinert, SC, PhD, RN, FAAN, is a Professor in the College of Nursing, Montana State University-Bozeman. For the past 15 years she has taught undergraduate and graduate nursing students and conducted research in social support measurement, family adaptation to chronic illness, and rural health. She received a BSN from the College of Mt. St. Joseph, a MS from the Ohio State University, and a MA and PhD in Sociology from the University of Washington.

Carolyn Wenger, RN, MSN, is a faculty member at Montana State University-Bozeman, Billings campus. She received her BSN from the State University of New York at Buffalo and her MSN from Case Western Reserve University. She is Past President of the Yellowstone County Homeless Board, a coalition of service providers to the homeless. She is a member of Sigma Theta Tau, American Nurses Association, and the American Public Health Association.

Ellen F. Wirtz, MN, RNC, is the Patient Travel Program Coordinator for Fort Harrison Veterans Administration Medical Center in Helena, MT. She is developing, implementing, and managing a pilot program to facilitate interfacility and intrafacility patient travel. She has taught as Associate professor at Montana State University-Northern and has thirteen years of nursing experience. She holds ANA certification in medical surgical nursing. She earned her BSN and MN degrees from Montana State University-Bozeman.

Preface

This book is an attempt to provide a conceptual basis for the practice of rural nursing. It reflects the work of over 20 years by the Rural Nursing Theory Special Committee at the College of Nursing, Montana State University-Bozeman. This work was initiated through the vision of Anna Shannon who came to the sparsely populated state of Montana in 1975, and who developed the initial project at MSU. The project is ongoing, and is enhanced by the continued involvement of graduate nursing students.

To set the stage for reading the content of this book, let me take you on a drive through the area where I live—rural Montana. We are driving on Highway 200 from Missoula east to Great Falls. Missoula is a thriving university city of approximately 50,000. After leaving Interstate 90 a few miles east of Missoula, we drive the two lane highway through two small towns, one of which contains a lumber company. After that, the houses become fewer; the next gathering of buildings is Clearwater Junction, 40 miles away from Missoula. This gathering consists of a gas station, a restaurant, and the State of Montana truck weighing station. We then begin the gradual ascent toward the Continental Divide. We continue east to the small town of Lincoln, 40 miles further down the road. The scenery is beautiful—mountains, sometimes close at hand and always within view—and valley floors with cultivated hay crops and grazing animals. It is a pastoral scene; however, the controversial clear cutting of evergreens is evident on many mountain sides.

We arrive at Lincoln (the recent home of the Unibomber suspect), 10 miles to the west of the Divide. There are several motels and gas stations, all ready for the summer tourists, the hunters in the fall, and the snowmobilers during the winter. We stop at the Conoco station to refresh ourselves. We have a sense of being outsiders in this small town that thrives on people passing through and yet, simultaneously, feel like insiders because we are greeted by familiar faces at the station.

Back in the car, the ascent to Roger's Pass continues gradually. Then, suddenly, we are on top of the Divide and begin descending rapidly through a series of switchbacks. A few miles down this steep incline, we note two or three homes nestled up against the mountainside. Soon we come to the Montana Highway Department sand and gravel site. Two homes are there; since it is spring, the activity is nil. their busy time starts when the snow flies, and, believe me, the winter storms can bring with them some wicked driving conditions.

As we travel east, the mountain scenery is gradually replaced with that of the high mountain plains. A saying heard frequently in Montana, "On a clear day, you can see forever," is truly applicable. At times during this stretch of the drive in the high mountain desert, one can only see fence posts and barbed wire lining each side of the road and an occasional herd of grazing Black Angus cattle. There are no visible ranches or telephone poles. If one scans the landscape the full radius of 360 degrees, the fence and the cattle and an occasional vehicle on the ribbon of highway in front and behind us are the only signs of humanity. What would happen if we had car trouble? How long would it be before someone came along? Would they stop and help or would they pass by, thinking that someone else would eventually come along? Would the car phone I recently acquired have enough power to transmit to a towing service, wherever the nearest one is? Would someone be available at that service? How long would it take for them to reach us?

As we continue east, there are a couple of missile sites off each side of the highway. The sites are both serviced by Malmstrom Air Force Base in Great Falls. A 4-wheeled vehicle is the only evidence that one of the sites is manned. Soon, we descend into the valley formed by the Sun River; homes and ranches begin appearing. Small towns with pasted speed limits appear. Rolling plains replace the mountains. Irregular land shapes like square buttes appear in the horizon. The ranching activity (grazing cattle and hay fields) is now combined with the raising of small grain crops.

We soon become aware that we are approaching the city of Great Falls because of increasing numbers of visible homes and billboard signs along the highway. For the last 11 miles into Great Falls we are again able to drive on the Interstate. Soon we arrive at Great Falls—another pocket of civilization (60,000 population) in this scarcely inhabited state.

Obviously, the drive of 170 lonely miles through a wild and beautiful and nearly empty landscape provides only a brief glimpse of the rural environment to which Anna Shannon came in 1975. This environment stimulated Anna and her cohorts, Jacqueline Taylor and Ruth Ludemann, to ask questions about what was different about nursing in such a place. What was different about the people who live in or chose to come to this environment? How does nursing provide care for rural people under circumstances different from those in an urban environment? How do nurses coming from different environments adapt to providing care? These questions stimulated the quest to search for ways to better meet the nursing needs of the people living in rural areas better.

This book reports on the continued quest to provide theoretical structure, a seeking of patterns which ultimately will help rural nurses provide better care for persons in rural environments. Part I contains background information on rural nursing theory development. The chapters in Part II give the reader an analysis of crucial concepts to rural nursing. Part III includes chapters reporting on the perspective of rural persons about health, self-reliance, independence, and hardiness. Rural nursing care is the focus of Part IV; selected rural clinical issues are covered in Part V. Many facets of health care resources are addressed in Part VI. The book concludes with suggestions for future direction in rural theory development.

All of us involved in this project hope that the work contained in the following pages sheds more light on how nurses can best bring the best of their knowledge and skills to meet the special challenges of practice in rural settings.

ACKNOWLEDGMENTS

A book such as this does not happen without the assistance of a great number of individuals. First, I wish to acknowledge the untiring efforts of the members of the editorial board—Jean Ballantyne, Janice A. Buehler, Barbara A. Derwinski-robinson, and Therese Sullivan. They came through for me many times, and sometimes on quite short notice.

The working group of the Rural Nursing Theory Special Committee who meet monthly by teleconference, three to five p.m., on the last Friday of each month, also deserve special thanks. They are Jean Ballantyne, Janice A. Buehler, Barbara A. Derwinski-robinson, Catherine D. Caniparoli, Doris Henson, A. Gretchen McNeely, Deborah D. Myers, Jane E. Scharff, M. Jean Shreffler, Therese Sullivan, Dena J. Sutermaster, and Carolyn H. Wenger. It seems pretty amazing that we were able to accomplish what we did considering the time of the week we were meeting.

I also wish to acknowledge a monetary grant received from the Montana Consortium for Excellence in Health Care. These monies came to us through the efforts of Jane E. Scharff. The Consortium funded two of the chapters (Buehler, chapter 26; Derwinski-robinson, Lee, Ballantyne, and Scharff, chapter 33) within the book and is helping to support publication of this book. It also lifted our spirits when they were beginning to lag.

Two persons really came through for me and quite often on short notice. Mary Snepenger, Office of Applied Research, scanned many chapters because of incompatible computer formats and did many statistical computer runs until the right information was obtained.

I

INTRODUCTION

This introduction contains three chapters that introduce the reader to the rural theory development. The first, is a seminal article published in 1989, which made the nursing community at-large aware of the rural nursing theory development activity at Montana State University-Bozeman. The second chapter is written by an individual who conducted an exemplary study of what is distinctive about rural nursing. The study involved rural nurses in western Montana, northern Idaho, and eastern Washington. In the third chapter, the authors describe a graduate nursing curricula used in educating the rural nursing generalist.

1

Rural Nursing: Developing the Theory Base*

Kathleen Ann Long and Clarann Weinert

A logger suffering from "heart lock" does not have a cardiovascular abnormality. He is suffering from a work-related anxiety disorder and can be assisted by an emergency room nurse who accurately assesses his needs and responds with effective communication and a supportive interpersonal relationship. A farmer who has lost his finger in a grain thresher several hours earlier does not have time during the harvesting season for a discussion of occupational safety. He will cope with his injury assisted by a clinic nurse who can adjust the timing of his antibiotic doses to fit with his work schedule in the fields.

Many health care needs of rural dwellers cannot be adequately addressed by the application of nursing models developed in urban or suburban areas but require unique approaches emphasizing the special needs of this population. While nurses are significant, and frequently the sole, health care providers for people living in rural areas, little has been written to guide the practice of rural nursing.

Acknowledgments: Qualitative data collected and analyzed by Montana State University, College of Nursing graduate students and faculty, form the basis for a substantial portion of this paper. Ethnographic data collection and analysis was supported, in part, by a U.S. Department of Health and Human Services, Division of Nursing, Advanced Training Grant to the Montana State University, College of Nursing (#1816001649AI). The project that provided the survey data was funded by a Montana State University Faculty Research/ Creativity Grant. This article is based partially on a paper presented at the Western Society for Research in Nursing Conference, Tempe, AZ, May 1987.

**Note.* From "Rural Nursing: Developing the Theory Base," by K. A. Long and C. Weinert, 1989, *Scholarly Inquiry for Nursing Practice: An International Journal, 3,* pp. 113–127.

The literature provides vignettes and individual descriptions, but there is a need for an integrated, theoretical approach to rural nursing.

Rural nursing is defined as the provision of health care by professional nurses to persons living in sparsely populated areas. Over the past 8 years, graduate students and faculty members at the Montana State University College of Nursing, have worked toward developing a theory base for rural nursing. Theory development has used primarily a retroductive approach, and data have been collected and refined using a combination of qualitative and quantitative methods. The experiences of rural residents and rural nurses have guided the identification of key concepts relevant to rural nursing. The goal of the theory building process has been to identify commonalties and differences in nursing practice across all rural areas and the common and unique elements of rural nursing in relation to nursing overall. The implications of developing a theory of rural nursing for practice have been examined as a part of the ongoing process.

The theory building process was initiated in the late 1970s. At that time, literature and research related to rural health care were limited and focused primarily on the problem of retaining physicians in rural areas and providing assessments of rural health care needs and prescriptions for rural health care services based on models and experiences from urban and suburban areas (Coward, 1977; Flax, Wagenfield, Ivens, & Weiss, 1979). The unique health problems and health care needs of extremely sparsely populated states, such as Montana, had not been addressed from the perspective of the rural consumer. No organized theoretical base for guiding rural health care practice in general, or rural nursing in particular, existed.

QUALITATIVE DATA

The target population for qualitative data collection was the people of Montana. Montana, the fourth largest state in the United States, is an extremely sparsely populated state, with nearly 800,000 people and an average population density of approximately five persons per square mile. One half of the counties in Montana have three or fewer persons per square mile, with six of those counties having less than one person per square mile. There is only one metropolitan center in the state; it is a city of nearly 70,000 people, with a surrounding area that constitutes a center of approximately 100,000 *(Population Profiles, 1985).*

Qualitative data were collected through ethnographic study by Montana State University College of Nursing graduate students. These data provided the initial ideas about health and health care in Montana. Since general propositions about rural health and rural health care did not exist, the gathering of concrete data was the first step toward subsequent development of more general theoretical propositions.

Graduate students used ethnographic techniques as described by Spradley (1979) to gather information from individuals, families, and health service providers. Interview sites were selected by students on the basis of specific interest and convenience. During a 6-year period, data were gathered from approximately 25 locations. In general, each student worked in depth in one community, collecting data from 10 to 20 informants over a period of at least 1 year. Data were gathered primarily from persons in ranching and farming areas and from towns of less than 2,500 persons. In some instances, student interest led to extensive interviews with specific rural subgroups, such as men in the logging industry or elderly residents in a rural town (Weinert & Long, 1987). Open-ended interview questions were developed using Spradley's (1979) guidelines. The questions emphasized seeking the informants' views without superimposing the cultural biases of the interviewer. The opening question in the interview was, "What is health to you . . . from your viewpoint? . . . your definition?" Interviewers used standard probes and a standard format of questions regarding health beliefs and health care preferences.

Spradley (1979) indicated that the goal of ethnographic study is to "build a systematic understanding of all human cultures from the perspective of those who have learned them" (p. 10). The goal of data collection in Montana was to learn about the culture of rural Montanans from rural Montanans. Emphasis in the cultural learning process was on understanding health beliefs, values, and practices. Rigdon, Clayton, and Diamond (1987) have noted that understanding the meaning that persons attach to subjective experiences is an important aspect of nursing knowledge. The ethnographic approach captured the meanings that rural dwellers ascribe to the subjective states of health and illness and facilitated the development of a rich data base.

As the data base developed, the following definitions and assumptions were accepted as a foundation for theory development. Rural was defined as meaning sparsely populated. Within this context, states such as Montana, which are sparsely populated overall, are viewed as rural throughout, despite the existence of some population centers within them. Further, based on this definition, rural regions or areas can be identified within otherwise heavily populated states. The assumption is made that, to some degree, health care needs are different in rural areas from that of urban areas. Also, all rural areas are viewed as having some common health care needs. Finally, the assumption is made that urban models are not appropriate to, or adequate for, meeting health care needs in rural areas.

Retroductive Theory Generation

Faculty work groups were developed to examine and organize the qualitative data. The work groups involved three to five nursing faculty members, each with rural nursing experience, but with varied backgrounds and expertise. Thus, a work group included experts from various clinical areas, as well as persons with direct experience either in small rural hospitals or in larger, metropolitan centers within rural states. Standard ethnographic content analysis (Spradley, 1979) was used to sort and categorize the ethnographic data. Groups worked toward consensus about the meaning and organization of specific data. Recurring themes were identified, and these were viewed as having relevance and importance for the rural informants in relation to their views of health.

A retroductive approach, as originally described by Hanson (1958), was used to examine the initial ethnographic data and build the theory base. Specific concepts and relational statements were derived from the data, and more general propositions were induced from these statements. The new propositions were then used to develop additional specific statements which could be supported by existing data or which were categorized for later testing. The retroductive approach was literally a "back and forth" process that permitted persons familiar with the data to move between the data and beginning-level theoretical propositions. The process was orderly and consistent and required group consensus about data interpretation and the relevance of derived propositions. The retroductive process continued in work groups over several years as additional ethnographic data were gathered. Consultants participated at key points in the process, in order to raise questions, add insights, and critically evaluate the group's theory building approach. Walker and Avant (1983) have noted that the retroductive process "adds considerably to the body of theoretical knowledge. It is, in fact, the way theory develops in the 'real world' " (p. 176).

QUANTITATIVE DATA

Following several years of ethnographic study, the faculty members involved in theory development wished to enrich the qualitative data base by collecting relevant quantitative data. Kleinman (1983) stated, "Qualitative description, taken together with various quantitative measures, can be a standardized research method for assessing validity. It is especially valuable in studying social and cultural significance, e.g. illness beliefs interaction norms, social gain, ethnic help seeking, and treatment responses" (p. 543). Hinds and Young (1987) noted, "The combination of different methodologies within a single study promotes the likelihood of uncovering multiple dimensions of a phenomenon's empirical reality" (p. 195).

A survey developed by Weinert in 1983 attempted to validate some of the rural health concepts that had emerged from the ethnographic data. These concepts were: health status and health beliefs, isolation and distance, self-reliance, and informal health care systems. Survey instruments with established psychometric properties were selected to measure the specific concepts of interest. A mail questionnaire completed by the respondents included the Beck Depression Inventory (Beck, 1967) and the Trait Anxiety Scale (Spielberger, Gorsuch, & Lushene, 1970), to tap mental health status, and the General Health Perception Scale (Davies & Ware, 1981), to measure physical health status and health beliefs. A background information form assessed demographic variables, including length of residence and geographic locale. The Personal Resource Questionnaire (Brandt & Weinert, 1981) assessed use of informal systems for support and health care.

The convenience sample of survey participants was located through the Agricultural Extension Service, social groups, and informal networks. All participants lived in Montana, completed the questionnaires in their homes, and returned them by mail to the researcher. The 62 survey participants were middle-class whites, with an average of 13.5 years of education and a mean age of 61.3 years, who had lived in Montana an average of 45.6 years. The survey sample consisted of 40 women and 22 men residing in one of 13 sparsely populated Montana counties. The most populated county has a population density of 5.9 persons per square mile and one town of nearly 6,000 people. In the most sparsely populated county, there is one town of 600 people and an average population density of 0.5 persons per square mile.

Findings from the quantitative study were used throughout the theory development process to support or refute concept descriptions and relational statements derived from the ethnographic data. Survey findings are discussed in the following section as they relate to key concepts and relational statements.

REFINING THE BUILDING BLOCKS OF THEORY

To order the data and foster the formation of relational statements, an organizational scheme for theory development was adopted. Using the paradigm first described by Yura and Torres (1975) and later by Fawcett (1984), ethnographic data were categorized under the four major dimensions of nursing theory: person, health, environment, and nursing. The data were then ordered from the more general to the more specific. This process led to the identification of constructs, concepts, variables, and indicators.

An example helps to illustrate this process. Ethnographic data had been gathered from "gypo" loggers. These men are independent logging contractors from northwestern Montana who work in rugged isolated areas, usually living in trailers or tents while working. Examples of quotes from these loggers and their associates as found in the data are: A logger states, "We worry about the here and now"; a local physician says, "Loggers enter the health care system during times of crisis only"; the public health nurse in the area says, "Loggers don't want to hear about health care problems; they don't return until the next accident."

Table 1.1 shows the scheme used to organize these data. The concepts "present time" orientation and crisis orientation to health are identified. These are placed under the person dimension. In this example, the constructs are not fully developed, but are viewed as psychological and/ or sociocultural. The important variables identified thus far are definitions of time and of crisis. Possible indicators are measures of time, such as hours or seasons, and measures of crisis, such as numbers of illnesses or injuries.

TABLE 1.1 Data Ordering Scheme

Component	Examples
Dimension	Person
Construct	Psychological/sociocultural
Concept	"Present time" orientation
	Crisis orientation to health
Variable	Definitions of time
	Definitions of crisis
Indicators	Hours, minutes, days
	Seasons, work seasons
	Number of injuries
	Number of illnesses

Key Concepts

In the process of data organization it was noted that some concepts appeared repeatedly in ethnographic data collected in several different areas of the state. In addition, aspects of several of these concepts were supported by the quantitative survey data (Weinert, 1983). Using Walker and Avant's (1983) model of concept synthesis, these concepts were identified as key concepts in relation to understanding rural health needs and rural nursing practice. These key concepts are as follows: work beliefs and health beliefs, isolation and distance, self reliance, lack of anonymity, outsider/insider, and old timer/newcomer.

As key concepts in this theory, work beliefs and health beliefs are viewed as different for rural dwellers as contrasted with urban or suburban residents. These two sets of beliefs appear to be closely interrelated among rural persons. Work, or the fulfilling of one's usual functions, is of primary importance. Health is assessed by rural people in relation to work role and work activities, and health needs are usually secondary to work needs.

The related concepts of isolation and distance are identified as important in understanding rural health and nursing. Specifically, they help in understanding health care-seeking behavior. Quantitative survey data indicated that rural informants who lived outside of towns traveled a distance of almost 23 miles, on average, for emergency health care and over 50 miles for routine health care. Despite these distances, ethnographic data indicated that rural dwellers tended to see health services as accessible and did not view themselves as isolated.

Self-reliance and independence of rural persons are also seen as key concepts. The desire to do for oneself and care for oneself was strong among the rural persons interviewed and has important ramifications in relation to the provision of health care.

Two key concept areas, lack of anonymity and outsider/insider, have particular relevance for the practice of rural nursing. Lack of anonymity, a hallmark of small towns and surrounding sparsely populated areas, implies a limited ability for rural persons to have private areas of their lives. Rural nurses almost always reported being known to their patients as neighbors, part of a given family, members of a certain church, and so on. Similarly, these nurses usually know their patients in several different social and personal relationships beyond the nurse-patient relationship. The old timer/newcomer concept, or the related concepts of outsider/insider, is relevant in terms of the acceptance of nurses and of all health care providers in rural communities. The ethnographic data indicated that these concepts were used by rural dwellers in organizing their view of the social environment and in guiding their interactions and relationships. Survey data revealed that those who had lived in Montana over 10 years, but less than 20, still considered themselves to be "newcomers" and expected to be viewed as such by those in their community (Weinert & Long, 1987).

Relational Statements

In an effort to move from a purely descriptive theory to a beginning level explanatory one, some initial relational statements were generated from the qualitative data and were supported by the quantitative data that had been collected thus far. The statements are in the early stages of testing.

The first statement is that rural dwellers define health primarily as the ability to work, to be productive, to do usual tasks. The ethnographic data indicate that rural persons place little emphasis on the comfort, cosmetic, and life-prolonging aspects of health. One is viewed as healthy when able to function and be productive in one's work role. Specifically, rural residents indicated that pain was tolerated, often for extended periods, so long as it did not interfere with the ability to function. The General Health Perception Scale indicated that rural survey participants reported experiencing less pain than an age-comparable urban sample (Weinert & Long, 1987). Further, scores on the Beck Depression Inventory and the Trait Anxiety Scale (Weinert, 1983) revealed that they experienced less anxiety and less depression.

The second statement is that rural dwellers are self-reliant and resist accepting help or services from those seen as "outsiders" or from agencies seen as national or regional "welfare" programs. A corollary to this statement is that help, including needed health care, is usually sought through an informal rather than a formal system. Ethnographic data supported both the second statement and its corollary. Numerous references were found showing, for example, a preference for "the `old doc' who knows us" over the new specialist who was unfamiliar. Data from the Personal Resource Questionnaire (Weinert, 1983) indicated that rural dwellers relied primarily on family, relatives, and close friends for help and support. Further, the rural survey respondents reported using health care professionals and formal human service agencies much less frequently than did comparable urban respondents in previous studies.

A third statement is that health care providers in rural areas must deal with a lack of anonymity and much greater role diffusion than providers in urban or suburban settings. This statement has marked significance for rural nursing practice. Although limited ethnographic and survey data have been collected from rural nurses thus far, some emerging themes have been identified. In addition to identifying a sense of isolation from professional peers, rural nurses emphasize their lack of anonymity and a sense of role diffusion. There is an inability to keep separate the activities and behaviors of the individual nurse's various roles. In a small town, for example, the nurse's behavior as a wife, a mother, and a church attendee are all significantly related to her effectiveness as a health care professional in that community. Further, in their professional role, nurses reported experiencing role diffusion. Nurses are expected to perform a variety of diverse and unrelated tasks. On a single shift, a nurse may work in obstetrics delivering a baby, care for a dying patient on the medical-surgical unit, and initiate care of a trauma patient in the emergency room. Likewise, on evening shift or weekends, a nurse may be required to carry out tasks reserved for the pharmacist or dietitian on the day shift.

RELATIONSHIP OF CONCEPTS AND STATEMENTS TO THE LARGER BODY OF NURSING KNOWLEDGE

How people define health and illness has a direct impact on how they seek and use health care services and is a key concept in understanding client behavior and in planning intervention.

Definition of Health

The rural Montana dwellers primarily define health as the ability to work and to be productive. The work of other researchers supports the finding that residents of sparsely populated areas view health in terms of ability to work and remain productive. Ross (1982), a nurse anthropologist, studied the health perceptions of women living in the Lake District along the coast of Nova Scotia. She conducted in-depth interviews with 60 women of both British and French backgrounds in small coastal fishing communities. Similar to the rural dwellers in Montana, these women described good health as being "able to do what you want to do" and to "be able to work." Lee's (1987) recent work in Montana supports earlier findings on which the rural nursing theory was built. She found that work and health practices were closely related among farmers and ranchers; health is viewed as a functional state in relation to work. Scharff's (1987) interviews with nurses practicing in small rural hospitals in eastern Washington, northern Idaho, and western Montana indicated that they viewed the health needs of rural people as overlapping those of people living in urban situations in many instances. The nurse informants, however, noted that rural people equate health with the ability to work or function in their daily activities. Rural people were viewed as delaying health care until they were very ill, thus often needing hospitalization at the point of seeking care.

Self-Reliance

The statement derived from the Montana data that "rural dwellers resist accepting help from outsiders or strangers" has been supported in data from research in rural Maryland (Salisbury State College, 1986). People living in the rural eastern shore area were described as highly resistant to care from persons viewed as outsiders, and rural shore residents often refused to go "across the bridge" to Baltimore to seek health care, even though this was a trip of less than 100 miles and would allow access to sophisticated, specialized treatment. Like the rural people in Montana, these Maryland residents sought health care information and assistance from local, and often informal, sources. The self- reliance of rural persons and their resistance to outside help were also reported by Counts and Boil (1987) in relation to residents of the Appalachian area. Self-reliance was noted as a major feature that must be considered in planning nursing care services for this population.

The rural Nova Scotia women studied by Ross (1982) indicated informal personal networks of family, friends, and neighbors as important sources of health information who also provided the physical, financial, emotional and social support that contributes to well-being. When these women were asked what connection there was between health and the availability of hospitals, doctors, and other medical care, 42% indicated that it was the individual's responsibility for health knowledge and care; 25% thought professionals were useful to a certain point in providing advice and services such as routine physical exams; 19% indicated that these services were for sick persons, not healthy persons; and 9% felt the formal health care system had no relationship to health (Ross, 1982, p. 311). One woman commented, "Health is not a topic to discuss with doctors and nurses" (Ross, 1982, p. 309).

Rural Nursing

The Montana data and the theory derived from it indicate that nurses and other health care providers in rural areas must deal with a lack of anonymity. Nurses are known in a variety of roles to their patients and, in turn, know their patients in a variety of roles. Most of the nurses interviewed by Scharff (1987) felt that by knowing their patients personally they could give better care. Other nurses, however, noted that providing professional care for family or friends can be a frightening experience. Nurses indicated that there was no anonymity for them in the rural community, which, at times, was reassuring and, at other times, constricting (Scharff, 1987).

The concept of role diffusion in the rural hospital setting was very apparent in Scharff's (1987) work. She reported that a rural hospital nurse must be a jack-of-all-trades who often practices within the realm of numerous other health care disciplines, including respiratory therapy, laboratory technology, dietetics, pharmacy, social work, psychology, and medicine. Examples of the intersections between rural nursing and other disciplines include doing EKGs, performing arterial punctures, running blood gas machines, drawing blood, setting up cultures, going to the pharmacy to pour drugs, going to the local drugstore to get medications for patients, ordering x-rays and medications, delivering babies, directing the actions of physicians, and cooking meals when the cook gets snowed in. As Scharff (1987) noted, some of these functions are carried out by urban nurses practicing in particular settings such as a trauma center or intensive care unit. Rural nurses, however, are usually not circumscribed by assignment to a particular unit or department and are expected to function in multiple roles, even within one work shift.

This generalist work role and the lack of anonymity of rural nurses are substantiated by findings and descriptions from several other rural areas of the United States (Biegel, 1983; St. Clair, Pickard, & Harlow, 1986). A study of nurses in rural Texas noted, "Nurses play roles as nurse, friend, neighbor, citizen, and family member" within a community; further, rural nurses in their work roles were described as needing to be "all things to all people" (St. Clair et al., 1986, p. 28).

Generalizability

The issue of a situation or locale-specific theory and its relationship to the larger body of nursing knowledge needs serious consideration. The work of Scharff (1987) indicated that the core of rural nursing is not different from urban nursing. The intersections, however, those "meeting points at which nursing extends its practice into the domains of other professions"; the dimensions, that is, the "philosophy, responsibilities, functions, roles, and skills"; and the boundaries, which "respond to new and growing needs and demands from society" (American Nurses Association, 1980), appear to be very distinct for rural nursing practice.

Questions still remain as to how generalizable findings from Montana residents are to other rural populations. Clearly, there is a need for more organized and rigorous data collection in relation to rural nursing before these questions can be answered. A sound theory base for rural practice requires continued research, conducted across diverse rural settings.

IMPLICATIONS FOR NURSING PRACTICE

The findings from the Montana research about people living in sparsely populated areas have implications for nursing practice in rural areas. Since work is of major importance to rural people, health care must fit within work schedules. Health care programs or clinics which conflict with the rural economic cycle, such as haying or calving, will not be used. Since health is defined as the ability to work, health promotion must address the work issue. For example, health education related to cardiovascular disease should highlight strategies for preventing conditions that involve long-term disability, such as stroke. These aspects will be more meaningful to rural dwellers than preventive aspects that emphasize a longer, more comfortable life.

The self-reliance of rural dwellers has specific nursing implications. Rural people will often delay seeking health care until they are gravely ill or incapacitated. Nursing approaches need to address two distinct aspects: non-judgmental intervention for those who have delayed treatment and a strong emphasis on preventive health teaching. If the nurse can provide adequate health knowledge, the rural dweller's desire for self-reliance may lead to health-promotion behaviors. With a good information base, rural people can make appropriate decisions about self-care versus the need for professional intervention.

Health care services must be tailored to suit the preferences of rural persons for family and community help during periods of illness. Nurses can provide instruction, support, and relief to family members and neighbors, who are often the primary-care providers for sick and disabled persons. The formal health care system needs to fit into the informal helping system in rural areas. A long-term community resident, such as the drugstore proprietor, can be assisted in providing accurate advice to residents through the provision of reference materials and a telephone back-up system. One can anticipate greater acceptance and use by rural residents of an updated but old and trusted health care resource, rather than a new, professional, but "outsider" service (Weinert & Long, 1987).

Nurses who enter rural communities must allow for extended periods prior to acceptance. Involvement in diverse community activities, such as civic organizations and recreational clubs, may assist the nurse in being known and accepted as a person. In rural communities acceptance as a health care professional is often tied to personal acceptance. Thus it appears that rural communities are not appropriate practice settings for nurses who prefer to maintain entirely separate professional and personal lives.

The stresses that appear to affect nurses in rural practice settings have particular importance. Rural nurses see themselves as cut off from the professional mainstream. They are often in situations where there is no collegial support to assist in defining an appropriate practice role and its boundaries. The educational preparation of those who wish to practice in rural settings needs to emphasize not only generalist skills, but also a strong base in change theory and leadership techniques. Nurses in rural practice need a sound orientation to techniques for accessing diverse sources of current information. If the closest library is several hundred miles away, for example, can all arrangement for interlibrary loan and access to material via telephone, bus, or mail be arranged? Networks that link together nurses practicing in distant rural sites are particularly useful, both for information exchange and for mutual support.

SUMMARY

It is becoming increasingly clear that rural dwellers have distinct definitions of health. Their health care needs require approaches that differ significantly from urban and suburban populations. Subcultural values, norms, and belief's play a key role in how rural people define health and from whom they seek advice and care. These values and beliefs, combined with the realities of rural living—such as weather, distance, and isolation—markedly affect the practice of nursing in rural settings. Additional ethnographic and quantitative data are needed to further define both the common and the locale-specific conditions and characteristics of rural populations. Continued research can provide a more solid base for the nursing theory that is required to guide practice and the delivery of health care to rural populations.

REFERENCES

American Nurses Association, (1980). *Nursing. A social policy statement* (No. NP-63 20M 9/82R). Kansas City MO: Author.

Brandt, P., & Weinert, C. (1981). The PRQ: A social support measure. *Nursing Research, 30,* 277–280.

Beck, A. (1967). *Depression: Causes and treatment.* Philadelphia: University of Pennsylvania Press.

Biegel, A. (1983). Toward a definition of rural nursing. *Home Health Care Nursing, 1,* 45–46.

Counts, M., & Boyle, J. (1987). Nursing, health and policy winner a community context. *Advances in Nursing Science, 9,* 12–23.

Coward, R. (1977). Delivering social services in small towns and rural communities. In R. Coward *(Ed.), Rural families across the life span: Implications for community, programming* (pp. 1–17). West Lafayette, IN: Indiana Cooperative Extension Services.

Davies, A., & Ware, J. (1981). *Measuring health perceptions in the health insurance experiment.* Santa Monica, CA: Rand.

Fawcett, J. (1984). *Analysis and evaluation of conceptual models of nursing.* Philadelphia: F. A. Davis.

Flax, J., Wagenfeld, M., Ivens, R., & Weiss, R. (1979). *Mental health and rural America: An overview, and annotated bibliography.* Rockville, MD: U.S. Government Printing Office.

Hanson, N. (1958). *Patterns of discovery.* Cambridge: Cambridge University Press.

Hinds, P., & Young, K. (1987). A triangulation of methods and paradigms to study nurse-given wellness care. *Nursing Research, 36,* 195–198.

Kleinman, A. (1983). The cultural meanings and social uses of illness: A role for medical anthropology and clinically oriented social science in the development of primary care theory and research. *Journal of Family Practice, 16,* 539–545.

Lee, H. (1987). *Relationship of hardiness and current life events to perceived health and rural adults.* Manuscript submitted for publication.

Population profiles of Montana counties: 1980. (1985). Bozeman, MT: Montana State University Center for Data Systems and Analysis.

Rigdon, I., Clayton, B., & Diamond, M. (1987). Toward a theory of helpfulness for the elderly bereaved: An invitation to a new life. *Advances in Nursing Science, 9,* 32–43.

Ross, H. (1982). Women and wellness: Defining, attaining, and maintaining health in Eastern Canada. *Dissertation Abstracts International, 42,* DEO 82–12624.

Salisbury State College (1986, June). *Discussion of Salisbury Slate College rural health findings.* Presented at the Contemporary Issues in Rural Health Conference, Salisbury, MD.

Scharff, J. (1987). *The nature and scope of rural nursing: Distinctive characteristics.* Unpublished master's thesis, Montana State University, Bozeman, MT.

Spielberger, C., Gorsuch, R., & Lushene, R. (1970). *STAI manual for the State-Trait Anxiety Questionnaire.* Palo Alto, CA: Consulting Psychologist.

Spradley, J. (1979). *The ethnographic interview.* New York: Holt, Rinehart, and Winston.

St. Clair, C., Pickard, M., & Harlow, K. (1986). Continuing education for self actualization: Building a plan for rural nurses. *Journal of Continuing Education in Nursing, 17,* 27–31.

Walker, L., & Avant, K. (1983). *Strategies for theory construction in nursing.* Norwalk, CT: Appleton-Century-Crofts.

Weinert, C. (1983). [Social support: Rural people in their new middle years"]. Unpublished raw data.

Weinert, C., & Long, K. (1987). Understanding the health care needs of rural families. *Journal of Family Relations, 36,* 450–455.

Yura, H., & Torres, G. (1975). *Today's conceptual frameworks with the baccalaureate nursing programs* (NLN Pub. No. 15-1558, pp. 17–75). New York: NLN.

2

The Distinctive Nature and Scope of Rural Nursing Practice: Philosophical Bases

Jane Ellis Scharff

LOOKING BACK

Plenty and little have changed in ten years. Rural nursing practice seemed a dichotomous set of the routine and the extraordinary to me back then, as it does now. I was an insider, if not an old-timer, and my findings, although remarkable to some, seemed simply confirmatory to me. Already a budding pragmatist and not yet fully a scientist, I thought, at the time, it was enough to have empiric validation for the practice that I had known and in which my former workplace colleagues continued. For that reason and so many others, I did not publish the findings of my master's thesis in 1987. Subsequently, I have been cited frequently, misrepresented occasionally, and poached a time or two when it comes to references about the world of rural nursing. It is time to uphold my responsibility to nursing science and to set the record straight. The nature and scope of rural nursing IS distinctive. I am now willing to be quoted on that. Furthermore, rural nursing can now be given a definition based on that distinctiveness.

Rural nursing practice, be it hospital practice, private practice, or community health practice, is distinctive in its nature and scope from the practice of nursing in urban settings. It is distinctive in its boundaries, intersections, dimensions, and even in its core. Ten years ago I was loath to claim distinctiveness within rural nursing's core. It seemed too bold to proclaim that at the very level of essence, and not attributable to setting alone, rural nursing could be so different. Today, I am determined to claim it: The core of all nursing is care, and care is the substance of the relationship between nurse and patient; consequently, what happens at the core of rural nursing is something apart from what happens at the core of nursing anywhere else.

Still a pragmatist, my job is to get readers as close to the experience as I can. Thankfully, my growth as a scientist makes the job easier than it was some years back. Although no longer in the practice, I understand rural nursing better today than I did then. The importance of rural nursing has not decreased as my world view has expanded. On the contrary, the more I dissect and reconstruct my thoughts about life and truth and nursing science, the more clearly I see the beauty emanating from the nature and scope of rural nursing, and the more clearly I appreciate its relevance to all of nursing science.

From an ontological viewpoint, I will share some information about what it means to "be" a rural nurse, and from an epistemological viewpoint, I will express a little of what it means to "know" rural nursing practice. What came as primary expression to me, because I lived it, breathed it, and studied it, is secondary expression as I write it, and I will do my best to translate the experience through common language. However, the story I tell will require imagination to transcend time and space and to gain a sense of the reality of rural nursing practice. The information for this chapter comes from my ethnographic study of rural hospital nurses in the Inland Northwest completed in 1987, from dialogue with key informants before then and up until today, and from my personal experiences within rural health care systems over the past 20 years.

In the last 10 or 15 years, I have made some presentations about portions of this work to nurse clinicians, nurse researchers, and non-nurse health care audiences. Inevitably, following such presentations, I am approached by one or two individuals who have been rural nurses who want to tell me that the presentation struck a chord. I understand their need, which stems from the human desire to be recognized and understood. It stems from the frequent, albeit unintended, distortion of truth about rural nursing communicated by those who do not fully understand what it means to walk a mile in a rural nurse's duty shoes. I may not be able to change that, but I offer my perspective nonetheless.

CONCEPTUALIZING RURAL NURSING PRACTICE

Being Rural

There was a wonderful line in the 1984 science fiction film, *The Adventures of Buckaroo Banzai: Across the Eighth Dimension* (Rausch). The line was delivered by the main character, Buckaroo, a multiskilled neurosurgeon, particle physicist, rock musician, and Zen warrior who, in the midst of chaos matter-of-factly declared, "No matter where you go, there you are." If this sounds simple, I would caution that it is hardly simple. Buckaroo was talking about being in the moment, so imagine for a moment what it means to have *gone* rural. What of rural nursing identity? While the imagery may seem silly or surreal, the truth is real, authentic, important, credible, respectable, and as serious as any nursing practice anywhere. However, as indicated earlier, rural nursing practice is also distinctive from nursing anywhere else. Although I use the analogy of Buckaroo Banzai hoping it will bring a smile, rural nurses will recognize the script of playing a cool and noble professional, simultaneously enacting multiple roles, and managing the continual transition from one part to another with the frankness of Buckaroo.

Being rural means being a long way from anywhere and pretty close to nowhere. Being rural means being independent or perhaps just being alone. Being a rural nurse means that when a nurse saves a life, everyone in town recognizes that she or he was there, and when a nurse loses a life, everyone in town recognizes that she or he was there. Being rural means turning inward for answers, because there may be nobody to turn to outward. Being rural means that when a nurse walks into the emergency room, it may be her or his spouse or child who needs a nurse and, at that moment, being a nurse takes priority over being anyone else. Being a rural nurse means being able to deal with what she or he has got, where she or he is, and being able to live with the consequences.

Knowing Rural

Certainly every reader has heard that a little knowledge can be a dangerous thing. The adage was probably modified from what Alexander Pope said in the 17th century: "A little learning is a dangerous thing." I dispute it now and say that a little knowledge can be a lifesaving thing. The demarcation between danger and safety is the difference between *having* knowledge and *using* knowledge. From time to time, I have had conversations with academic colleagues about dangerous nurses. In these conversations, we have agreed that dangerous nurses are not those who know they do not know what they are doing—although there is certainly an element of danger in that scenario, which ultimately must be addressed. The greater danger, however, emerges with those nurses who think they do know, but actually do not know, what they are doing. Although I have no statistics on the prevalence of such nurses, it is my belief that they hide more easily in urban settings than they do in rural settings.

Knowing rural means knowing that what one knows may be all one has. Knowing rural means personally knowing everyone with whom one works and having knowledge about nearly everyone for whom one cares. As a rural nurse, knowing means sharing knowledge in an informal, yet crucially important exchange, with other professionals, where the addition of one mind can mean expanding the knowledge base by 100 percent. Although *who* one knows can be important in any setting, the distinction between rural and urban dynamics of whom one knows, is that in the urban setting who one knows is more likely to be related to competitive advantage, whereas in the rural setting who one knows is more likely to be related to cooperative advantage. Knowing rural means that knowledge can mean the difference between perishing, surviving, and thriving and, therefore, knowing is inextricably connected to being when one is rural.

THE NATURE AND SCOPE OF NURSING

For practicality, a framework for the study of the nature and scope of rural nursing practice was sought to identify and describe the distinctive characteristics of practice in rural settings. The American Nurses' Association (ANA) Social Policy Statement (1980) provided the framework for a logical sequence of investigation into details of rural nursing practice. The policy statement includes an organized and systematic approach to studying nursing nature and scope.

1. *Nursing's Nature.* Within the policy statement, the nature of nursing is characterized as a relationship between the nursing pro-

fession and society that is mutually beneficial, and nursing itself is deemed an essential outgrowth of the society that it serves. Nursing is described as existing in response to society's needs. From that standpoint, my study of rural nursing was based on assumptions that rural nursing emerges from and is essential to rural society, and distinctions of rural nursing are due, in part, to distinctive interests and needs of rural society.

2. *Nursing's Scope.* The scope of nursing includes four definitive characteristics that are intersections, dimensions, core, and boundary (ANA, 1980). These four characteristics became conceptual foundation blocks for my study of rural nursing.

   a. *Intersections.* Nursing intersects with other professions involved in health care. These intersections are points at which nursing meets and interfaces with other professions as well as expands its practice into the domain of other professions as necessary.

   b. *Dimensions.* Characteristics such as philosophy, ethics, roles, responsibilities, skills, and authority are examples of nursing dimensions. These are qualities that add depth to nursing practice. They are characteristics underscored and influenced by interpersonal relationships and intimacy as well as the intrapersonal quality of nursing.

   c. *Core.* The concept of the core of nursing is complex and somewhat more difficult to discuss than are the other concepts. It is oversimplification to say that the needs of people are the core of nursing, although such is true. Nursing exists to deal with human response to health issues, and human response can be equated to human need with respect to health. The patients' *needs* and their *responses* are outgrowths of whom they are as human *beings.* The nursing care we provide is an outgrowth of whom we are as human beings. The core of nursing is the dynamic of nursing care juxtaposed with human response.

   d. *Boundaries.* Nursing's boundaries change and expand in direct reflection of the intersections, dimensions, and core of practice. Boundaries are nebulous, unseen, intangible lines of demarcation between what is clearly within the nature and scope of nursing and what is questionably within nursing's scope. Unlike physical boundaries, nursing's boundaries are metaphysical, relationally and contextually based, and sometimes have origins outside the control of nursing.

METHODS

In an effort to describe the nature and scope of rural nursing, it was determined that an ethnographic method, using participant observation and interviewing techniques, would yield the most pertinent data for analysis. Data were gathered throughout several stages of conceptualization concerning rural nursing phenomena. Field notations, printed news media, and taped interviews were employed. The study of rural hospital nurses included an exploratory phase in which 8 rural nurses from northwest Montana were interviewed. These interviews were audio tape recorded, and from initial open-ended questions, a more refined interview guide was developed that contained both closed-and open-ended questions. Twenty-six rural hospital nurses in one of four rural towns in eastern Washington, northern Idaho, or western Montana were interviewed. All interviews were audio taped and then transcribed verbatim. The findings reported in this chapter are related to many aspects of rural nursing practice and are based on the responses of all 34 rural nurses, as well as several other key rural informants and my own observations. All samples were convenience, and all informants elected to be included in the studies.

FINDINGS

Informant Demographics

All of the informants were women ranging in age from 25 to 61 years with an average age of 40 years. The number of years actively employed as a registered nurse was 3 to 35 years. The mean number of years spent working in rural hospitals was 8 years and, for most informants, was roughly half the total active nursing years. Most informants were originally diploma-prepared, 7 were baccalaureate graduates, and 4 were associate graduates. Two informants had achieved a master's degree in nursing. Although informants were not asked about marital or parental status, nearly all said during the interview that they were married and were parents.

Most of the informants worked full-time, and those who worked part-time averaged 23 hours per week. In addition, many were placed on call if they were not working. On call status could be attributed to low census, high census, operating room call, cardiac care call, or emergency department call. Most informants reported one or two days of overtime per month. In almost every case, informants indicated a need to be flexible about their working schedules with regard to the events of the rural practice setting. Turnover rates were low at all facilities, and the most senior nurses had been on staff from 16 to 25 years.

Hospital Demographics

Information about the hospitals was obtained through interviews with nursing, fiscal, administrative, or other personnel, as well as from public records and the participant observation process. The hospital organizations were between 20 and 60 years in existence, the present structures were between 3 and 35 years old, and all had undergone some renovation over time. Ownership of the hospitals was stated as nonproprietary, public district, or community. Each hospital was governed by a board of directors of three to ten individuals who held fiduciary responsibility, decision-making authority, and to whom the administration was accountable. Board membership was either self-perpetuating or community elected. One facility was accredited by what was then the Joint Commission on Accreditation of Hospitals (JCAH). Administrative personnel said that there was little to be gained by small rural hospitals having JCAH accreditation, especially in light of what the JCAH charged for the process.

The hospitals had licensure ranging from 20 to 44 acute care beds, 0 to 3 intensive or cardiac beds, 5 to 7 newborn bassinets, and 3 to 5 swing beds for extended care. In every case, occupancy was at a fraction of licensure, and occupancy figures averaged to be about 20% to 40% for acute care beds. There was some variability in the use of the other services at each facility. Two had fairly active use of the cardiac or intensive care beds. Two had fairly active obstetrical departments. Three had active surgical departments. Emergency cases at these hospitals ranged from 3 to 13 per 24 hour day during the previous fiscal year. One relied on the constant occupancy of swing beds to maintain financial solvency. The number of physicians on medical staff ranged from a low of 3 to a high of 17. Typically, physicians who held admitting privilege at a given facility did not necessarily live within the community. Undoubtedly, the variety of medical practitioners on staff impacted the occupancy of each facility. Usually, nurses were expected to be able to float from medical–surgical areas to emergency, obstetrical, and intensive care areas but not to the operating room, which seemed to be the one sacrosanct specialty area.

The Rural Communities

At the time of the study, I spent several weeks traveling to and about four separate communities in western Montana, northern Idaho, and eastern Washington to gather information regarding the nature and scope of rural nursing. Each of these towns fit the operational definition of being geographically isolated and of having less than 5,000 residents. Upon arrival in each community, time was taken to drive about, observe the local terrain, look for indicators of economy, walk around town to observe the pace and lifestyle, note the casual conversations taking place in public areas, and read each community's local weekly newspaper.

There were many similarities and few differences between the communities in terms of how they appeared to the outsider. Each town was located near railroad tracks, all of which were currently used. Three of the towns were on a river in forested mountain terrain and were logging or lumbermill towns. The fourth town was on an expansive plain and was an agricultural community. Each town was inhabited mostly by Caucasian people and each was laid out in typical western fashion with one main street and several auxiliary streets at which the center of the business district was found. Each town boasted the typical hardware stores, grocery stores, restaurants, farm or logging machinery shops, tool shops, post office, drug store, employment office, beauty shops, ice cream stands, feed stores, junk shops, small motels, bars, and churches. Each town had a well-kept appearance, although each had a few empty buildings or storefronts in the business district.

Residents in these communities were friendly and helpful. They recognized me as an outsider and, although willing to answer my questions, were curious and wanted to know the purpose of my presence in their town. When I explained myself, the residents registered sincere interest and pleasure that their community had been targeted for this study. They acted like they felt privileged and eagerly conveyed their high regard for nurses in general and *their* nurses specifically. Never did these residents express animosity toward the community of nurses. Most of them had a story to tell about how a friend's or relative's life was saved at the local hospital.

Rural Hospital Nurses

The rural nurses I observed and interviewed were a dynamic group of women who could certainly be called expert generalists. They moved quickly and, for the most part easily from one role to another as circumstances required. They explained that most rural nurses have a great deal of knowledge regarding a variety of nursing practice areas. When beginning work in a rural hospital, many nurses suffer reality shock due to the variety of demands placed on them. One seasoned nurse told me, "Although you might start out and you don't have that wide knowledge, you better get it quickly." A relative newcomer nurse expressed admiration about the knowledge level of her rural colleagues, calling them "impressive." The nurses I interviewed routinely worked in three or four different specialty areas of nursing practice every week and, sometimes, every day. When talking with one respondent about this phenomenon and how easy certain nurses made it look, she said, "The ones who are experienced in rural nursing seem to be very comfortable in switching back and forth between specialties."

Nursing Staff Tenure and Group Acceptance

At all facilities nurses were heard to use the terms "new" or "newcomer" and "old" or "old-timer" in reference to a given nurse's tenure on the staff. There was no particular time limit identified when a nurse makes the transition from new to old, nor how one arrives at a level of acceptance. However, tenure of less than two years was apparently definitely considered new, and tenure of three to five years in combination with competence generally constituted acceptance. Tenure beyond ten years was considered seasoned and, in special cases of achieving high proficiency or social acceptance, one of these nurses might be called an old-timer, but usually this term was reserved for someone who had been around for twenty or more years. What I discerned was some gray area depending on a nurse's tenure, level of proficiency, and sociability related to group fit. It seemed that a nurse who was very skillful, flexible, and likeable might reach old-timer status sooner than a nurse who was lacking one of those characteristics.

Although I cannot pinpoint a "typical" rural nurse, certain characteristics were confirmed as traits of distinctive advantage for a rural nurse's success. For example, good common sense, good judgment ability, the ability to set priorities, good physical assessment skills, and physical and emotional strengths were considered of survival significance to these nurses, due, in part, to the aloneness of their practices. They made comments such as, "You have to make all your own decisions. There's no one to do that for you." "You have to be able to be autonomous." "You can't go to somebody for concurrence with decision making." "At any time during your shift, your assignment may change drastically." "You can make the difference between life or death—the judgement calls are yours." All informants were adamant that the prevalent feeling of aloneness and serious responsibility were distinctive to the rural setting. None would concede that the feeling was anything like that experienced in an urban setting. These nurses expressed a very real and pervasive sense of responsibility which rural nurses bear for their patients. The nurses who do not have the ability consistently to carry the burden of such decisional responsibility are the ones who do not survive as rural nurses. Old-timers claimed they could often tell right away, or within a few weeks, if a newcomer was going to catch on or not. Old-timers based such predictions on their assessments of a newcomer's characteristics as mentioned above, combined with evidence of adaptation to the new environment.

Education and Professional Development

The burden for self-responsibility of education is greater in the rural setting than in the urban setting, and most rural nurses accept this burden in stride. There are a wide variety of sources from which rural nurses receive their continuing education, such as out-of-town workshops or conferences, in-service education, journals, textbooks, practice sessions, physicians, and other nurses. The greatest educational needs voiced were in cardiac, trauma, maternal-child, and complex medical nursing.

Informants indicated a thirst for knowledge in accredited professional continuing education. Several respondents reported attending more than ten continuing education events in a year. Most attended between three and ten events annually. These events were either developed and held locally, developed elsewhere but held locally, or developed and held in urban settings. Although expenses were a factor, they were not the central factor in respondents' attending continuing education events.

Nearly all informants also relied on journals for new information, read journals regularly, and reported the most popular journals to be *Nursing, American Journal of Nursing, RN, Journal of Nursing Administra-*

tion, and *Nursing Management,* in that order. Current journals were visible in each facility, and notations were seen hanging on bulletin boards in nursing report rooms or locker rooms with a suggestion from one nurse to others that everyone review a given recent journal article germane to a given current case.

Rural nurses, in fact, identify one another as their most important single source of information and education. This was often explained as information being imparted from a peer when it was needed most, so that learning occurred while doing, which tended to heighten the memory. Comments that supported these phenomena included, "We try to share everything we can with each other." "New nurses sometimes come in with great new information or real current ideas. It helps a lot." "Sometimes the new girls expect you to know things, and I don't, and it can be embarrassing. So we look it up together." "When you've been around for awhile, you develop a comaraderie. We know what we can expect from each other."

Out of town workshops were identified as the next most important source of continuing education to rural nurses. Informants qualified this by stressing that the topic or presentation needed to be relevant to the rural environment. One informant said, "It's got to be meaningful. You know, you go up to the city and they tell you how to do something, and they don't realize how different the setup is."

Interpersonal Relationships and Nursing Practice

Rural nurses know everyone who works at the hospital, all of the physicians, and most of their patients. Rural nurses say that the interpersonal closeness of knowing everyone with whom they work, and for whom they care, generally has a positive influence on their practice. The intensity of this interpersonal dynamic is unique to the rural setting. Although it is likely that nurses in any setting develop close relationships, rural nurses are in a distinctive situation of being personally acquainted with all of those around them, so that the depth of interaction is potentially greater, and the accountability for interpersonal exchange is a constant that is simply not present in other settings. An informant explained the bond she felt with coworkers by saying, "It's nice to know the people you're working with. You work more together, you try harder, and you work closer." Another nurse shared that among many rewarding qualities of rural nursing, "The cooperation of the other nurses and the cohesiveness of the group is probably the biggest."

An old-timer at one hospital said, "I don't have to explain when I say something. They believe me, and they do it without wasting time." It was easy to verify this through observation. Certain old-timers could communicate a virtual reassignment of responsibilities through the tone of their voices as they disappeared momentarily to deal with arisen crises, such as the admission of trauma victims in the emergency room. On occasions it was like watching a dance, the motions of which were so well understood, each dancer so valued and respected, that without missing a step, workers would change places based on available expertise and would back each other up without visible cues. Even physicians were seen deferring to old-timer nurses at such times. Yet, the choreography depended heavily on the direction of the one in charge, and on other occasions, with an inexperienced newcomer directing, the dance was frantic, and the flow chaotic.

Practicing Medicine

Rural nurses are understandably reluctant to admit that they practice medicine, but they know their boundaries are sometimes stretched by circumstance. "You take it upon yourself and do what has to be done to make sure the patient's stable before you can call the doctor," said one nurse to me. When patient crises occur, calling the physician is considered important, but it simply does not rank at the top of the list. The nurses I interviewed and watched used a standard A-B-C (airway, breathing, circulation) order of setting priorities to respond to patient needs. Thus, they often began written or unwritten medical protocols while the aide would be sent to summon the physician. Physician response times varied from 5 to 30 minutes at the rural hospitals, resulting in nurses being responsible for considerable decision making during the time lapse. At each site, I heard or saw variations on the themes of nurses stabilizing cardiac or trauma victims and nurses managing precipitous births without benefit of physicians present. In interviews, nurses were adamant that they had a responsibility to patients to do whatever was required during an emergency, and that although it sometimes felt uncomfortable, inaction would have constituted neglect. The words of one nurse summarize the collective opinion, "We do it because we have to, because it would be wrong if we didn't."

There were also circumstances of newcomer physicians relying on seasoned nurses for insight into or even direction regarding a given patient case. Per physician request, the nurse would literally advise what medications and treatments to order in cases where the doctor did not have the familiarity with a patient's history that the nurse did. This was especially true in after-hours situations of physicians covering for another's patients. My assessment of these circumstances is that each party acted within unseen lines of mutual trust and understanding with the dynamic of trust specific to a given relationship.

Another observation I made at these facilities, which struck me then and which I have informally reconfirmed on multiple occasions since, is that rural physicians seem more likely to read and respond to nurses' notes about patients than do urban physicians. Doubtless there is great individual variability, yet it is tempting to hypothesize that rural professionals have a better grasp than do their urban counterparts of pertinent information that is necessary to communicate to the health care team. Certainly, further study would be required to confirm the probability.

Rural Expertise: Aces, and Pinch Hitters

Rural nurses generally believe that no one can be an expert in every area of rural nursing practice. However, a few nurses are extremely proficient in all clinical areas, and these nurses become role models and mentors to the other nurses with whom they work. At two study sites many informants identified a colleague or two who fit this category. Interestingly, those who were identified by others as *aces* did not identify themselves as such. Each nurse was very modest about her own capability, but the pride toward aces among the staff was obvious. I was aware that talking to or watching these aces in action was as much an honor for the locals as it was for me as an investigating outsider.

All rural nurses interviewed agreed that they must be competent in more than one clinical area to be considered an acceptable staff member. The top four clinical areas deemed to be most important for competency were emergency nursing, obstetrical nursing, intensive or coronary nursing, and medical-surgical nursing. A supervisory nurse told me, "There's a difference between competent and expert. I think everybody who works in this hospital should be able to walk into any specialty area and function." But there was an expectation held by all informants that they be clinically strong, if not expert, in at least two of the above-named areas and be able to float to any other department and still function well in a pinch.

With regard to functioning in a pinch, in the early 1980s two rural Montana nurse executives who are admitted baseball fans coined the *Pinch Hitter Theory of Rural Nursing*. One of those persons, Jean Shreffler, now an academic, is author of other chapters in this text. The second person, Maura Fields, was then and remains today the nurse executive at a rural hospital in Montana and is arguably one of the most innovative and masterful nurse leaders I have ever had the good fortune to know. Her rendition of the theory went like this:

In rural nursing, you have to be like a pinch hitter. You may not perform a task or procedure or work on a very specialized case but once a year. But when you go to do it, you have to do it like you do it every day. In baseball, a batting average of 300 is good. But the pinch hitter, well, you want them to be better than that, really, you want them to bat a thousand. That's what it's like for a rural nurse, when they go to work, you want them to bat a thousand. (Personal conversation, Maura Fields, 1983.)

For those readers who are doubting that there can be that many instances in which the above theory becomes important, rest assured that it happens all the time. Industrial and recreational traumas are frequent in these communities. Rural citizens experience their share of severe burns, drug overdoses, cardiac arrests, head injuries, freak accidents, and critical illness. Although transfer to larger medical centers is sometimes preferred, stabilization is first necessary, and transfer is sometimes not possible. One hospital in this study is 90 road miles from the nearest medical center of any size and 150 road miles from a trauma center. Rotary blade or fixed wing aircraft are often used to transport cases that require more care than can be delivered locally, but northwest mountain weather conditions can be a significant factor in keeping aircraft grounded.

Although rural nurses do not expect an easy routine, frustration is common surrounding the conflict of trying to achieve expertise in such a complex practice. Boredom is rare as they face the constant variety of demands. One informant related the example of the prior day's evening shift. The informant was one of two RNs on duty at the time, assisted by one aide. The scenario she described began after change of shift report and went like this:

Just yesterday evening there were seven patients in the house with nothing going on. Within an hour, there was one admitted with a depression state,

> *an OB came in, and there were four or five cases in the ER, one being a child with rectal bleeding, which makes you wonder about child abuse.*

Although two nurses and an aide would have no difficulty caring for seven stable medical surgical patients, the admission of the depressed patient was a wrench in the works. Mental health diagnoses are among those which rural nurses feel least appropriately prepared for, and they lack confidence in rural physicians' ability to treat mental health patients appropriately, as well. The depressed patient required suicide precautions for a period of time which meant that the aide was assigned to remain with the patient at all times. The pediatric patient in the emergency room required careful documentation, delicate interaction, and a social services consultation. The obstetrical patient admission required nurse assessment and individual care until it was determined that the patient was in early labor. One nurse moved back and forth between the emergency room and the general care unit; the other moved back and forth between the labor room, the depressed patient, and the general care unit.

Here is an account from another informant about another evening shift where three RNs were on duty but without assistance from an aide:

> *Not long ago we had an OB with a bad baby, small for gestational age, and at the same time we got two ambulances five minutes apart, and they were both cardiacs with chest pain. While that was happening, there was surgery going on, and there was somebody in the unit. I don't know if God is watching you or what, but, for the most part, things seem to come out okay in the end.*

In this case, one nurse was already assigned to the intensive care unit, and one was required to remain with the obstetrical patient to do monitoring and other procedures. When the first ambulance arrived, the third nurse was dispatched to the emergency room. Fortunately, some ambulance crew members were emergency medical technicians and could help with continued patient monitoring and calling in the physician, laboratory, and respiratory personnel. Also fortunately, the physician arrived within ten minutes and was designated to care for both patients. The final good fortune is that nothing went wrong on the general care unit while hell was breaking loose elsewhere.

Knowing Patients Personally

Most rural nurses subscribe to the belief that when they know patients personally, they can give better care. The possibility of experiencing fear when caring for family members or best friends notwithstanding, the rewards are considered rich. A gradual loss of anonymity occurs to rural nurses as they become immersed in and assimilated into rural society, making anonymity nonexistent for old-timers. "I can be more supportive emotionally when I know them," one said, and another elaborated, "Let's say in the ER, with chronic lungers, you know them, and they feel secure because they know we remember them." I saw instances of rural nurses informally calling to check on patients after discharge. As far as I know, patients were always glad to have these calls. The loss of anonymity is generally considered reassuring for those professionals who are comfortable with rural life, but it can be constricting as well. It should not be assumed, however, that negative aspects of anonymity loss are necessarily related to poor patient outcomes. On the contrary, one informant told me,

> *I know of several situations where knowing my OB patients who had poor outcomes made a difference to them, where I was really able to help them get through the experience. It's a real emotional drain, but you're ahead of the game, because the trust is there.*

The argument could be made that patients perceive their care to be better based on the close personal contact that is often made in the rural setting. A nurse who believes that her relationship to a patient made a difference in the patient's outcome said,

> *I recovered my little neighbor girl after her surgery. Most little kids are scared when they wake up, but when she woke up she knew me and wasn't afraid and recovered really fast. Because fear generates pain, but she wasn't afraid, she recovered faster than usual.*

It is a cultural expectation of many rural people to be taken care of by someone they know. This differs from the expectation in urban settings. For the most part, informants agreed that rural people do expect to have their medical needs met, even though they live far from a major medical center. However, one informant said that rural patients often wait until they are "half dead" before they seek intervention and are "grateful for what they get." Another nurse said,

"People have told me they were glad I was on when they were here, that if I said it was going to be okay, then it was going to be okay."

Nearly all rural nurses could confirm that sometimes they had patients from out of town who had previously experienced urban hospital admissions. These patients, whether vacationing in the rural setting or passing through the rural area, ended up in rural hospitals for reasons not important to this story. Their comments about the care they received in rural hospitals are important. The nurses were told by these patients that the care was of better quality, that they felt more cared for, that the rural nurses took more time to listen, that care was accomplished more quickly and smoothly, and that they felt more like people and less like numbers in the rural hospital than they did in any urban hospital. The outsider patients often expressed surprise at the high level of competence they encountered in the rural setting.

DISCUSSION

Rural Nursing's Distinctive Nature and Scope

Analyses of the reports of rural nurses show that the nature and scope of rural nursing are clearly distinctive. Using a framework to focus the discussion, the distinctions can apparently be categorized as those pertaining to rural nursing's nature, as well as the four components of rural nursing's scope, those being intersections, dimensions, core, and boundary.

The Nature of Rural Nursing

Most rural nurses have difficulty defining their practice, although they can describe it. Their descriptions are a variety of rich, thoughtful, colorful, and articulate responses. Rural nursing is generalist nursing, not to be mistaken for mundane, and includes an intensity of purpose which makes it distinctive. Rural nurses may feel misunderstood and poorly recognized by the larger nursing community, but they are nonetheless a proud lot.

The Scope of Rural Nursing

The intersections of rural nursing are distinctively marked and fluid. Rural nurses consistently and necessarily practice well within the realm of other health care disciplines, the most notable being respiratory therapy, pharmacy, and medicine. The intersection between nursing and medicine has the most extensive implications. It is a gray area that hinges on circumstances and relationships, and the most complex intersections occur during emergent situations; "until the doctor gets there." Some rural nurses embrace this intersection more willingly than others, but none do it casually. Reflective concern is apparent in comments related to this intersection. One informant said, "It means putting your neck out there on the line, but you have to make the judgment and go on." Another told me, "It sometimes feels uncomfortable, but it's part of my responsibility to the patient."

It is evident that the practice of rural nursing is dimensionally distinctive. Rural nurses embrace an ethic of openness and honesty that is pervasive. The dimension of interpersonal knowing is viewed as a positive feature of rural practice, and it exists between nurses and patients as well as among coworkers. A nurse administrator shared with me that, "in terms of practice outcomes, your accountability is right in front of your face." Rural nurses talked about being able to accomplish goals more quickly with their patients and said that guidance, teaching, and counseling behaviors are automatic to their practice in the rural environment. Communication patterns in the rural setting are more direct and suffer less obfuscation than do those in urban settings. There are fewer barriers to go through when imparting messages from one to another. As a result, there are probably fewer errors of omission and commission related to practice in the rural setting than there are in the urban setting. Confronting and managing conflict is more common in the rural setting, avoidance being an unacceptable dynamic for group cohesiveness that stems from mutual concern and regard for one another. Independent decision making is a given in rural practice, but rural nurses are aware of their limitations. One said, "You have to know when you don't know, and you have to know where to go to find out." Rural nurses are mindful, if not fully informed, about the legal dimensions of their practice. However, with respect to questions of patient safety and survival, rural nurses sometimes decide their ethical obligation to do what is right for their patients carries more weight than their legal responsibility to uphold the law. These cases generally become lessons of learning, are scrutinized and discussed by the group, and are entered into memory for future reference.

Human responses, which nurses diagnose and treat, are the core of nursing. Some sources have suggested, and informants in this study agreed, that rural dwellers are known to delay health seeking, and tend to define health as the ability to get out of bed and go to work. Thinking in terms of nursing diagnosis, one might call this behavior "dysfunctional perceptual orientation to health" which requires distinctive intervention at nursing's core. Rural nurses are faced with determining an appropriate line of demarcation between a rural dweller's rugged individualism and stubborn disregard for health. Inextricable from rural nursing's core are the relational issues of what it means to be rural. As introduced earlier in this chapter, from an ontological standpoint, rural nursing is distinctive at its very core.

Boundary being dependent on the intersections, dimensions, and core of nursing, there can be no question as to rural nursing's distinctive boundary. Rural nursing is constantly changing in response to complex intersections and dimensional intricacies distinctive to rural society. The boundary is, therefore, neither smooth nor even static. When nurses come to a rural setting from an urban setting they are very aware that the boundary of their practice changes. The transitional period for these nurses is not always easy, and boundary expansion can be accompanied by ambivalence, anxiety, and frustration. Newcomers must become adjusted to the rural culture to function effectively, and not all survive. Rural experts can play a key role in the success of newcomer transition, and those "aces" who invest themselves in the orientation and mentoring of newcomers know the importance of the payoff.

Defining Rural Nursing

Rural nursing is a special variety of nursing in which the nurse must have a wide range of advanced knowledge and ability, in combination with commitment, to practice proficiently in multiple clinical areas simultaneously along the career trajectory. The practice requires constant and continual personal and professional adaptation in developing identity. A rural nurse has both an ontological sense of being and an epistemological sense of knowing that connect the nurse with the surrounding community, and through which the rural nurse creates a reality of rural professional nursing practice. In no other setting is a nurse's practice so thoroughly and integrally a constant factor in a nurse's life. In a society where separating one's private life from one's professional life is considered obligatory, rural nurses are singularly challenged, stripped of their own anonymity while simultaneously charged with protecting their patients' privacy.

Closing Thought

The newcomer practices nursing in a rural setting, unlike the old-timer, who practices *rural nursing.* Somewhere between these spectral extremes lies the transitional period of events and conditions through which each nurse passes at her or his own pace. It is within this temporal zone that nurses experience rural reality and move toward becoming professionals who understand that having gone rural, they are not less than they were, but rather, they are more than they expected to be. Some may be conscious of the transition, and others may not, but in the end, a few will say, "I am a rural nurse."

REFERENCES

American Nurses' Association (ANA). (1980). *Nursing: A social policy statement* (Publication No. NP-63 20M 9/82R). Kansas City, MO: Author.

Rausch, E. M. (Screenplay Author). (1984). *The adventures of Buckaroo Banzai: Across the eighth dimension.* [Film]. (Available through Vestron Video.)

Alexander Pope. (1711). Essay on criticism. Cited in B. Evans (Ed.), *Dictionary on Quotations* (1978). New York: Avenel Books, Delecort Press.

3

Advanced Education for the Role of Rural Nurse Generalist*

Kathleen Ann Long, Jane Ellis Scharff, and Clarann Weinert

INTRODUCTION

Health care in rural areas has unique requirements and challenges, and the provision of appropriate and adequate health care requires models of delivery tailored to the rural environment. Likewise, rural practitioners need to have educational preparation that enhances their ability to understand and address the health care needs of rural dwellers. This chapter describes a graduate nursing program at Montana State University which has been designed to prepare nurses to effectively deliver health care to Montanans and other rural dwellers.

For the past fifteen years, the graduate program at the Montana State University College of Nursing has focused on the delivery of nursing and health care in sparsely populated areas. Prior to that time, the nursing master's program emphasized preparation for nursing education. However, as similar nursing education programs developed regionally, the nursing faculty were able to examine ways in which their graduate program could address the unique needs of

Acknowledgment. The authors wish to acknowledge the work of Montana State University College of Nursing graduate students and faculty. Qualitative data collected and analyzed by them form a basis for portions of this article. Ethnographic data collection and analysis were supported in part by a U.S. DHHS Division of Nursing Advanced Training grant (1816001649A).

Montana and the rural West. A decision to develop a program focusing on graduate-level preparation in rural nursing was seen as fitting well with the University's land grant mission of service to the people of the state and region. The program was begun at a time when there was a relatively sparse literature about the special health needs of rural populations, and almost nothing written about rural nursing. Recognizing the need for a theory base for practice, the graduate program was developed in such a way that it facilitated pioneering work in the development of rural nursing theory (Long & Weinert, 1989). The program is now nationally recognized for its leadership in the field of rural nursing, and was cited in a Health Resources and Services Administration report to the United States Congress as one of two national model graduate programs preparing nurses for rural practice (National Rural Health Association, 1992).

RURAL HEALTH AND HEALTH CARE

In contrast to the popular notion of rural dwellers "living the simple life," the problems associated with rural lifestyles are complex. Crises, which affect the nation's health care system in general, affect the rural system in a more pronounced way. Although rural mortality rates are lower in general than those of urban areas (U.S. Congress, 1990), two notable exceptions are death due to accidental injury, which is dramatically higher in the rural population, and infant mortality (U.S. Congress, 1990). Incidence of occupational injury is higher for the rural work force and rural workers are more likely to be exposed to job-related health hazards (U.S. Congress, 1990). Additionally, chronic illness and disability are experienced at higher rates in rural populations, and the numbers are increasing (U.S. Congress, 1990). These health problems are exacerbated for people in the frontier areas of Montana and other parts of the rural West by extreme difficulty in accessing appropriate health care services.

Over a decade ago, Rosenblatt and Moscovice wrote: "... rural dwellers tend to be poorer and older than their urban counterparts," "... both private and public insurance programs are deficient in rural America," and " .. the need for health care is higher in rural America despite the deficient resources." They also stated: "... this disjunction between need and supply is a major challenge to the creation of workable, accessible rural health care systems" (Rosenblatt and Moscovice, 1982, p. 77). The rural health situation has not improved, and the literature documents continuing and worsening problems related to inadequate preventive and primary health care for rural residents (Bushy, 1991; U.S. Congress, 1990). Distance is becoming a greater barrier to health care access as economic pressures force the closure of many rural health care facilities. In addition, many rural areas are dealing with an exodus of younger, healthier residents.

THE NEED FOR RURAL GENERALISTS

Rosenblatt and Moscovice (1982) noted that "... rural professionals must be comfortable with uncertainty, challenged by diversity, and flexible in their skills, working hours, and interpersonal style," and that "... each individual must be willing and able to cover for a colleague along the entire breadth of ... practice" (p. 273). The need for rural health care providers and, specifically, rural nurses to be prepared as generalists is well documented (National Rural Health Association, 1992; Lassiter, 1985). The hallmark of rural nursing practice is the diversity of knowledge expected and the diversity of practice experiences encountered (Bushy, 1991; Lassiter, 1985). Scharff's (1987) study of nurses in rural Montana documented the variety of clinical experiences encountered in a single day, and the need for broad-based knowledge and generalist skills.

Part of the health care tradition in rural Montana is that nurses, both within formal practice settings and informally as local community residents, are relied upon to meet diverse health care needs and function in a variety of roles. Often nurses are the only resident providers in small, rural communities. In rural hospitals and health care agencies, they are expected to function in all clinical areas—medical, surgical, obstetrical, psychiatric, etc.—often in a single day. In addition numerous activities, including for example, health education, infant delivery, medication prescription, patient transportation, and even snow shoveling are, by default or design, performed by rural nurses (Scharff, 1987). Aspects of rural nursing practice, such as nurses "substituting" for physicians, pharmacists, or hospital maintenance personnel, may be ineffective, inefficient or unsafe. However, they are often accepted and even covertly encouraged within rural health care systems (Lassiter, 1985; Scharff, 1987). In order to provide leadership in system reform and improvement, rural nurses must understand organizational dynamics and the economics and politics which affect care delivery. Thus, the delivery of high quality rural nursing care requires not only a broad base of nursing knowledge and skills, but also a sophisticated ability to assess communities and provide leadership for change.

THE RURAL NURSING EDUCATION PROGRAM

The graduate program at the Montana State University (MSU) College of Nursing addresses the preparation of nurse generalists with advanced education in rural clinical practice, leadership, and research. There is emphasis on the assessment and management of health needs and the delivery of health care services in sparsely populated areas. In conjunction with the overall rural emphasis, students select a specific clinical focus area such as family-child nursing or community health nursing, and take support courses from related disciplines designed to enrich an individual plan for future practice. Frequently selected course areas include management and administration, family and rural sociology, and adult education. Each student in the program completes independent research leading to a master's thesis or additional course work and a professional project. An emphasis area in education is available, and the College faculty are actively considering the development of a specific track in nursing administration/leadership. A family nurse practitioner option has recently been added, and complements the program's overall emphasis on rural nursing.

The major objective of the program is to prepare graduates who are able to practice professional nursing in rural settings with an understanding of the traditional and expanded roles of the nurse. This includes the ability to provide quality care as related to stabilization, transport, and coordination in environments that are characterized by the lack of highly specialized health care resources. Graduates are expected to apply systems theories as a framework to analyze, modify, and plan for rural nursing services, and to synthesize concepts that contribute to the development of nursing theory especially as it relates to health care delivery in sparsely populated areas.

Curricula

The program's nursing course work falls into three main areas: theory and research; health care assessment and intervention; and the assessment, management, and change of health care delivery systems. Students acquire a strong base in nursing theory and research. Specialized work in ethnography focuses on helping students understand the perspectives of rural clients, and how these can and should affect the delivery of health care. Advanced clinical courses emphasize the application of clinical knowledge within rural practice settings. Specific course work in systems, leadership, and change provides students with knowledge and experiential opportunities, enhancing the ability to work with rural people and within rural health care systems to effect needed reforms. A major difference from traditional advanced practice graduate programs is the emphasis on advanced *generalist,* rather than specialist, knowledge and application. While students focus their work with particular client groups (e.g., maternal/child), there is continual reference to how knowledge from a broad array of nursing specialties must be integrated in order to meet diverse client needs. Students are prepared for practice in rural areas where they are often unable to rely on consultation or referral processes because 'experts' in specialty fields are unavailable or inaccessible.

Currently, the program is small, admitting no more than 15 students per year. Size is limited in order to accommodate individual student goals and in keeping with available financial, clinical, and faculty resources. The full-time program is four semesters, including one summer term, in length. However, most students are employed in nursing and attend on a part-time basis, usually completing the program in approximately three years. Program delivery makes use of the College's four campus sites and an interconnecting teleconference system. Thus, students may access courses through any one of four population centers in Montana. Additional outreach sites are periodically evaluated and added as resources permit. Several face-to-face classes of all students and each course instructor are held throughout the semester. These meetings allow for peer support, "live" discussion, faculty role modeling, and opportunity for direct faculty–student guidance and support. Direct supervision of clinical learning experiences is provided by faculty members, and includes on-site visits and participation in clinical care. While agency preceptors are often utilized to assist students in the clinical setting, faculty members retain responsibility for overall supervision and evaluation.

Unique Features

Several unique features have contributed to the College's success in recruiting nurses interested in rural nursing, preparing them for leadership roles in rural health, and engendering an enthusiasm which causes graduates to seek out and remain in rural health care settings. The rural focus of the program is clearly identified in the recruiting of students and is specifically discussed in pre-admission interviews and at the onset of each student's course of graduate study. Recruitment of students targets rural areas, particularly Montana. In addition, the College has established an informal national network of those interested in rural nursing, and prospective students from other rural parts of the United States are also recruited. An underlying premise has been that students *from* rural areas are most likely to return *to* rural areas and practice there after graduation. The experience of the National Health Service Corps has shown that providing urban dwellers with rural learning experiences and/or requiring post-graduation service in rural areas have generally not been successful in the long-term retention of providers for rural settings (Pathman, Konrad, & Ricketts, 1992).

Faculty members in the College are enthusiastic about the rural nursing focus, and many are active in rural practice. In addition, a faculty committee in the College focuses specifically on rural nursing theory building, research, and curricular enhancement. Graduate students are actively encouraged to participate in and contribute to this committee's work.

Another unique feature of the program is a specific course which engages students in reexamining their thinking about health care in rural areas. Through ethnographic interviews, students learn first-hand about how rural dwellers view health, and about consumer-defined health care needs and preferences. In addition, a variety of supervised clinical experiences in rural areas are offered to students. These experiences are designed around each student's preference for a clinical practice area (medical–surgical, family–child, etc.), type of practice (primary care, in-patient, long-term, etc.), and client group (elderly, children, Native American, etc.). Through these experiences students are provided opportunities to blend their own clinical interests into rural settings.

OUTCOMES

Educational Outcomes

From its inception, the rural generalist graduate program was intended to be a blend of education, theory development, and research designed to address the unique health care needs of persons living in sparsely populated areas. Graduates from the program have made significant contributions to the health care of people in Montana and other rural states. They hold leadership positions in rural health care facilities including acute and long-term care, home care and hospice agencies, the Indian Health Service, and state agencies. The program has also provided an educational base for those who have elected to continue their education at the doctoral level. A uniquely successful feature of the program has been the retention of graduates in rural practice settings. As indicated earlier, most students are from Montana, and most remain in practice in Montana after completing the program. The College has tracked graduates since 1985. In the period 1985–92 there were 38 graduates, and the location and practice of 33 were known. Of these, 85% (25) were working in a rural state, predominantly Montana, or in a rural section of a more populated state. Of the 28 graduates in rural areas, the vast majority were in direct practice settings, while a small number were in nursing education settings. The practice settings of graduates were almost evenly divided between population centers within rural states (50,000–85,000 pop.) and smaller towns (< 50,000 pop.). Three graduates were working in isolated rural areas on or near American Indian reservations.

Research and Theory Outcomes

The curriculum has a strong research focus with a particular emphasis on qualitative methods. An ethnographic approach is used in course assignments and provides students with opportunities to interact directly with a wide array of persons in small town and farm-ranch areas. Involvement in rural communities is reflected by students in their selection of thesis topics. Students have used a variety of methodologies to explore issues related to the health of rural dwellers including such topics as the self-reliance of rural dialysis patients, preventive health behaviors and attitudes of rural people, childbearing in the Hutterite culture, Crow Indian women's childbearing practices, the effects of transfer from rural to urban health care institutions, lifestyles and alcohol use among rodeo participants, the nature and scope of rural nursing, and the use of herbs and health foods by rural families. In addition, publications by faculty members and graduates have made significant contributions to the rural nursing literature (Bushy, 1991; Lee, 1989; Long & Weinert, 1989; Snyder, 1981; Weinert & Long, 1991).

A unique aspect of the graduate program is the opportunity which students have to directly contribute to the building of a rural nursing theory. The College's Rural Nursing Theory Committee is a pivotal force in maintaining a core of interested faculty members and students working on various stages of rural nursing theory development, research, and publications. The theory development process is carried out by the committee, using both student- and faculty-generated data. Several major concepts significant for health and rural nursing have been examined. These include work beliefs and health beliefs, isolation and distance, self-reliance, lack of anonymity, and the "outsider/insider" phenomenon. Graduate students and faculty members have conducted research to validate the rural health concepts elicited from ethnographic data. Lee (1991), for example, explored the health perceptions of men in rural Montana. Weinert (1987) conducted a study using survey methodology to validate the concepts of health status, isolation and distance, self-reliance, and use of the informal care systems. In addition, findings by researchers studying other rural populations, such as women in fishing villages in Nova Scotia (Ross, 1982), Maryland's eastern shore dwellers (Salisbury State College, 1986), and farmers and oil field workers in Texas (Walker and Mountain, 1988) have been used to further develop and enrich the knowledge base for rural nursing theory. Continuing development of rural nursing theory and of the graduate program curriculum are reciprocal, linked processes within the College.

SUMMARY

The Montana State University College of Nursing has developed a master's degree program which prepares nurses as generalists with advanced knowledge for understanding and addressing rural health care needs. The program is clear about its goals and objectives and does not attempt to be "all things for all people." The emphasis is on rural nursing, and this emphasis is present in recruiting, teaching, research, and publication at the College. Classroom and clinical experiences challenge students to develop a broad range of skills, and most importantly to enhance critical thinking and problem-solving abilities. Since delivering high quality health care in rural areas requires the ability to understand health care from the consumer's perspective, both data collection and clinical experience in rural communities are required. The enthusiasm for rural nursing—practice, teaching, and research—displayed by faculty members, alumnae, and students—is both a major factor in, and an indication of, the program's success.

REFERENCES

Bushy, A. (Ed.). (1991). *Rural Nursing,* Vol. 1. Newbury Park, CA: Sage.

Lassiter, P. G. (1985). Education for rural health professionals. Nurses. *The Journal of Rural Health, 1,* 23–28.

Lee, H. J. (1989). *Quantitative validation of health perceptions in rural persons.* Unpublished manuscript, Montana State University, College of Nursing, Bozeman, MT.

Lee, H. J. (1991). Relationship of hardiness and current life events to perceived health in rural adults. *Research in Nursing and Health,* 14, 351–359.

Long, K., & Weinert, C. (1989). Rural nursing: Developing a theory base. *Scholarly Inquiry for Nursing Practice, 3,* 113–127.

National Rural Health Association (1992). *Study of models to meet rural health care needs through mobilization of health professions education and services resources.* (Report of HRSA Contract 240–89–0037). Washington, D.C.: Author.

Pathman, D. E., Konrad, T. R., & Ricketts, T. C. (1992). The comparative retention of National Health Services Corps and other rural physicians. *Journal of the American Medical Association, 268,* 1552–1558.

Rosenblatt, R. A., & Moscovice, 1. S. (1982). *Rural Health Care.* New York: Wiley.

Ross, H. (1982). Women and wellness: Defining, attaining, and maintaining health in Eastern Canada. *Dissertation Abstracts International, 42,* (University Microfilm No. DE0822624).

Salisbury State College (1986, June). *Discussion of Salisbury State College rural health findings.* Presented at the Contemporary Issues in Rural Health Care Conference, Salisbury, MD.

Scharff, J. (1987). *The nature and scope of rural nursing: Distinctive character-*

istics. Unpublished master's thesis, Montana State University, Bozeman, MT.

Snyder, T. (1981, September). Home care. Role of distance to the home training center. *Contemporary Dialysis,* 42–52.

U.S. Congress Office of Technology Assessment (1990). *Health care in rural America* (OTA-H-434). Washington, D.C.: U.S. Government Printing Office.

Walker, M., & Mountain, K. (1988, Spring/Summer). The rural Texan environment and its stressors: A comprehensive model for stress management. *Texas Journal of Rural Health,* 39–45.

Weinert, C., & Long, K. A. (1991). The theory and research base for rural nursing practice. In Bushy, A. (Ed.) *Rural Nursing,* Vol. 1. Newbury Park, CA: Sage.

Weinert, C. (1987). Social support: People living in rural areas. [Abstract]. *Communicating Nursing Research, 20,* 42.

II

ANALYSIS OF KEY CONCEPTS IN RURAL NURSING

In this part of the book, we look at several key concepts identified as important in providing care for persons living in and nurses providing care for persons in rural environments. With exception of chapter 13, the authors for all of the chapters in this section used the Wilsonian process for concept analysis as explicated by Walker and Avant (1983, 1988, 1995). Within those chapters, the attributes of the analyzed concept are based on review of pertinent literature from nursing and related disciplines. The first chapter (chapter 4) is an analysis of distance, a concept now considered less of a problem with more sophisticated vehicles; however, distance remains an issue in rural environments because of the time and resources needed to travel to access resources. In the second chapter (chapter 5), one aspect of the construct of isolation, geographic isolation, is addressed. Because of the arrival of more sophisticated technology (televisions, computers), this concept may seem less applicable to rural areas than in previous times. On the other hand, geographic isolation may never truly disappear in sparsely populated states.

Lack of anonymity and familiarity are the topics for the next two chapters (chatpers 6 and 7). These two concepts are closely related yet different. A compilation of four closely related concepts—oldtimer, newcomer, insider, and outsider—and a comparison of those four concepts is contained in the next five chapters (chapters 8, 9, 10, 11, and 12). Each concept chapter is written by different persons. A comparison was then done by the Rural Nursing Theory Special Committee (RNTSC) working group. We look forward to the rural nursing community's response to the comparison.

Qualitative research methodology was used to identify the characteristics of self-reliance in chapter 13. Chafey, Sullivan, and Shannon determined that, while there is a large body of literature about self-reliance, the concept is "murky with many implicit assumptions" (Morse, 1995). They interviewed rural elderly women and allowed the characteristics of self-reliance to emerge from the gathered data. Their findings, outlined in this chapter, are illuminating.

Chapter 14 on health resources contains a concept analysis followed by a case study in which the author has eloquently captured the essence of what frequently happens in rural settings.

The last two chapters in this section (chapters 15 and 16) are analyses of two closely related concepts important to care of rural persons—lay care network and informal networks. Both were written by graduate students while enrolled in the Family Nurse Practitioner program. The chapter on lay care network ends with suggestions for further refinement of the concept.

REFERENCES

Morse, J. M. (1995). Exploring the theoretical basis of nursing using advanced techniques of concept analysis. *Advances in Nursing Science 17* (3), 31–46.

Walker, L. O., & Avant, K. C. (1983, 1988, 1995). *Strategies for theory construction in nursing* (1st, 2nd, 3rd ed.). Norwalk, CN: Appleton & Lange.

4

Distance

Doris Henson, Teresa Sadler, and Sarah Walton

The purpose of this chapter is to analyze and to clarify the concept of distance as it applies to rural nursing theory. Guidelines suggested for concept analysis in Walker and Avant (1989) are used. This analysis includes examining the definitions and origin of the word "distance," looking at use of the concept in nursing and other disciplines, identifying critical attributes, developing model cases and examining the antecedent and consequences of distance.

DEFINITION

The word distance originates from the Latin verb *stare,* meaning to stand, and the Latin prefix *dis.,* meaning apart (Partridge, 1966). Guralnik (1970) gives the following definitions of the noun distance. "1. Being separated in space or time; remoteness. 2. An interval between two points in space or time. 3. Remoteness in behavior; reserve. 4. A faraway place. 5. In music, an interval between two tones" (p. 139). Synonyms for distance include gap, interval, remoteness, span; nouns describing behavior include restraint, aloofness, and coolness (Kipfer, 1992). In summary, "distance" implies a degree of separation between two or more entities. The nature of separation may be in space, time, or behavior.

Use of the concept of distance is found in many disciplines. The following review of the literature includes uses of distance in the disciplines of exercise physiology, education, psychology, sociology, literature, and the provision of health care, including those in rural nursing.

Exercise Physiology

Exercise physiologists often measure the success of runners by their ability to run certain distances. The aptitudes necessary for distance running include endurance, muscle strength, cardiovascular conditioning, and mental determination of the runner (Fixx, 1977). These attributes will develop and increase over time with proper training. Hydration, proper nutrition, and a good pair of running shoes also influence the ability of a person to run a longer distance. Improper conditioning results in tiredness and possible injury that disrupt the ability to run.

Mathematical models of human running are used to predict racing performance. The Hill–Keller theory states that a runner's speed for a specific distance depends on the balance between the force created by the runner, negative forces such as wind resistance, and the muscle energy both used and furnished from fuels such as glucose. Long-distance running performance also depends on balance between the body's internal heat generation and external heat dissipation (Pritchard & Pritchard, 1994).

Education

"Distance education" is a topic that has become popular in education journals (Shomaker, 1993). Distance education is a means to educate students who are unable to attend classes in a traditional classroom. In this instance, distance denotes the separation of the teacher or institution from the student. Some causes of this separation are geographical remoteness combined with excessive demands on time to travel, debilitating disease, or incarceration (Cadigan, 1993).

In the past, distance education took the form of correspondence schools. Postal services were the link between student and school. Today, with the arrival of fax machines and computer modems, telecommunications has become a major means of communication in distance education (Stevens, 1994). Although distance education is not without problems, the benefits are great. Working people and those with family obligations may receive an education without needing to move. A world of opportunities is opened for those who otherwise might be unable to pursue an education.

Sociology and Psychology

Within the disciplines of sociology and psychology, distance is often discussed as social distance. Social distance describes a level of interaction and intimacy between individuals or the lack thereof. The literature described an example of social distance from a study of students. The students indicated on a rating scale that they preferred greater social distance from patients with psychiatric disorders than from those with physical disorders. Students were uncomfortable with psychiatric patients, especially those who were violent, and were more likely to form less intimate relationships with them (Lyons & Hayes, 1993).

Many factors may influence social distance. Some of these factors are mental and physical disability or disfigurement, race, role, language, and situational uncertainty (Bernsten, 1976; Goto, 1996; Lee, Sapp, & Stephen, 1996; Lukins, 1977; Sayles-Cross, 1993).

Distance concerning relationships can be measured directly in feet and inches. For example, the distance a lower ranking military office stands from a superior officer when speaking to him is greater than it is for civilians interacting while conducting normal business. An interesting example of physical distance is found in an early work on this subject (Hall, 1959). Hall reports that North Americans consider 12 to 20 inches to be a "near distance" for speaking to someone confidentially. However, Latin Americans consider this too great a distance for speaking to someone in a confidential voice. Because comfort level with physical distance varies in different cultures, this can lead to interesting reactions. For example, the South American may not understand why the North American is alway backing away from him when they are in a social conversation. In fact, the North American is seeking a comfortable distance. He is not showing dislike or disinterest, a common misinterpretation. Similar factors that influence physical distance also influence social distance (Bernstein, 1976).

The idea of distance is also used in approaches to family psychotherapy. As an imbalance or remoteness in relationship develops within a family system, one member may manifest symptoms by distancing himself from another member or members. Increased distance is viewed as a decreased level of emotional involvement with other family members to preserve self. It is used as a coping mechanism, but does not resolve the underlying conflict. An example would be the husband who turns his attention to his golf game or a relationship with another woman rather than to a marital conflict with his wife. Emptiness and emotional distance develop between husband and wife. The goal of the family therapist would be to work toward closing this gap (Fogarty, 1976).

Health Care Provision

In health care, the distance of the patient from the health care facility often influences the delivery and receipt of services. Rahaman, Aziz, Munshi, Patwari, and Rahman (1982) studied the impact of distance on use of diarrhea treatment centers in rural Bangladesh. They found that 90% of the people living within one mile of the clinics attended the clinics. The attendance rate of those living greater distances away dropped sharply. Attendance at the clinic "required considerable physical effort if the distance was long" (p. 1127). They also found that the "higher requirement of intravenous solutions in patients reporting from a longer distance was due to longer duration of diarrhea resulting in more severe dehydration" (p. 1127).

Rueben (1993) studied pregnant African women and their attendance at mobile prenatal clinics to receive chemoprophylaxis against malaria. She found that "underprivileged women are generally loaded with household chores and the care of young children. They are therefore less likely than men to attend clinics or hospitals at a distance from their homes . . ." (p. 476).

In the United States medical doctors Valenzuela, Copass, Luna, Rice, and registered nurse Criss (Valenzuela, Criss, Copass, Luna, & Rice, 1990) reviewed aeromedical transport services. They asked the question: "Does long distance transport adversely affect survival?" (p. 169). They compared the mortality of critically injured patients who required aeromedical transport from a distance averaging 340 miles with that of patients transported by ground ambulance within the city limits of Seattle.

> *The range of distances flown by airlift Northwest afforded the opportunity to examine the hypothesis that critically injured patients could be transported by air over long distances without adverse effect as indicated by in-hospital mortality at the receiving regional center (p. 170).*

The aircraft used for transport in the study was equipped to resemble the capabilities of the intensive care unit of the receiving hospital. The results of the study showed that "the size of the distance flown had no significant effect subsequent death or survival" (p. 170). "A carefully configured aeromedical transport system can safely extend the area served by a regional trauma center to at least 800 miles" (p. 172).

Registered nurse Rae Memmott (1991) discussed the difficulties of providing hospice services in the homes of rural patients living in sparsely populated areas. She stated that the distance the nurse has to travel "may impede the delivery of services" (p. 73). In this example, the distance between the nurse and patient may be too difficult to overcome. A study by Buehler and Lee (1992) of home care resources for rural caregivers of a family member with cancer inferred that distance from formal resources limits assistance to the family and the patient. Hospices, home health care, respite, and homemaker services were less available to rural families than to those in more populated areas.

Bushy (1991), a registered nurse, also wrote of the need to consider rural peoples' perception of distance in provision or seeking of health services. "Couched in other terms, a family living five miles from the nearest neighbor may be perceived as close, and traveling 100 miles to the obstetrician may not seem like a great distance" (p. 138).

A study by Snyder (1981) illustrated the variation in perception. She reported that home dialysis patients living in a sparsely populated western state traveled an average of 415 miles to the home dialysis training center. Nine of the 15 subjects regarded the accessibility as "close" or "convenient" if the center was one-half or a day drive or could be reached in two to three hours by plane. Six of the subjects viewed the distance as "far away" but not particularly bothersome.

American Literature

Wallace Stegner (1992) wrote eloquently about the American West. He expressed the perception that the west is about great distance. Mobility is the condition of life if one is to live there. Mobility is necessary to cover great distances. Distance enforces mobility and westerners, especially rural westerners, adapt to it. Traveling is an adaptation—the result of living in the large, remote rural west. The human inhabitants travel as far for recreation, groceries, or health care as "antelopes go for a drink of water . . ." (p. 51).

ESSENTIAL ATTRIBUTES

Three essential attributes became evident from the review of literature. These attributes are mileage and/or time and perception variation.

1. *Mileage.* "Total number of miles traveled" (Guralnik, 1970, p. 474).
2. *Time.* Measurement in minutes it takes to travel from one place to another.
3. *Perception.* Variation in awareness of data that is different from others' awareness of the same data.

These essential attributes help clarify the concept of distance as it relates to health care in a rural environment.

CONSTRUCTED CASES

To clarify a concept, Walker and Avant (1989) advise developing model cases. Cases show the use of the concept with all of its essential attributes and no attributes of another concept. To clarify the concept even more, additional cases are used, such as related, borderline, or illegitimate cases, to explain how they do not define the concept. Related and borderline cases were constructed for this analysis.

Model Case

Hearing a chilling scream, Jane ran outside to find her six-year-old son, Don, laying unconscious on the ground under a tree. Unable to wake him, she ran inside and dialed 911, informing them that she was bringing her son to the local doctor's office. She quickly drove him over the five miles of dirt road and found the doctor waiting anxiously at the door. By this time, her son was starting to thrash around, screaming out at times as if having a nightmare. The doctor did a quick assessment and immediately made arrangements for transfer to the nearest trauma center, 90 miles away. During the next 30 minutes, while waiting for the medical flight plane, Jane called her husband, Joe, to notify him of the accident. They decided that flying with their son would be best for Jane, and Joe would drive to the transferring hospital. It took Joe 75 minutes to drive there, since the road was Interstate all the way. Jane's sister, Pat, lived in the city where the trauma center was and met Jane when she arrived. After Sam's complete recovery, when they were leaving to go home, Pat made the comment, "I would be afraid to raise children being such a distance from adequate health care." Jane responded, "The distance doesn't bother me because we still have access to as much health care as you; it just might take a little longer."

This model case demonstrates all the essential attributes identified for the concept of distance. Distance was described in terms of mileage and time. Perception variation was shown in the discussion between Jane and her sister Pat.

Borderline Case

John lives out in the country by himself and goes into town only monthly to buy groceries. He cut his hand recently with a dirty saw and washed it out and bandaged it himself. When a friend came over to visit, John showed him his hand. His friend remarked, "That cut looks infected. Why don't you go in to see the doctor?" John remarked, "It's too far." The friend replied, "It's not too far if you want to save your hand." John did not go in to see the doctor.

This case uses only one essential attribute of distance, the variation in perception. It does not use the attributes of time or mileage to describe the distance to health care access. Thus, this is a borderline case providing an example of how the concept is not illustrated.

EMPIRICAL REFERENTS

The last step in development of the concept of distance is to determine the empirical referents for critical attributes of mileage, time, and perception. Mileage or the time it takes to reach health care in a rural environment may be greater than in an urban environment and is objective. The MSU Rurality Index, a research tool, uses distance to emergency care as one of its two key variables. This tool has been developed to measure rurality of families residing outside urban locations (Weinert & Boik, 1995). Travel time is also used to express the difference between frontier, urban, and rural service areas (Elison, 1986). Miles and time are objective attributes of distance. However, the way in which distance is perceived is highly subjective. Families and clients determine perceptions; distance is "too great" and thus prohibitive in reaching care or "far away" but not a problem.

Implications for Rural Nursing

The concept of distance has great implications for nurses serving rural areas. Rural patients may be separated by significant distances from health care facilities and services. Depending on the resources and the perceptions of the rural patient, overcoming distance may be difficult. Therefore, assessing the influence of distance on patients and their care is important for nurses. With this information, nurses can help patients use available resources to reduce the impact of distance.

ANTECEDENTS AND CONSEQUENCES

An antecedent for distance as it pertains to health care in the rural environment is access. The consequence is the potential for compromised health care. In the review of the literature, a consequence of distance is revealed. This consequence is as follows: to alter the distance between two or more entities, energy or resource is necessary. One entity must use the available energy or resource to modify the distance between itself and the other entity.

SUMMARY

This analysis contributes to the explanation of the concept of distance as it relates to accessing health care in a rural environment.

The use of the concept was identified through sources from the disciplines of exercise physiology, education, sociology, psychology, American literature, and health care. A literature review of the sources previously listed provided support in selecting the essential attributes of miles, time, and perception. The essential attributes and constructed cases clarified distance. Implications for rural nursing were outlined.

REFERENCES

Bernstein, N. (1976). *Emotional care of the facially burned and disfigured.* Boston: Little, Brown.

Buehler, J., & Lee, H. (1992). Exploration of home care resources for rural families with cancer. *Cancer Nursing, 15* (4), 299–308.

Bushy, A. (1991). Rural determinants in family health: Considerations for community nurses. In A. Bushy (Ed.), *Rural nursing: Vol. 1* (pp. 133–145). Newbury Park, CA: Sage.

Cadigan, J. (1993). Report from Alaska. *Journal of Research in Rural Education, 9* (1), 32–34.

Elison, G. (1986, September/October). Frontier areas: Problems for delivery of health care services. *Rural Health Care, 8* (5), 1, 3.

Fixx, J. F. (1977). *The complete handbook of running.* New York: Random House.

Fogarty, T. F. (1976). System concepts and the dimensions of self. In Guerin (Ed.), *Family therapy, theory, and practice* (pp. 144–153). New York: Gardner Press.

Goto, S. (1996). To trust or not to trust: Situational and dispositional determinant. *Social Behavior and Personality, 24* (2), 119–131.

Guralnik, D.B. (Ed.). (1970). *Webster's new world dictionary: Modern desk edition.* Cleveland, OH: World.

Hall, E. (1959). *The silent language.* New York: Doubleday.

Kipfer, B.A. (Ed.). (1992). *Roget's 21st century thesaurus.* New York: Dell.

Lee, M. Y., Sapp, S. G., & Ray, M. C. (1996). The reverse Social Distance Scale. *Journal of Social Psychology, 136* (1), 17–24.

Lukens, J. (1977, May). *Bridging the communication gap: Understanding communicative distances and cultural differences.* Paper presented at the annual meeting of the International Communication Association, Berlin, Germany.

Lyons, M., & Hayes, R. (1993). Student perceptions of persons with psychiatric and other disorders. *The American Journal of Occupational Therapy, 47* (6), 541–547.

Memmott, R. (1991). Developing hospice programs in frontier communities. In A. Bushy (Ed.), *Rural nursing: Vol. 2* (pp. 63–75). Newbury Park, CA: Sage.

Partridge, E. (1966). *Origins: A short etymological dictionary of modern English.* New York: Macmillian.

Pritchard, W., & Pritchard, J. (1994). Mathematical models of running (noting the effect of wind speed). *American Scientist, 82,* 546–553.

Rahaman, M. M., Aziz, M. S., Munshi, M. H., Patwari, Y., & Rahman, M. (1982). A diarrhea clinic in rural Bangladesh: Influence of distance, age, and sex on attendance and diarrheal mortality. *American Journal of Public Health, 72* (10), 1124–1128.

Reuben, R. (1993). Women and malaria: Special risks and appropriate control strategy. *Social Science Medicine, 37* (4), 437–480.

Shomaker, D. (1993). A statewide instructional television program via satellite for RN-to-B.S.N. students. *Journal of Professional Nursing, 9* (3), 153–158.

Sayles-Cross, S. (1993). Perceptions of familial caregiver of elder adults. *Image, 25* (2),88–92.

Snyder, T. (1981). Role of distance to the home training center, Part I. *Comtemporary Dialysis,* September, 42–52.

Stegner, W. (1992). *Where the bluebird sings to the lemonade springs.* New York: Random House.

Stevens, K. (1994). Australian developments in distance education and their implications for rural schools. *Journal of Research in Rural Education, 10* (1), 78–83.

Valenzuela, T.D., Criss, E.A., Copass, M.K., Luna, G.K., & Rice, C.L. (1990). Critical air transportation of the severely injured: Does distance transport adversely affect survival? *Annals of Emergency Medicine, 19* (2), 169–172.

Weinert, C., & Boik, R. (1995). MSU rurality index: Development and evaluation. *Research in Nursing and Health, 18,* 453–464.

Walker, L. O., & Avant, K. C. (1989). *Strategies for theory construction in nursing* (2nd ed.) (pp. 35–50). Norwalk, CT: Appleton & Lange.

5

Isolation

Helen J. Lee, Brett R. Hollis, and Kathleen A. McClain

INTRODUCTION

The use and meaning of the concept, "isolation" varies with its context as found in health care literature. Rural isolation is presumed to be different from isolation in a large urban area. Within the rural setting one might suppose a differentiation between geographic, social, and professional isolation. The formal definition of the concept remains elusive and confusing. Walker and Avant (1995) state that defining the attributes of a concept promote understanding and communication among colleagues. Therefore, the purpose of this chapter is to analyze the concept of isolation as it pertains to providing health care for clients in sparsely populated areas.

The model of Walker and Avant (1995) is used for the analysis. To clarify the meaning of isolation, various definitions and etymologies are examined. The use of the word is examined across several disciplines. Then, essential attributes of the concept are identified. A case illustrating application of the essential attributes is provided.

DEFINITIONS

The noun, isolation, is defined in Webster's unabridged dictionary (McKechnie, 1983) as the act of isolating or being isolated. Definitions for the verb, isolate, include

> *1. to set apart from others; to place alone. 2. in bacteriology, to grow a pure culture of (a specific bacterium). 3. in chemistry, to separate (an element or compound) in pure form from substances with which it is combined or mixed. 4. in medicine, to place (a patient with a contagious disease) apart from others to prevent the spread of infection. (p. 974)*

The source of *isolate* is derived from the French, *isole,* which comes from the Latin word, *insulatus,* meaning "made into an island" (Flexner, 1993, p. 783). *Insulatus* was transformed by removing the Latin "-atus" and adding the suffix, "-ate." The final form, isolation, was reached with the addition of "-ion," "a suffix appearing in words of Latin origin denoting action or condition, used in Latin and English to form nouns from stems of Latin adjectives, verbs, and part participles" (p. 777). Synonyms include "separation, dissociation, disconnection, detachment, segregation, sequestration, insulation, quarantine" (Rodale, 1978, p. 607).

In *Mosby's Medical and Nursing Dictionary* (Mullens, 1986), isolation refers to the separation of a seriously ill patient from others to prevent the spread of infection either to the patient or to other patients. Isolation may also protect the patient from irritating environmental factors. In a biological science dictionary, isolation means the segregation of organisms (Gray, 1967). Variations from this core definition of isolation are ecoclimatic (isolation due to the climate), ecogeographic (isolation because of geographic location), and ecological (isolation of populations because of living conditions). Bates and Jackson (1980) provide a composite biological definition: isolation is "any process or condition by which a group of individuals is separated for a considerable length of time from other areas or groups as the result of geographic, behavioral, or ecologic factors" (p. 330).

USES OF THE CONCEPT

The concept of isolation was found in many disciplines. Included in this review of literature are biology, education, geography, psychology, sociology, and health care. In some articles reference was made to the root form of the term, isolate or isolated. These have been considered synonymous with isolation for the purposes of this chapter.

Biology

In discussing evolutionary adaptations, Colbert (1969) reported the success of marsupial mammals in Australia because of "isolation from the rest of the world" (p.264) and the lack of competition from placental mammals. He stated that South America "once isolated . . . became a haven for the marsupials since there was not opportunity for advanced placentals to enter the continent from the north" (p. 264). The barriers to random interbreeding affecting isolated populations can have dramatic effects on the genetic make-up and organic evolution of that group.

In microbiology differential centrifugation of culture fluids allows the isolation of viral and bacterial materials necessary for study (Jawetz, Melnick, & Adelberg, 1987). Once separated, the individual specimens, sometimes individual cells, are cultivated so that the resultant progeny remains isolated. A semisolid gelled medium is often used which immobilizes the individual cells and allows each to grow into an isolated colony.

Education

Authors in educational literature mention isolation concerning teachers and students both in relation to environment and academia but do not define the concept. Bell and Sigsworth (1987) use the term "professional isolation" interchangeably with teacher isolation, which is characterized as focusing inward on the school rather than outward to wider professional issues. Isolation is further promoted by the reclusiveness in the rural setting. The most common isolation endured by educators is self-imposed (isolated in one's own concerns); it may be experienced when surrounded by teachers, administrators, and students. Another form of isolation is displayed by departments insulating themselves from other curricula (Sears, 1991). Similarly, in geographic and emotional terms, academic isolation is identified as a key word in an article by Norrell and Ingoldsby (1991) who present strategies for success for new professionals. However, the authors did not provide further interpretation of the concept.

Students may encounter boredom, yearn for greater contact with peers, and more extracurricular activities because of the isolation of the one-room school (Jordan, 1991). The rural school typically holds events that facilitate social interaction in an attempt to preclude social isolation for both adults and students (Bell & Sigsworth, 1987). Rural teachers in many Montana regions must endure winters in isolation, frequently in cramped quarters attached to the schoolhouse, which may contribute to the high turnover rate of teachers in rural areas (Jordan, 1991).

The above articles predominantly view teacher isolation as a self-imposed insulation from the profession. However, isolation can be discussed as a consequence of geographic location, notably in rural settings.

Geography

Geographers are concerned with physical and cultural processes which forge the man–environment system (Cohen, 1967). The study "of rural settlement and the process of rural settling has been an important part of the discipline" (Stone, 1967, p. 221). In a book chapter focused on providing guides for new rural settlements, Stone noted that the more isolated people are from each other, the more dependent they are on each other. Therefore, he proposed a first measure of isolation to be the availability of persons for "emergency or short-time aid to each other" (p. 222). His second measure of isolation was "the location of the residences with regard to existing transport routes" (p. 223).

To introduce the issues pertinent to the writing a rural geography text, Gilg (1985) discussed the difficulties related to the "internal and infernal discussions about the definition of rural areas" (p. 4). One definition he explicated was from rural sociologists Miller and Luloff (1981). They noted that "the term 'rural' is conventionally employed to denote a delimited geographical area characterized by a population that is small, unconcentrated and relatively isolated from the influence of large metropolitan centres" (Miller and Luloff, 1981, p. 609–10).

These geographical references about isolation focus on populations residing within the rural environment. Further, their definition of isolation is relative to the availability of resources (human and transport) and the influence of urban populations.

Psychology

As a broad psychological concept, isolation is described as "a reduction in level of normal sensory and social input without necessarily involving a limitation in physical space or freedom of movement" (Rasmussen, 1973, p .3). Rather than a consequence of the physical environment, isolation may be the result of the individual's perception of a response to the surroundings. Berezin (1980, as cited in Hagerty, Lynch-Sauer, Patusky, & Bouwsema, 1993) indicates that isolation can be an experience to promote growth and renewal. Certain forms of isolation, e.g., lack of involvement, may contribute to creativity, focused concentration, and rest.

Rural Sociology

In their discussion of the ecological component of rurality, Bealer, Willits, and Kuvlesky (1965) define isolation as the lack of "accessibility of one region to others, most particularly to the larger population centers"(p. 341). Historically, the more isolated segments of rural America had little connection with more densely populated areas. Today, "absolute isolation for any geographical area is rare" (p. 341). However, relative isolation currently exists because transportation involves costs and communication is not immediate. Rural and frontier youth may need to travel more than 50 miles to attend school; older individuals who need the health care of a specialist may need to drive 100 miles or more to the city to meet an appointment. These sociologists ask "should isolation be construed in terms of physical distance, commuting costs, availability of communication media, some other factors or combination of factors? Which population centers should be taken as points of reference in determining accessibility?" (p. 342).

Rural Health Care

Although articles in the health care literature included discussion of the causes and effects of isolation, they fail to define the concept. Long and Weinert (1989) reported the analysis of ethnographic data collected from rural residents by graduate students. They found that despite the distance rural residents must travel to receive emergency and routine health care, they did not view themselves as isolated. These rural residents also thought health care services were accessible. However, Long and Weinert did note that rural professionals often reported some degree of isolation.

Gessler, Hartwell, Rickets, and Rosenberg (1992) specify "degree of isolation of health care components" (p. 21) as one of eight geographic themes influencing health care services and delivery in North America. Isolation is discussed in terms of a) definitions of rural, b) providing mental health services to children, and c) emergency medical services.

The first element of the isolation theme was defining what is rural. Concepts of "rural" and "urban" now exist as part of a continuum (Hewitt, 1992). The extremes of the continuum are easy to understand—Los Angeles is an example of the urban end while an isolated farming community in Montana is an example of the rural end. However, determining the cutoff between rural and urban on the continuum becomes much more difficult.

Besides the two well-known definitions of the United States Bureau of the Census and Metropolitan Statistical Areas established by the Office of Management and Budget, several county-based urban/rural typologies exist. Hewitt (1992) says that most of the typology schemes incorporate these measures: a) population size and density, b) adjacency to metropolitan areas, c) degree of urbanization, and d) principle economic activity. For the purposes of health care services planning and research, different designations may be used by the same agency. Hewitt further states that "visual aids such as maps can effectively serve as an analytic device to illustrate geographic variation in health status and access to health care resources . . ." (p. 54). In spatially large western counties, "subcounty geographic units need to be employed to help identify health service areas with special characteristics, such as those which are frontier [i.e., have six or fewer persons per square mile]" (p. 54).

In the second element related to the isolation theme (providing mental health services to children), Hall, Parlour, Nelson, and Walsh (1992) focused on the issue of providing adequate services for children's mental health in a remote province of Ontario. Three major systems impact the social context of children's mental health—the geosocial (the patterning of socioeconomic indicators in geographic space), the sociocultural (norms, values, and traditions of rural families and communities), and the planning, policy, and service delivery (formal health, social, and education system). Geographically speaking, most Canadian provinces are characterized by vast stretches of sparsely populated lands. The economy is dependent on the extractive industries (mining, logging, & farming); therefore, employment opportunities are scarce. Socioculturally, the communities display a strong sense of belongingness, community identity, mutual aid, self-sufficiency, and strong social controls over individual and community behavior. If professionals are able to set aside urban oriented misconceptions and develop sensitivity to cultural differences, their practice can include elements "of community participation, integration of services, and health promotion and prevention" (Bell, 1980 as cited in Hall et al., 1992, p. 144). However, the communities lack cultural opportunities and "communication and access to services . . . are hampered by distance, as well as cultural, experiential, and linguistic differences" (p. 144). Twenty percent of the total population in the northern part of the province is French-speaking; these people are becoming more isolated as many communities are officially declaring themselves unilingual in English. Inadequate data bases were established because the on-reservation Native American (Metis, Ojibway, and Cree) children were not included in a province-wide child's mental health study sample. The authors conclude that while "programs receptive to the needs of children in northern communities are slowly beginning to emerge . . . unhealthy current and sociocultural environments for children do not bode well for their future health as adults" (p. 150).

For the third element of the isolation theme (emergency medical services), Rutledge, Rickets, & Bell (1992) iterated several problems in providing emergency medical services (EMS) for rural areas. Specific problems include a) poor roads, causing EMS transport delays, and b) "difficulty in public access because of limited implementation of 911 systems throughout the states" (p. 227). In many rural areas long-distance calls must be made to obtain emergency assistance. Even in today's world, some rural areas do not have telephone service. "Rural and frontier EMS crews will continue to be at risk, because they are out of radio contact when on difficult runs" (Anderson, 1992, p. 130). Many rural EMS systems are limited because their prehopsital care providers are volunteers who have only basic levels of training. Maintaining specialized EMS skills is difficult because of the low volume of emergencies. Rural physicians and nurses may not have advanced EMS training. Rural hospitals may not have developed EMS protocols, or have the necessary equipment. "Rural areas often lack the resources (basically financial) needed to address EMS systems" (Rutledge et al., p. 227).

MEDIA

Three recent newspaper articles point out experiences with the isolation of rural living. The first addresses living on an American Indian reservation. The second discusses the realities of rural living for prospective residents of a rural county. The third speaks to the need for rural parents to move to provide opportunity for their child to participate in sports.

American Indian

Every year Giago (1997) interviews elders for a special tabloid called "Many Winters" for his newspaper, *Indian Country Today,* a national weekly newspaper on American Indian issues. He noted the importance of absorbing the knowledge elders have to offer as Indian culture, language, and traditions are being lost. He wrote

> *Quite often I read about an elder of a tribe located in the East who was the last left in the tribe who could speak the language. This is a real shame. Out in the Midwest it will never be a problem. Because of the isolation of tribes such as the Sioux or the Navajo, the language continued to be an important part of the day-to-day conversation. It is to this day. (p. A10)*

Rural Living

To educate prospective residents seeking "spectacular views, a sense of solitude and wide open spaces" (Thayer, 1997, p. B1), Larimer County (Colorado) Commissioner, John Clarke wrote a booklet titled, *The Code of the West.* In it he outlines specific differences between city and country living. Emergency response time may be longer; maintenance of some roads may be the responsibility of private road associations rather than the county. "Water, sewer, electric, telephone and other services may be unavailable or [not] operate at urban standards. Repairs can often take much longer than in towns and cities. . . . trash removal can cost more in rural areas than in a city" (p. B2).

Sports Participation

The front page of the *Missoulian* carried the story of the parents of three University of Montana Lady Griz players who drive from Malta, a town in north central Montana close to the Canadian border, to Missoula for home game nights (Merriam, 1997). The distance is 366 miles one way; only the last 10 miles are interstate. The parents of a senior player, Greta Koss, made it to every game during the 1996–1997 season except one; that game was missed because of a snow storm. Greta's mom shared with the news reporter that the Kosses lived 50 miles out in the country and Greta attended a "little room country school" (p. A2). For Greta to become active in school basketball required that the family move to Malta, a community of 2,500 population.

ESSENTIAL ATTRIBUTES

The examination of various disciplines' uses of the concept "isolation" revealed "characteristics of the concept which appear over and over again" (Walker and Avant, 1995, p. 41). These characteristics or attributes differentiate the meaning of "isolation" from other, similar concepts, and, as such, are essential to its understanding. These attributes are identified as (a) separation, (b) relativeness, and (c) perception.

Separation refers to "being divided from the rest" (McKechnie, 1983, p. 1653). This condition can occur for many different reasons.

Relativeness says that isolation is "something dependent on external conditions for its specific nature . . . existing or having its specific nature only by relation to something else; not absolute or independent" (McKechnie, 1983, p. 1211).

Perception means "consciousness or awareness" (McKechnie, 1983, p. 1330). Depending on one's background, a person may or may not be aware of the experience of isolation.

Antecedents and Consequences

Necessary for the condition of isolation to occur is the presence of indicator(s). An indicator will "point out . . . (or) direct attention to" (McKechnie, 1983, p. 724) the condition of isolation. Examples of indicators are geographical terrain, distance, changes imposed by weather (e.g., snow storm, black ice, floods), economic costs, time, or personal preference.

One consequence of isolation is decreased communication or interaction with other persons. This may lead to social isolation and, for health care personnel, professional isolation. Additional consequences of isolation in client health care situations are the potential loss of life, limbs, and health.

MODEL CASE

Cases promote further understanding of a concept. "A model case is a 'real life example' of the use of the concept that includes all the critical attributes on the concept" (Walker & Avant, 1995, p. 42). This case is of an individual, JB, who shared her experiences growing up in eastern Montana.

Isolation is pretty much the story of my early life. I was born in Miles City, Montana, which was 80 miles from my home, a ranch in Carter County. The ranch was located in the community of Hammond which was our address. The Hammond post office was 32 miles away; mail was delivered on a rural route twice a week. For prenatal care my mother obviously needed to go to a larger community to have her babies. Miles City was where she did that. She needed to move there and stay for two weeks before both my brother and I were born. I went home in an airplane, my first trip home. My dad had a four-seater, single engine plane. At that time the roads were all gumbo and there was no upgrading of those roads until I was nine or ten years old. So my early years were spent in that ranch community with our nearest neighbor two or three miles away. The nearest town was Ekalaka, a town of 700–800 people about 50 miles away. Going to town used to be a really big treat!

While growing up, the only interaction I had with kids was when there were community social events. Otherwise, families pretty much stayed to themselves. You played with your siblings or did whatever you could think of to do. Kids had to entertain themselves. Your parents didn't have a lot of time to be fooling around with you, playing with you, that sort of thing. There wasn't anything like an organized baseball league. So you had your siblings and yourself and an occasional visitor.

I had imaginary playmates. My imaginary playmates were my dresses. Interestingly, I had quite a few nice dresses. The reason I had so many nice dresses was because of a neighbor and her husband. They didn't have any children. She was from Mississippi; she had married this guy when he was in the service and they ended up in Carter county. She liked me and always bought me dresses for special occasions like Easter, Christmas, my birthday. So I always had dresses, nice dresses. I named them and they were my friends. We would have parties. I would sit them erect in the living room and they would be on hangers and I would put them around and we would play. I did have dolls but they were not as real to me as the dresses. More interesting to me than dolls was old catalogs. I'd take them and cut out families. I'd have a mother and a father and the little kids. And then I'd cut out clothes and fix houses. Mostly they would be books on the floor and I'd put towels on them for carpeting. I would do that by the hour.

There was a really strong sense of community in this area. Community social events included a week of community bible school in the community hall during the summer. They had an event in the summer called Box Elder Day that was a picnic and a dance at the community hall. There was much visiting when you could get around. The community hall was six miles away. When it rained, before we had gravel, you just didn't go to school or you road horseback. You've never seen gumbo like gumbo in Ekalaka; I mean, it will hang six inches off your overshoes!

There was always a concern about whether somebody was getting sick or hurt and whether you were going to be able to get out of there. Mud was the worst; next to that was no visibility with snow. I don't remember that cold ever stopped us from going anywhere. I remember my parents having discussions about whether they should take one of us to the doctor. Of course, we never wanted to go. I had an appendicitis when I was seven years old. It came on real suddenly and my mom first thought I had a stomachache from eating too many raisin cookies! I got sick in the night. Somehow my mom did pretty well at knowing when we needed to go (which wasn't very often!). My folks took me to town the next day in the car; they took me to Belle Fouche (South Dakota) which was 75 miles. I had surgery there in Belle Fouche.

The incident with the appendicitis was the only time I can remember being taken to the doctor when I was sick. I can remember having terrible flu, vomiting and fever and getting off the couch and feeling like the floor is coming up at you. I mean really, really sick and my mother never considered that to be that serious. And we always did come out of it. I have several scars that obviously would not look like they do if I had had stitches. We just didn't do that; I don't know why we didn't die of tetanus. I don't remember having a tetanus shot unless I had it when I was a baby, and that's not likely. In the fourth grade I cut one of my fingers really really badly. It took a long long time for that to heal. I have one scar on my knee that should have been sutured.

My brother and I attended a country school five miles from the ranch. This was a one room school house. There was one teacher and about ten kids in several grades. When we got to the age for my brother and I to begin high school (my brother had graduated from the eighth grade and I was in the sixth grade), my dad began to think about moving. My parents didn't want us to be raised by somebody else, farmed out with other people during the week. He looked for a different ranch. We sold our two ranches in Carter county and brought one in Glendive, 24 miles away. At that point we had a house in town and a house on the ranch. My dad would go out every day and my mom stayed in town.

I know that some bad roads still exist for some of those families, even to this day. The last time I was in the area I visited a family out on their ranch. Their ranch is three or four miles off the main gravel road and the road into their house was still gumbo. And it rained while I was there and we had quite a time getting out to the main road. We actually had to drive out into the main pasture where you could get on the sod and kind of work your way out of there. The weather certainly is a huge factor in making it difficult to actually get physically from one place to another. They need to get to the doctor. They need to get their kids to school. They are boarding their high school students in a town during the week. Getting them on weekends, getting them back can be a real problem. If families don't move to town when their kids are in high school they may make them ride the bus (there were no busses when I was growing up). But, if you ride the bus you don't have any opportunity to participate in anything, the extracurricular activities.You move to town with your kids or you farm them out with family and friends.

I've never had any desire to go back and live in that environment (presently lives in Billings, the largest city in the state of Montana). I've had enough of not having access to services, of not having 'real' people. Once I had a taste of that, once I realized the way other people lived, I was sort of like the Mississippi woman. But while I was there, it didn't bother me. Once I had something to compare it to, then I didn't want to go back.

The model case interview with JB reveals the attributes, the antecedents, and the consequences of the concept of isolation. Growing up in a remote rural area of Montana, JB experienced *separation* from other children her age and from health care services. She encountered the *relativeness* of isolation when her parents moved from one rural site to another. Her *perception* of isolation also changed with experience. The antecedent indicators present in JB's story include geographical terrain, distance, changes imposed by the weather, and time. A major consequence for her was the decreased interaction with other potential playmates during her early years of growing up.

SUMMARY

This analysis of the concept of isolation resulted in the identification of the essential attributes of separation, relativeness, and perception. Clarification of the ambiguity of the concept through definitions and a case illustration may contribute to rural nursing theory development by enhancing communication and understanding between professionals. Further study aimed at identifying and decreasing the effects of isolation in rural health care settings is needed.

REFERENCES

Anderson, P. B. (1992). Rural EMS system development: Innovative technological approaches. In L. A. Straub & N. Walzer (Eds.). *Rural health care: Innovation in a changing environment.* Westport, CN: Praeger.

Bates, R. J., & Jackson, J. A. (Eds.) (1980). *Glossary of geology* (2nd ed.). Falls Church, VA: American Geological Institute.

Bealer, R. C., Willits, F. K., & Kuvlesky, W. P. (1965). The meaning of "rurality" in American society: Some implications of alternative definitions. In R. D. Rodefield, J. Flora, D. Voth, I. Fujimoto, & J. Converse (1978), *Change in rural America* (pp. 338–351). St. Louis, MO: Mosby.

Bell, A., & Sigsworth, A. (1987). *The small rural primary school: A matter of quality.* London: Falmer Press.

Cohen, S. B. (Ed.). (1967). *Problems and trends in American geography.* New York: Basic Books.

Colbert, E.H. (1969). *Evolution of the vertebrates* (2nd ed.). New York: John Wiley.

Flexner, S. B. (Ed.) (1993). *Random House Unabridged Dictionary* (2nd ed.). New York: Random House.

Gesler, W. M., Hartwell, S., Ricketts, T. C., & Rosenberg, M. W. (1992). Introduction. In W. M. Gesler & T. C. Ricketts (Eds.), *Health in rural North America: The geography of health care services and delivery* (pp. 1–24). New Brunswick, NJ: Rutgers University Press.

Giago, T. (1997, March 28). Voices of elders speak loudly in "Many Winters." *Missoulian,* p. A10.

Gilg, A. (1985). *Introduction to rural geography.* London: Edward Arnold.

Gray, P. (Ed.). (1967). *The dictionary of the biological sciences.* New York: Reinhold.

Hagerty, B. M. K., Lynch-Sauer, J., Patusky, K. L., & Bouwsema, M. (1993). An emerging theory of human relatedness. *Image:Journal of Nursing Scholarship, 25* (4), 291–296.

Hall, G. B., Paulour, S. J., Nelson, G. B., & Walsh, R. T. (1992). In W. M. Gesler & T. C. Ricketts (Eds.). *Health in rural North America: The geography of health care services and delivery* (pp. 131–152). New Brunswick, NJ: Rutgers University Press.

Hewitt, M. (1992). Defining "rural" areas: Impact on health care policy and research. In W. M. Gesler & T. C. Ricketts (Eds.). *Health in rural North America: The geography of health care services and delivery* (pp. 25–54). New Brunswick, NJ: Rutgers University Press.

Jawetz, E., Melnick, J., & Adelberg, E. A. (Eds.) (1987). *Review of medical microbiology* (17th ed.). Norwalk, CN: Appleton & Lange.

Jordan, S. (1991). The schoolhouse on the prairie. *Time, 137,* 56.

Long, K. A., & Weinert, C. (1989). Rural nursing: Developing the theory base. *Scholarly Inquiry for Nursing Practice, 3,* 113–127.

McKechnie, J. L. (Ed.). (1983). *Webster's new universal unabridged dictionary* (2nd ed.). New York: Simon & Schuster.

Merriam, G. (1977, March 8). Driving the lane. *Missoulian.* pp. A1–2.

Miller, M. K., & Luloff , A. E. (1981). Who is rural: A typological approach to the examination or rurality. *Rural Sociology, 46,* 608–625.

Mullins, N.L. (Ed.). (1986). *Mosby's medical & nursing dictionary* (2nd ed.). St. Louis, MO: Mosby.

Norrell, J., & Ingoldsby, B. (1991). Surviving academic isolation: Strategies for success. *Family Relations, 40,* 345–347.

Rasmussen, J.E. (Ed.). (1973). *Man in isolation and confinement.* Chicago: Aldine.

Rodale, J. I. (1978). *The synonym finder.* Emmaus, PA: Warner.

Rutledge, R., Rickets, T. C., & Bell, E. (1992). Emergency medical care in rural areas. In W. M. Gesler & T. C. Ricketts (1992). *Health in rural*

North America: The geography of health care services and delivery (pp.226–248). New Brunswick, NJ: Rutgers University Press.

Sears, S. (1991). The isolated teacher. *English Journal, 80,* 15–16.

Stone, K. H. (1967).Geographic aspects of planning for new rural settling in the free world's northern lands. In S. B. Cohen (Ed.). *Problems and trends in American geography.* New York: Basic Books.

Thayer J. (1977, March). Living the code of the west. *Missoulian,* p. B1.

Walker, L. O., & Avant, K.C. (1995). *Strategies for theory construction in nursing* (3rd ed.). Norwalk, CT: Appleton & Lange.

6

Lack of Anonymity

Helen J. Lee

A key concept identified for persons living and working in a rural environment is "lack of anonymity" (Long & Weinert, 1989). For persons living in rural areas, the concept suggests a lack of privacy about their personal lives. For nurses working in sparsely populated areas, "lack of anonymity" means taking care of clients who are known through associations other than the nurse/client relationship. While the term lack of anonymity is frequently mentioned in rural and rural nursing literature, a clear definition of the concept was not found. Therefore, the aim of this chapter is to analyze lack of anonymity to refine and clarify the concept. "Careful concept development is the basis for any attempt to describe or explain phenomena" (Walker & Avant, 1994, p. 36). Wilson's method of analysis as explicated and modified by Walker and Avant was used. The steps followed include identification of uses of the concept in various disciplines, determination of attributes, identification of antecedents and consequences, development of cases, and determination of empirical referents.

DEFINITIONS

The concept, lack of anonymity, consists of two terms linked with a participle. The dictionary definition of the noun anonymity is "the quality or state of being anonymous" (McKechnie, 1979, p. 75). Webster' Dictionary (1983) includes these definitions for anonymous: "1. without any name acknowledged, as that of author, contributor, or the like: an anonymous pamphlet. 2. of unknown name; whose name is withheld; an anonymous author" (p. 61). The source of the adjective anonymous is from the Latin *anonymus* and Greek *anonymos*; *an-* means without, *onym* (a) refers to name, and *-os* is a suffix forming adjectives (Barnhart, 1988, p. 37). Synonyms for anonymous include nameless, unidentified, unknown, and unsigned (Corel, 1996).

The noun lack has these definitions:

> *1. deficiency or absence of something needed, desirable, or customary:* lack of money or skill. *2. something missing or needed:* After he left, they really felt the lack.*-v.t. 3. to be without or deficient in:* to lack ability; to lack confidence; to lack the necessities of life *(Webster, 1983, p. 800).*

Lack is derived from the "Middle English *lak* (and); the Middle Dutch *lac,* 'deficiency, fault' which is related to Old Norsk, *lakr,* 'lacking' " (Klein, 1966, p. 857). Synonyms for lack include dearth, scarcity, paucity, shortcoming, deficit, and insufficiency (Webster, 1983). "Lack emphasizes the void or deficiency that results from the absence of the thing in question . . ." (*American Heritage Dictionary,* 1992, p. 1006). Therefore, lack of anonymity refers to a condition in which one cannot remain nameless or unknown.

USES OF THE CONCEPT

The concept of anonymity was found in several disciplines including psychology, sociology, social work, research, and agricultural history. The concept lack of anonymity was found in a few articles describing the discipline of professional practice within rural settings and with rural clients. This review reflects literature for both concepts.

Psychology

In an essay reflecting on anonymity, social psychologist Williams (1988) described two categories, inevitable and exploitive. Inevitable anonymity relates to the number of people normally encountered during a week; "the anonymity of individuals is overcome for us primarily because we know them by name" (p. 761). The second category, exploitive, "is regarded as a condition that frees individuals from social evaluation or scrutiny" (p. 765).

Several experimental studies have been conducted with students comparing the condition of anonymity with a public or identifiable condition. Findings show that students acting in a current situation in which they are anonymous are less self-conscious and less inhibited (Nadler, Goldberg, & Jaffe, 1982) and are less willing to do prosocial behaviors (i.e., donations to a worthy cause) (Bontempo, Lobel, & Triandis, 1990; Nadler et al., 1982). Findings from a human development study were that all the children (kindergartners through eighth graders) shared more in public than through secret balloting. However, eighth graders were more likely to share with friends than with acquaintances and disliked peers than the younger children (Buhrmester, Goldfarb, & Cantrell, 1992). Retrospectively examining the condition of anonymity, Quigley-Fernandez (1983) found that female college students were more likely to develop explanations for success or failure when public knowledge of their performance existed.

Reams (1987) described a case study in which darkness was used as a facilitator of disclosure in play therapy. The child "had repeatedly hit other children, his mother, and his teachers. He had no friends" (Reams, 1987, p. 112). When the therapy room was initially darkened, the child spoke of his fears; however, with the second episode of darkness, the child hugged the therapist for more than 15 seconds. "Darkness confers an anonymity on the people it surrounds . . . [and] allows him [the child] to shed any stigma from his out-of-role behavior [the hug]" (Reams, 1987, p. 113).

Solomon, Solomon, and Maiorca (1982) reviewed three studies that provided evidence that anonymity reduces helping behaviors for persons (emergency, low economic status, information) in urban settings. They suggested that living in large cities encourages anonymity as a response to a sensory overload. They also implied that anonymous big city dwellers may further attempt to adapt to overload by ignoring low priority inputs such as low status victims and ambiguous requests for help.

Sociology

Tittle and Stafford (1992) defined an anonymous individual as one who "feels so free of surveillance by others that he or she conceives little chance that potential misbehavior will be discovered, much less responded to in a negative way" (p. 732). In their three-state survey that compared urban, suburban, and rural residents on items reflecting potential misbehavior, they found that perceived levels of anonymity rose with increasing population density with the least amount of anonymity in the rural dwellers.

Social Work

While health care, law enforcement, and school personnel are mandated by law to report suspected abuse, many agencies will also accept accounts of abuse from nonmandated sources. Many nonmandated accounts of abuse are anonymous. "Intuitive belief is that these (anonymous) reports are generally less serious" (Adams, Barone & Tooman, 1982, p. 4). However, two studies found that while anonymous accounts of suspected abuse were more likely to be unfounded, those reports substantiated were equally serious as to physical abuse (Adams et al., 1982; Zuravin & Watson, 1987).

Research

Williams (1988) says that ". . . anonymity of the subjects in research studies has always been an essential aspect of research" (p.764). Anonymity, one of several types of privacy (Westin, 1970, & Peterson, 1979 as cited in Williams, 1988) is the strongest method of ensuring privacy. Privacy means that persons can maintain control over information about themselves (Sobel, 1992). The researcher should not know and be able to trace the identity of persons agreeing to be research subjects. Conducting qualitative research demands paying special attention to protecting the identity and confidentiality of participants.

Agricultural History

"Privacy as an asserted legal right is a development of the last 100 years . . . [it] is a part of the right to life, within which is a right to be left alone" (Peterson, 1990, p. 3). However, with respect to voting, Peterson states that the

> *... culturally homogeneous rural community does not easily accommodate personal anonymity.... Lacking anonymity, the rural voter was known to his neighbors. They knew whether or not he participated in political matters, whether he voted, what party he favored, what views he held. A secret ballot would do little to give him real privacy in political association. (p. 6)*

Peterson (1990) further said that:

> *... agricultural labor was often performed in the company of other family members or hired labor. Nor did the farmer have any economic privacy: his crops stood for all to see, the numbers and health of his livestock could be inspected by anyone passing by, the prices he got were routinely known in the local community where the elevator operator and the stock buyer worked. (p. 6)*

Rural Clients

In a presentation at the Annual National Institute on Social Work and Human Services in Rural Areas, Link (1988) discussed the lessons learned from a project designed to increase use of mental health services among persons affected by the farm crisis. One service delivery issue was that satellite offices needed to be available but not near the clients' home community. "Clients were willing to go some extra miles to an office where they felt they had less chance of being identified by their own community members" (Link, 1988, p. 5). A recent study conducted by Rost, Smith, and Taylor (1993) examined rural-urban differences in stigma and the use of care for depressive disorders. They found that, in comparison to urban persons, rural persons with a history of depressive symptoms labeled people who sought help for symptoms more negatively and were also less likely to seek professional help themselves.

Jones (1981), a social worker, identified several characteristics of the rural poor; included were rugged individualism, low use of services, and the potential for those asking for help being held up to community scorn. He showed that the rural poor do not have the protective anonymity of the urban area; social workers reported having lost clients because they ran into acquaintances in the waiting room.

Long (1986), a clinical nurse specialist and educator, identified lack of anonymity as one risk factor for suicide in Native American adolescents living on reservations. She notes that people know each other well in sparsely populated geographic areas. Influenced by peer behaviors, the individual suicide action "becomes a role model of coping behavior for many persons in the community. The contagion effect of suicide is greatly enhanced because it is not happening to strangers" (p. 250).

Craig (1994) was interested in older individuals conception of health and how this conception was supported by the rural community where they resided. Older community residents, their families, community members, community leaders, and health care professionals residing in a small Great Plains farming community were interviewed for her ethnographic study. Themes evolving from her data analysis appear closely related to the concept of lack of anonymity. Relationship was the key theme found; reciprocal relationships provided benefits for the older residents and the community. "Younger people helped older ones with shopping, transportation, and household chores, whereas older residents contributed volunteer time in community organizations and schools" (p. 244). Sometimes, however, elders were overwhelmed with the decreased privacy and the stigma encountered by persons from a different culture or when welfare was accepted.

Rural Professional Practice

Professional practice in rural communities has a different flavor than practice in an urban setting. Jennings (1992), a psychologist who practiced in both rural and urban settings, describes the ethical problems he encountered when practicing psychotherapy in a rural environment. Included is the

> *extent to which lack of anonymity, and considerable public scrutiny (and knowledge), about the psychologist's personal life often creates major difficulty in rendering professional services. The emphasis both in training programs and in the tenor of ethics statements is toward maintenance of a certain amount of*

anonymity in the delivery of professional services. The writer would argue that this ideal is flatly impossible to achieve in most rural settings (p. 96).

In an article addressing issues in the development of quality assurance programs in rural hospitals, Bushy (1991), a nurse educator, stated that

the small town's informal social structure, better known as the 'main street grapevine' facilitates professional disagreements becoming public knowledge . . . Concerns related to confidentiality and anonymity . . . stem from the reality that most persons who live in a small community are (at least) fairly well acquainted. Many residents are blood relatives or have become a member of an extended family through marriage . . . the small, local hospital often is one of the largest employers within a rural community . . . contribute[ing] to leaks of hospital-related information among local residents (p. 36).

While a graduate nursing student, Saunders (1992) gathered perceptions of nurses practicing in frontier medical assistance facilities (MAF) in Montana. Examples of lack of anonymity from her thesis narrative follow.

Nurses reported that everyone knows who you are and where you are and will call you. One nurse explained the only 'vacation' from nursing that she takes is during the 'lambing season.' She went on to explain when she did not answer her telephone while on vacation . . . 'they'll drive out and come up to the lambing shed looking for me.' One nurse participant described a lack of anonymity during an emergency situation then 'they found me at the court house and asked me to hurry to the MAF.' (p. 41–42)

Martinez-Brawley (1991), a social worker, says people move to small towns because they do not want to be anonymous. They value "being recognized and treated as people with names at the grocery store, the school, or the playground" (p. 224). For elderly individuals, the "lack of anonymity of the small community is usually a safeguard or asset and can be transformed into a major component of care in the community" (p. 224). She notes that while lack of anonymity may be positive in certain situations (providing services to older people), it also may be negative because of the stigma attached to particular services (welfare).

"While not systematically taught or regarded as bona fide in many circles . . . a different kind of practice has always been required in small towns" (Martinez-Brawley, 1991, p. 216). Martinez-Brawley suggested that "professional commitments to anonymity, definitions of confidentiality, and reliance on lay helpers all require modification in the less formal and bureaucratic context of small towns" (p. 215). The modifications needed include principles that are the basis of "community-oriented social work" (p. 216). The principles are

> *(a) the provision of care by members of the community, to each other, in mutually supporting relationships and by social workers and other human services personnel working in the community, in partnership with friends, neighbors, and volunteers . . .*
> *(b) the reinterpretation of confidentiality to suit the context;*
> *(c) the use of nonprofessional helpers in many varied tasks; and*
> *(d) greater reliance on neighbors and churches. (p. 216)*

ESSENTIAL ATTRIBUTES

Three essential attributes were identified through examination of the use of the concepts of anonymity and lack of anonymity in available literature. The attributes for lack of anonymity are (a) visible, (b) identifiable, and (c) diminished personal/professional boundaries.

- *Visible*: that which can be seen, is apparent or obvious.
- *Identifiable*: being able to recognize or establish the condition or character of a person.
- *Diminished personal/professional boundaries*: borders or perimeters through which one functions are smaller, more circumscribed.

ANTECEDENTS AND CONSEQUENCES

Lack of anonymity occurs in an environmental context characterized by a low level of stimulation. It contains fewer numbers of individuals and/or objects (e.g., automobiles, buildings) needing to be considered in the normal deliberation of one's activities.

An overall consequence for lack of anonymity is a relationship. In this relationship, one's actions are visible and readily observed. Because of the relationship, there is greater difficulty in maintaining personal and professional privacy.

CASES USING IDENTIFIED ATTRIBUTES

Two cases are presented. The first case is a model case; it contains all the identified attributes for the concept of lack of anonymity. The second case is a borderline case containing most but not all of the attributes.

Model Case

Alice Brown is a nurse who lives in a community of 11,000 population and works at the local combined 24-bed community hospital and 50-bed nursing home. On the Saturday of her weekend off, she goes to pick up groceries at the local store. While there, she meets Mrs. Larson who was her patient Monday of the previous week. In response to the usual question, "How are you?" Mrs. Larson reports of her progress since her dismissal. In addition, she asks Alice Brown for advice about a health problem that is currently bothering her husband. Alice gives Mrs. Larson a response, and they part to continue their grocery shopping.

This case meets all the attributes of lack of anonymity. Alice Brown is *visible* and *identifiable* within the rural community in which she lives and works as a nurse in the local hospital. Because of her identification as a nurse within the rural community of which she is a part, she has *diminished professional role boundaries.* This is evident in the expectations of her former patient to provide professional information in a public and not a professional setting.

Borderline Case

Jane Wood comes from a small town of 200 people. Currently she is a nursing student at a hospital campus in a nearby city of 70,000.

While participating in her clinical experience she encounters Juanita Jones, a 46–year-old woman from her hometown who is hospitalized for a bleeding ulcer. A week later during a visit home, Jane's mother shares with Jane that Mrs. Jones had been in the hospital and wants to know if Jane saw her. Jane said that she did see Mrs. Jones. Jane's mother immediately responds with the question, "Why didn't you tell us?" Jane replies, "That information was for Mrs. Jones to share."

This case partially meets the essential attributes for lack of anonymity. Because the two individuals came from the same town, the nursing student was *visible* and *identifiable* to the hospitalized Mrs. Jones. However, the attribute of *a diminished professional role boundary* was not met because Jane Wood could follow her professional ethical code by not discussing Mrs. Jones' hospitalization until Mrs. Jones came home and told others.

SUMMARY

The concept of lack of anonymity was analyzed using the dictionary and literature about anonymity and lack of anonymity from several disciplines. Essential attributes, antecedents, and consequences of the concept were identified. Two cases, model and borderline, were constructed.

The available rural literature and the literature from other disciplines infer that the presence of lack of anonymity does make a difference for persons living and working in rural areas. For example, rural clients may not feel comfortable accessing mental health services with others knowing. Obviously, this leads to reduced use of those services. The obvious practice implication is that health care services need to be provided in a manner or place where privacy can be respected.

Within the seminal theory development article by Long and Weinert (1989), a descriptive statement ". . . that healthcare providers must deal with lack of anonymity . . ." (p. 120) is made. What does that mean for rural nurses and their clients? Does lack of anonymity make rural nurses more accountable? Does this view influence the kind of nursing care delivered because the rural nurse and the client know each other? Does lack of anonymity interfere with being able to make an objective client assessment? Does the presence of lack of anonymity result in providing better quality of nursing care for clients? In what way does lack of anonymity affect the care given to clients from diverse ethnic groups? And how does lack of anonymity affect the retention and turnover of nurses?

Many of the above questions raised about lack of anonymity bear a close relationship to the concept of familiarity. How are these two concepts related and how are they different? Based on this question and the questions raised in the previous paragraph, the concept analysis of lack of anonymity has generated further work for rural nursing theory developers!

REFERENCES

Adams, W., Barone, N., & Tooman, P. (1982). The dilemma of anonymous reporting in child protective services. *Child Welfare, 61,* 3–14.

American Heritage Dictionary of the English Language. (1992). Boston: Houghton Mifflin.

Barnhart, R. K. (Ed.). (1988). *The Barnhart dictionary of etymology.* Bronx, NY: Wilson.

Bontempo, R., Lobel, S., & Triandis, H. (1990). Compliance and value internalization in Brazil and the U.S.: Effects of allocentrism and anonymity. *Journal of Cross-Cultural Psychology, 21,* 200–213.

Buhrmester, D., Goldfarb, J., & Cantrell, D. (1992). Self-presentation when sharing with friends and nonfriends. *Journal of Early Adolescence, 12,* 61–79.

Bushy, A. (1991). Quality assurance in rural hospitals. *Journal of Nursing Administration, 21*(10), 34–39.

Corel Word Perfect. (1996). *Thesaurus,* Version 6.1. Ottawa, Ontario, Canada: Corel Corporation.

Craig, C. (1994). Community determinants of health for rural elderly. *Public Health Nursing, 11*(4), 242–246.

Jennings, F. L. (1992). Ethics of rural practice. *Psychotherapy in Private Practice, 10*(3), 85–104.

Jones, L. P. (1981). Distinctive features of mid-west rural poverty: Implications for social work practice. *ERDS, ED 261 816,* 22.

Klein, E. (1966). *A comprehensive etymological dictionary of the English language.* Amsterdam: Elsevier.

Link, E. A. (1988). Mental health services to rural consumers: Lessons learned from a four year Iowa farm crisis project. *ERDS, ED 313 202,* 6.

Long, K. A. (1986). Suicide intervention and prevention with Indian adolescent populations. *Issues in Mental Health Nursing, 8,* 247–253.

Long, K. A., & Weinert, C. (1989). Rural nursing: Developing the theory base. *Scholarly Inquiry for Nursing Practice, 3*(2), 113–127.

Martinez-Brawley, E. E. (1990). *Perspectives on the small community: Humanistic views for practitioners.* Silver Spring, MD: National Association of Social Workers Press.

McKechnie, J. L. (1979). *Webster's new universal unabridged dictionary* (2nd Ed.). New York: Dorcet & Baber.

Nadler, A., Goldberg, M., & Jaffe, Y. (1982). Effect of self-differentiation and anonymity in group on deindividuation. *Journal of Personality and Social Psychology, 42,* 1127–1136.

Peterson, T. (1990). Rural life and the privacy of political association. *Agriculture History, 64*(3), 1–8.

Quigley-Fernandez, B. (1983, 16–20, 1983 April). Self-service biases: Private perceptions or public distortion. *Paper presented at the annual meeting of the Western Psychological Association, San Francisco, CA.* 1–9.

Reams, R. (1987). Darkness in play therapy: Anonymity and a sense of control as facilitators of disclosure. *Journal of Child and Adolescent Psychotherapy, 4*(2), 112–115.

Rost, K., Smith, Gr. R., & Taylor, J. L. (1993). Rural-urban differences in stigma and the use of care for depressive disorders. *Journal of Rural Health, 9,* 57–62.

Saunders, N. N. (1992). *Frontier nursing: Nursing practice in medical assistance facilities staffed by physician assistants.* Unpublished master's thesis, Montana State University, Bozeman.

Sobel, J. (1992). Research ethics in nutrition education. *Journal of Nutrition Education, 24,* 234–238.

Solomon, L. Z., Solomon, H, & Maiorca, J. (1982). The effects of bystanders' anonymity, situation ambiguity, and victims' status on helping. *Journal of Social Psychology, 117,* 285–294.

Tittle, C. R., & Stafford, M. C. (1992). Urban theory, urbanism, and suburban residence. *Social Forces. 70,* 725–744.

Walker, L. O., & Avant, K. C. (1994). *Strategies for theory construciton in nursing* (3rd ed.). Norwalk, CT: Appleton & Lange.

Webster's encyclopedic unabridged dictionary of the english language. (1983). New York: Gramercy.

Williams, R. (1988). Reflections on anonymity. *Perceptual and Motor Skills, 67,* 763–766.

Zuravin, S. J., & Watson, B. (1987). Anonymous reports of child physical abuse: Are they as serious as reports from other sources? *Child Abuse and Neglect, 11,* 521–529.

7

Familiarity

A. Gretchen McNeely and M. Jean Shreffler

INTRODUCTION

The saying, "familiarity breeds contempt," from *The Fox and the Lion* by Aesop in 550 BC (Bartlett, 1968, p. 76) is well known but is not always true. Indeed, Mark Twain (*Notebooks*) added that "familiarity breeds contempt—and children!" (Bartlett, 1968, p. 764). This saying is not always true either! Havelock Ellis, in *The Task of Social Hygiene,* remarked that "there are few among us who have not suffered from too early familiarity with the Bible and the conception of religion" (Bartlett, 1968, p. 850). There are those who would disagree with this saying as well. "Familiarity with danger makes a brave man braver, but less daring," is the thought of Herman Melville in his 1850 work *White-Jacket* (Bartlett, 1968, p. 695). Another lesser known quotation, "familiarity begets boldness," is from Shackerly Marmion's *The Antiquary,* Act 1 (Cumberlege, 1953). It could be argued that these last two quotations are not always true either. A college professor once told his class, "familiarity breeds confidence," referring to students' feelings after gaining some familiarity with calculus concepts.

The above examples of antithetical views of the concept are borne out in the dictionary definitions of familiarity. Funk & Wagnalls' *Standard Encyclopedic Dictionary* defines familiarity as "thorough knowledge of or acquaintance with something; friendly closeness, intimacy" (the perspective of the calculus professor). This dictionary also offers the opposing definition that familiarity is "offensively familiar conduct; unwarranted intimacy; an action warranted only by intimate acquaintance" (which supports the familiar quotation regarding contempt) (Landau, 1965).

AIM OF THE ANALYSIS

The purpose of this analysis is to clarify the meaning of the concept "familiarity" and to distinguish between its ordinary use and its use in a rural context. Eventually, familiarity will be added to a growing group of concepts that comprise rural nursing theory. The concept will be analyzed using the procedures outlined by Walker and Avant (1995). They include, but are not limited to

- determining the aims or purposes of analysis;
- identifying all uses of the concept one can discover;
- determining its defining attributes, and
- constructing a model case and borderline, related, contrary, or invented cases.

USE OF THE CONCEPT

Dictionary Definitions

Partridge (1983) presents the etymology of the word familiarity through its connections to the word "family" which comes from the Latin word, *familia.* This word includes "the servants and slaves of a great house, then the house itself with master, mistress, children—and the staff" (p. 199). *Familiaris,* the adjective of *familia,* includes the idea of intimacy of the family and close friends. Family is defined by Funk & Wagnalls (Landau, 1965) as a "group of persons or a succession of persons connected by blood, marriage, name, etc." (p. 229).

The word familiar includes the ideas of "well-known, customary, informal, unconstrained" and "a friend or close associate" (Landau, 1965, p. 229). Familiar is defined as

> *adj 1. commonly or generally known or seen: a familiar sight. 2. well-acquainted; thoroughly conversant: to be familiar with a subject. 3. informal, easy going, unceremonious, unconstrained: to write in a familiar*

> *style. 4. closely intimate or personal: a familiar friend; to be on familiar terms. 5. unduly intimate to personal taking liberties; presuming. 6. domesticated; tame. 7. of, or pertaining to, a family or household. noun 8. familiar friend or associate. (Flexner, 1987, p. 696)*

Synonyms for the fourth meaning include confidential and intimate. "Confidential suggests a sense of mutual trust that extends to the sharing of confidences and secrets: *a confidential adviser.* Intimate suggests a close acquaintance or connection, often based on interest, sympathy or affection: *intimate and affectionate letters*" (Flexner, 1987, p. 696). Synonyms for the fifth meaning include bold and forward.

Familiarity is defined as

> *noun 1. a thorough knowledge or mastery of a thing, subject, etc. 2. the state of being familiar; friendly relationship; close acquaintance; intimacy. 3. an absence of ceremony and formality; informality. 4. freedom of behavior justified only by the closest relationship; undue intimacy. 5. often familiarities (plural), an instance of such freedom, as in action or speech. 6. a sexual liberty or impropriety. (Flexner, 1987, p. 696)*

Synonyms include unconstrained, for the third meaning, and liberty, freedom, and license, for the fourth meaning (Flexner).

The dictionary definitions of the three words, family, familiar, and familiarity, combined with the origins and synonyms of familiarity, provide a fairly complete picture of the concept. Familiarity could be preliminarily summarized as an antithetical concept that includes the positive ideas of thorough knowledge of or acquaintance with and closeness and intimacy, such as one would find in a family or deep friendship, and the contrasting perspective of offensive, unwarranted, intimate conduct that might include behaviors such as flirting, sexual harassment, domestic violence, abusive relationships, or incest.

USE OF THE CONCEPT IN NON-HEALTH CARE DISCIPLINES

Rural Education

Ashley (1982) provides an exemplar of the use of familiarity in the field of rural education. As a professor of education at the University of New Hampshire, he suggests several steps that school boards can take to improve the quality of rural schools. Among these is the suggestion that educators can foster cooperation in the development and use of policies by capitalizing on the familiarity of the small town environments in which they are located. He points out that "in rural education, there is every reason to have wider community involvement" (p. 19) and then goes on to share the results of a study by another researcher who "urges schools to be open for community participation" in goal setting by "involving more parents and citizens (taxpayers)" (p. 20). Ashley concludes that "in rural settings . . . a common ingredient for successful educational change . . . is collaboration among all members of the educational community, including students, parents, administrators, college educators, and state education officials" (p. 21), in addition to teachers, principals, superintendents, and school boards. This article seems to show that these community participants are not strangers but know each other well, i.e., have a sense of familiarity with one another. This use of the concept is related to the ideas of intimacy and informality as noted in the dictionary definition of familiarity.

Another example of the use of the term familiarity within rural education is provided by O'Connell and Hagans (1985). They cite the climate of familiarity among teachers, students, principals, and community members as a key ingredient in being able to provide all students in rural schools (including the gifted) with unique opportunities to develop their intellectual, social and creative capacities. The authors stated that "a 'family atmosphere' often develops in which teachers create close, supportive relationships with all students and many parents" (p.4). This use of the concept is related to the ideas of intimacy and informality as noted in the dictionary definition of familiarity.

Communications

The field of communications offers another perspective on the concept of familiarity. Clausen (1985) presents a compelling argument for the use of a more formal approach to strangers by using their titles and last names in speaking to them for the first time. The example he cites is being called by his first name at the dentist's office by the new receptionist who does not know him. His response is to tell her his name is Mr. Clausen. He says "When everyone is a first name and intimacy is the sought-for ideal in all situations, both intimacy and judgment become harder to reach than ever. . . . That is the best reason for insisting that strangers not presume on one's first name" (p. 540). Clausen equates the informality of using first names with intimacy and the formality of titles and last names with strangers. This use of the concept is related to the ideas of intimacy and informality as noted in the dictionary definition of familiarity.

Professor Dudszak (1985) presented his research of communication with familiar and unfamiliar persons in terms of how one anticipates that situation. He commented that before meeting someone for the first time, one usually anticipates what the person will be like based on the available information about that person's traits and characteristics. How familiar one is with those traits and characteristics will determine what expectations one will have of that person. The assumption of the study was that "most persons will act differently in the manner they process information and form impressions about another person when the other is familiar than when the other is unfamiliar to them" (p. 2). One finding was that "children tended to represent friends through the description of their traits while more concrete behaviors were used in accounting for strangers" (p. 5). Children also reported more information about friends than strangers. Dudszak also mentioned that a function of the familiarity of groups is that "members feel more secure in interacting with each other than with strangers and they can predict each other's actions" (p. 6). His work seems to support the two previous examples from the field of communication in relating familiarity to friendship and close acquaintances and unfamiliarity with strangers.

Gerontology

The discipline of gerontology offers another perspective on familiarity. Atchley (1989) posited that, in making adaptive choices, older adults attempt to preserve and maintain existing internal and external structures in their lives, and they prefer to accomplish this by using continuity, that is "applying familiar strategies in familiar arenas of life" (p. 183). In Atchley's view, familiarity helps older adults to adapt to change, since they prefer to use strategies tied to their past experiences of themselves and their social world or strategies that make the changing circumstance seem more familiar. Atchley differentiated between internal and external continuity. Internal continuity is a healthy capacity to see inner change as connected to and supported by one's past; the new self is familiar. The older adult perceives a sense of external continuity "from being and doing in familiar environments, practicing familiar skills, and interacting with familiar people" (p. 185). External continuity accounts for the persistence of a structure of relationships in an older person's life and a set of typical overt behaviors. "[E]everyday life for most older people is like long-running improvisational theater in which the settings, characters, and actions are familiar and the changes are mostly in the form of new episodes rather than entirely new plays" (p. 185).

In a study of the meaning of home in later life, Sixsmith (1990) found that the attachment the elderly have to "home" is in part due to familiarity. Attachment to home was found to have many dimensions for the elderly such as "a warehouse for memories and historical continuity, as a familiar physical structure that provides stability, a sense of rootedness, and a feeling of being settled-in" (Cookman, 1996, p. 229). Fogel (1992) discussed the many benefits of helping the elderly to remain in their homes as they age. These included "benefits related to familiarity of a particular home environment, for example, ease of finding one's way around . . . and benefits related to residence in a specific neighborhood, including social network of friends and neighbors" (p. 15).

Rural Sociology and Rural Life

In a classic work on the values of community versus mass society first published in 1887, Tonnes made the distinction between *gemeinschaft,* translated as "community," and *gesellschaft,* translated as "society." Familiarity and close interpersonal relationships are some of the distinguishing characteristics of *gemeinschaft* in contrast to *gesellschaft* where large scale, impersonal, and contractual relationships prevail. "In *gemeinschaft,* community human relationships are intimate, enduring, and based on a clear understanding of where each person stands in society. A man's 'worth' is estimated according to *who* he is not *what* he has done" (Bell & Newby, 1972, p. 23). In *gemeinschaft,* the close interpersonal interactions result "in a personalizing of issues, events and explanations, because familiar names and characters inevitably become associated with everything that happens" (Bell & Newby, 1972, pp. 23–24). In a discussion of the attributes of small rural communities and how they exemplify the characteristics of *gemeinschaft,* Martinez-Brawley (1990) noted that a sense of personal identity is derived from the familiarity in small communities. "At the level of Gemeinschaft, people become familiar with each other's quirks. . . . Each person's identity becomes recognizably public and lives are shared experiences in all their facets" (Martinez-Brawley, 1990, p. 37).

In a study of the effect of rapid economic and demographic change on "neighboring" among residents of four rural western communities, Berry, Krannich, and Greider (1990) operationally defined neighboring activities as those involving both affiliation/familiarity with neighbors and social support. Familiarity with neighbors was measured by responses to the question: "Of the 10 houses nearest the respondent, how many has he or she been in?" (p. 178). Familiarity scores ranged from zero to 10. It was found that, in most instances, community change over time was accompanied by only minor shifts in neighboring activities. Several variables were positively associated with familiarity including length of residence and number of children.

Keyes (1973), an urban dweller temporarily living in a rural area, provided a classic example of familiarity in a small rural town:

> *Though I'd find it hard to live here the year round, several things impress me about Comptche. The store owner asks for no I.D. to cash a check. She knows who I am. Though the post office is tiny, and the postlady anything but a model of brisk efficiency, I find myself far more sure than in the city that she will get my letters where they're going. The postlady knows me, my name, where I live, why I'm here, and the fact that I'm always getting magazines Postage Due. I get a much greater feeling of trust from that than the brisk professionalism of the vaguely familiar faces at one of six counters of my post office in San Diego. One time, a sign appeared on the post office bulletin board saying: 'The wedding is on for July 21st.' The next day that sign was down and another had taken its place, reading 'The wedding is postponed till July 28th.' Nothing more.* That's *being known. (p. 173)*

USE OF THE CONCEPT IN RURAL NURSING AND HEALTH CARE

Familiarity, a characteristic of rural communities, influences the provision of nursing and health care services. Diamond and Van Dyke (1985) discussed the development of community-based support programs for residents with chronic psychiatric illness in three rural communities. Several factors simplified the development of the groups within the rural communities they studied, e.g., the familiarity of community residents with one another, the willingness to help one another, and the relative ease of communication within the community.

In a study of case management in rural areas, Parker et al. (1992) reported that informal social structures in a rural area enhanced case managers' abilities to provide consistent and effective follow-up care. The case managers know the clients and clients' families and see them in many different contexts and settings. "Because of the informal relationship between the client and case manager, and small town residents' familiarity with each other, however, confidentiality is easily compromised" (p. 56). In another study of case management in a rural community, it was found that familiarity between the case managers and clients affected the level of agreement on measures of client functioning (Widlak, McKee, Greenberg, & Greenley, 1992). The greater the familiarity, the more likely case managers' assessments of client functioning agreed with the clients' self assessments.

An editorial by a physician assistant provides an example of how familiarity can enhance medical practice. Davidson (1990) points out that the title "doctor" defines a formal relationship between a physician and the patient. However, physician assistants do not have such a title and often use their first names. He notes that "the familiarity is often reciprocated" (p. 16), and he believes that "such familiarity truly enhances my ability to provide care . . . and gives them permission to confide in me" (p. 16). Finally, he says that "When patients call and ask for 'Jim,' they know a friend will answer the phone" (p. 16). This use of the freedom of speech to use one's first name implies that informality and friendship are indeed important components of the concept of familiarity.

Although the term familiarity is not used, many publications about rural nursing practice describe what seems identical or similar to familiarity. Davis and Droes (1993) termed "in-depth interpersonal knowledge" a major characteristic of rural community health nursing practice. Their interviews with rural community-health nurses revealed that this in-depth interpersonal knowledge with their clients enhanced their effectiveness as providers. Some quotations cited by nurses in their study reveal characteristics and benefits of familiarity:

'Knowing your patient, knowing the life they lead, their usual habits, that helps me a lot in my approach.' 'I think my patients are more comfortable.' 'You start with a larger information base.' 'You get to know the patients

> *well and grow fond of them, become like a family . . . you can focus more on their total care because you get to know them like a person.' 'With some patients, you start with a level of respect that has already been earned in the past.' (p. 166)*

This study also noted some negative aspects of familiarity in rural practice such as incomplete assessments because the nurse assumed she knew the client, privacy concerns that made the client feel he or she must keep up an image in front of the nurse, confidentiality concerns, and additional stress for the nurse who knew and cared about her neighbors in distress.

Lassiter (1985) discusses the kin and friendship networks in rural communities that affect residents' health practices, both positively and negatively. These familylike relationships also influence nurses practicing in rural areas, who are themselves relatives and neighbors to the people they serve professionally. In a study of rural nursing administrators' practice, Henry and Moody (1986) found that highly personal care was an expectation of nursing administrators as well as of community residents. The patients admitted to the hospital were often friends, neighbors, or relatives; these personal relationships resulted in making rural nursing extremely personal. Long and Weinert (1989) termed "lack of anonymity" a major characteristic of rural nursing practice. This lack of anonymity limited the ability of nurses and residents to have private areas in their lives. "Rural nurses almost always reported being known to their patients as neighbors, part of a given family, members of a certain church, and so on. Similarly, these nurses usually know their patients in several different social and personal relationships beyond the nurse-patient relationship" (Long & Weinert, 1989, p. 117).

Summary of Uses of Familiarity in Different Contexts

The examples from various disciplines support the definition of the concept of familiarity related to informality, friendship, close relationships/acquaintances, and intimacy. They also support the antithetical nature of familiarity; at times it is welcomed by the recipient, and other times it is not. In the following section, the essential attributes of the concept of familiarity will be identified based on the dictionary definitions and the uses of the concept in different disciplines.

DETERMINING THE DEFINING ATTRIBUTES OF FAMILIARITY

From the dictionary definitions and etymology of the words family, familiar, and familiarity and from the uses of the concept in different disciplines, the attributes of the concept of familiarity were identified as (a) *friendly relationship or close acquaintance,* (b) *intimacy,* (c) *informality,* and (d) the *exhibited familiarity is welcome or unwelcome* depending on the perceptions of the receiver. Each attribute is relevant to the use of the concept of familiarity. The identified attributes are useful for rural living and rural nursing practice as well.

CASES

Model Cases

According to Walker & Avant (1995), "the model case is one that we are absolutely sure is an instance of the concept" (p. 42). The following model cases were developed from qualitative data gathered during a study of frontier residents' perceptions of their local health care services. Residents were asked during telephone interviews why they did or did not use their local health care services (Shreffler, 1996).

*One female resident explained the most important reasons why her family used the local primary health care provider for their regular health care: "Well you know everybody in a small town. I know (*provider's first name*), and he knows the kids. He's really down-home and treats us good. We like that." She went on to discuss the qualities she liked in this provider such as his caring, tender manner with her children. He knew her family members' medical histories, and they appreciated this continuity. She consistently called him by his first name. She also mentioned that her family and the provider's family were friends and attended social functions together.*

Other female residents explained the most important reasons why they or other women they knew did not use the local primary health care provider for their annual exams: "I go out of town for my yearly girly stuff. I don't like to go to someone I know or see around town." "In a town this small, everyone talks. If you have something you don't want everyone to know you're going to the doctor for, you go out of town. They joke that if you're pregnant, you'll know the results from the gossip before you get the test back." "A PA who works with a gynecologist in (town name) *comes down once a month for the female stuff; which is nice because* (provider's first name) *is a close personal friend so I wouldn't want to go to him for paps and things."*

These represent model cases of familiarity in that they all exhibit the attributes of friendly relationship or close acquaintance, intimacy, and informality. In the first case, the exhibited familiarity was welcome, and, in the second set of cases, it was not.

Contrary Case

"Contrary cases are those that are clear examples of 'not the concept' " (Walker & Avant, 1995, p. 44). The following contrary cases were also developed from qualitative data gathered during the same study referred to above. This set of cases was drawn from interviews with residents from one frontier community who had experienced a great deal of turnover of primary care providers (Shreffler, 1996).

Residents discussed their perspectives on the problems related to turnover of their local primary providers: "I've been in (town name) *only five years and they've gone through four P.A.s (physician assistants). I don't like going to somebody new each time. I don't know them when they're new and they don't know me. I didn't even know the last one's first name before he left." "We don't use the local care because of the turnover of the P.A.s. They don't stay long enough to get familiar with them. Familiarity is important to us." "I like to have a doctor that knows you and that only develops over years. They know your problems and if you call and say you're sick, they know you are because they trust you. They don't stay long enough here for that trust to develop. I think continuity and familiarity is important."*

These represent contrary cases of familiarity in that they exhibit none of the attributes of friendly relationship or close acquaintance, intimacy, and informality. The residents would have welcomed familiarity from their health care provider, but it was not exhibited from their perspectives.

SUMMARY

This analysis attempts to clarify the meaning of the concept of familiarity especially as it may be used in rural living and nursing practice. The analysis process has included the dictionary definitions of the words family, familiar, and familiarity, and the etymology of the word familiarity through its connections to the word family. In addition, the uses of the concept of familiarity in a variety of disciplines including nursing were identified. Based on the etymology, definitions, and uses, the defining attributes were identified: friendly relationship or close acquaintance, intimacy, informality, and the exhibited familiarity is welcome or unwelcome depending on the perceptions of the receiver. Cases were then presented—model cases, which displayed each of the identified attributes, and contrary cases in which none of the attributes were displayed.

REFERENCES

Ashley, C. H. (1982). Six points toward increased effectiveness in rural schools. In R. Fried (Ed.), *Effective schooling in a rural context: A New Hampshire view.* (pp. 17–24). Washington, DC: National Institute of Education, 17–24.

Atchley, R. C. (1989). A continuity theory of normal aging. *The Gerontologist, 29* (2), 183–190.

Bartlett, J. (1968). *Familiar quotations* (14th ed.). Boston: Little, Brown.

Bell, C., & Newby, H. (1972). *Community studies: An introduction to the sociology of the local community.* New York: Praeger.

Berry, E. H., Krannich, R. S. & Greider, T. (1990). A longitudinal analysis of neighboring in rapidly changing rural places. *Journal of Rural Studies, 6* (2), 175–186.

Clausen, C. (1985). Manners: A decent impersonality. *The American Scholar, 54,* 537–540.

Cookman, C. A. (1996). Older people and attachment to things, places, pets, and ideas. *Image, 28* (3), 227–231.

Cumberledge, G. (Ed.). (1953). *The Oxford dictionary of quotations* (2nd ed.). London: Oxford University Press.

Davidson, J. A. (March, 1990). What's in a name? *Physician Assistant, 16,* 21.

Davis, D. J., & Droes, N. S. (1993). Community health nursing in rural and frontier counties. *Nursing Clinics of North America, 28* (1), 159–169.

Diamond, R. J., & Van Dyke, D. (1985). Rural community support programs: The experience of three Wisconsin counties. *New Directions for Mental Health Services, 26,* 49–58.

Dudszak, C. A. (1985). *Anticipation of communication with familiar and unfamiliar persons.* Paper presented at the annual meeting of the Central States Speech Association, Indianapolis, IN (April 4–6, 1985), 1–27.

Flexner, S. B. (Ed.). (1987). *The Random House dictionary of the English language* (2nd ed., unabridged). New York: Random House.

Fogel, B. S. (1992). Psychological aspects of staying at home. *Generations, 16* (2), 15–20.

Henry, B. M. & Moody, L. E. (1986). Nursing administration in small rural hospitals. *Journal of Nursing Administration, 16* (7, 8), 37–44.

Keyes, R. (1973). *We the lonely people: Searching for community.* New York: Harper & Row.

Landau, S. E. (Ed.). (1965). *Funk and Wagnalls standard encyclopedic dictionary.* Chicago: J. G. Ferguson.

Lassiter, P. (1985). Education for rural health professionals: Nurses. *The Journal of Rural Health, 1,* 24–28.

Long, K. A., & Weinert, C. (1989). Rural nursing: Developing the theory base. *Scholarly Inquiry for Nursing Practice, An International Journal, 3,* 113–126.

Martinez-Brawley, E. E. (1990). *Perspectives on the small community: Humanistic views for practitioners.* Washington DC: NASW Press.

O'Connell, C., & Hagens, R. (1985). *High achievement in rural schools.* In Reports-Descriptive (141). Washington, DC: National Institute of Education, 1–17.

Parker, M., Quinn, J., Viehl, M., McKinley, A., Polich, C. L., Detzner, D. F., Hartwell, S., & Korn, K. (1992). Case management in rural areas: Definition, clients, financing, staffing, and service delivery issues. *Journal of Nursing Administration, 22* (2), 54–59.

Partridge, E. (1983). *Origins: A short etymological dictionary of modern English.* New York: Greenwich.

Shreffler, M. J. (1996). [Residents' views on access to care and medical assistance facilities.] Unpublished raw data.

Sixsmith, A. J. (1990). The meaning and experience of "home" in later life. In B. Bytheway & J. Johnson (Eds.), *Welfare and the ageing experience.* Aldershot, England: Averbury.

Walker, L. O., & Avant, K. C. (1995). *Strategies for theory construction in nursing,* (3rd ed.). Norwalk, CT: Appleton & Lange.

Widlak, P. A., McKee, D., Greenberg, J. R., & Greenley, J. R. (1992). An assessment of client function scales in the uniform client data instrument. *Psychosocial Rehabilitation Journal, 15* (4), 19–35.

8

Old-Timer

Catherine D. Caniparoli

In 1989, Long and Weinert identified some key concepts for rural nursing theory. These include "work and health beliefs, isolation and distance, self-reliance, lack of anonymity, outsider/insider, and old timer/newcomer" (p. 119). The purpose of this concept analysis is to clarify the meaning of "old-timer." The process used to analyze the concept of old-timer was developed by Wilson (1963) and modified by Walker and Avant (1995).

DEFINITIONS OF THE CONCEPT

Etymology:

Old-timer is defined in the Random House Dictionary (Flexner, 1987) as

> *1. A person whose residence, membership, or experience began long ago and has been continuing for a considerable length of time; veteran. 2. An old person. 3. An old-fashioned person or thing. 4. Sometimes offensive (as when used as a form of a familiar direct address to an elderly man). (p. 1003)*

According to this dictionary, the word originated between 1855 and 1860.

The word "old" appears in many languages, such as Celtic, Germanic, Gothic, Saxon, Old English, Greek, Sanskrit, Tocharian, and Indo-European languages with apparent common meaning. Meanings of the word old in these languages involve the use of terms such as grow, nourish, thrive, insatiable, father/grandfather/stepfather, increase, and fostering (Barnhart, 1988; Klein, 1967). In these languages, the word old is usually in the male gender of that language (Barnhart, 1988). The word old was attached to the word "time" around 1824. Mark Twain used the term old-time in his writings in 1870 (Partridge, 1970). Old-timer was first used around 1810 to describe one who is long established in a place or position. It was considered a colloquial term until around 1905 when its usage became standard English.

American slang

Dictionaries of American slang have several definitions of old-timer. These dictionaries identify the word old-timer as a term usually used in the American West. Chapman (1986) defines the term old-timer as having its origins in the "middle 1800's; Western" (p. 304). This word is also used to describe an "old man; often used in direct address, generally affectionately" (p. 304). In *Western Words: A Dictionary of the American West,* Adams (1968) says this about old-timer:

> *A man who has lived in the country a long time. Most old-timers had to fight many battles before the country became settled and it could be said of such a one that 'his scars was a regular map.' It was said of all good old-timer Texans that they were 'raised to vote the Democratic ticket, love good whiskey, and hate Mexicans. (p. 210)*

USES OF THE CONCEPT

The term old-timer appears infrequently in the literature of most disciplines. References to old-timer appear most often in historical literature. The disciplines of education, health care, psychology, and popular media have some articles that speak to the concept.

Education

The term old-timer was found in one newsletter in the educational literature. The purpose of the newsletter was to explore strategies that would increase community involvement in the school system (Winning Public Support, 1983). "Taping old-timer stories" was used as a strategy to involve senior citizens in a school system. Use of old-timers in a school system of the community illustrates the establishment of relationship within a community.

Health Care

In an article titled "My dream practice had everything, except patients," a physician described various issues involved in starting a practice in a small community (Anonymous, 1992). The term old-timer was used to describe the medical practice of the physician from whom the author bought his practice. The residents were "conditioned to accept outdated medicine. My efforts at change were not always appreciated, and at time were actively resisted" (p. 121). This situation describes the trust that rural dwellers establish with old-timers and their response to the changes the newcomers bring.

Weinert and Long (1987) and Long and Weinert (1989) identified the concept of old-timer/newcomer. Their articles explored perceptions of rural dwellers about health care. "If grandparents/parents settled in Montana, they most generally described themselves as a 'native.' If they did not have these roots in the state but had lived in Montana for 20 years or more, there was a 50–50 split between describing themselves as a 'native' or an 'old-timer'" (Weinert & Long, 1989, p. 454). Twenty years may be a magic number in achieving old-timer status. If individuals lived in an area for less than 20 years, they were viewed as newcomers to an area. A rancher described the relationship between old-timers and newcomers in this way: "Around here, a 'newcomer' is someone who's lived here from about three months to four years; an old-timer is someone who's ranched here at least one generation" (p. 455).

Psychology

The use of old-timer in the psychology literature appeared in relationship to roles within an alcohol abuse treatment group. Berliner (1987) identified eight roles within the group studied—one of those roles being "old-timer." The old-timer is described as

> *older than most others. He has used alcohol since his early years, attends group regularly but participates minimally; his manner toward the leader*

borders on the obsequious. He has no intention of changing in any way and seems to regard the group as an unavoidable imposition. He accepts this without apparent resentment or commitment. The younger members tend to regard him with disdain. (p. 47)

Popular Media

During 1996, newspaper headlines across the state screamed about the relationships between newcomers and long-time residents of Montana. The headlines and their related articles were based on a survey by the Rochester Research Group of Rochester, NY, commissioned by the *Great Falls Tribune* of Great Falls, Montana. The results of the survey described the attitudes of long-time residents toward quality of life, jobs, and importation of new ideas and innovations caused by newcomers to this rural state (Johnson, 1996). Johnson used the label "long-time Montanans" as those living in the state longer than 10 years. These individuals were more likely to criticize the impact of newcomers and to agree that the number of newcomers moving into the state would negatively affect the environment of the state. This is an example of old-timer and newcomer used as statuses within the social organization of communities.

In the "All Things Considered" program on National Public Radio (NPR), Wertheimer (1994) reported a segment called "Santa Fe Fighting Loss of Old Way of Life." Residents of Santa Fe, New Mexico were interviewed about the changes their community had undergone. Gloria Mendoza, a native of Santa Fe, grandmother, and community activist, discussed the impact of Anglos moving into this community. This long-time resident summed up her feelings about newcomers this way: "They put up their high walls, their gates; they don't want to get to know us. I think that has made the people here feel that they are no longer in the Santa Fe that they have always lived in."

On the NPR program called "Morning Edition," southern Idaho was the rural environment under discussion. Bob Edwards (1994), the host of the program, reported that many people regard Idaho as a land that is untouched and ideal for families. This caused an influx of newcomers. "Idaho has lived up to expectations, but old-timers are dismayed as newcomers move in and make changes." In the same segment, a writer, Clay Morgan, said that "old-timers fear the newcomers may be bringing with them the things they sought to escape." The theme in these references is that newcomers bring change and may not be aware of or respect the sensibilities of the old-timer residents.

History

Although the term old-timer was rarely used, historical Western literature depicting the 1800s is rich with descriptions of old-timers. Use of old-timer in Western folk lore generally focused upon the descriptions of local "characters." The statement by Burlingame (1942) for individuals fitting the image of old-timer seen in the early days of the West was insightful. "As the Americas had attracted the courageous, adventure-loving young men of Europe in an earlier century, so the West served to drain off the exuberant and irresponsible from the East in the middle 1800s" (p. 73). Perhaps the characteristics of exuberance and irresponsibility of persons learning to survive in the western environment led to the development of characters like Gabby Hayes pictured in Western folklore stories and films.

The vast majority of old-timers described in the Western literature were men. Historical literature published before the 1960s rarely discussed women at all. When women were mentioned, it was in relationship to the men in the stories, but they were rarely central to the story being told. As publication dates became more contemporary, some women fit the characteristics of old-timer. Shirley (1995) describes the axiom, "women *are* history, but men *make* history" (p. 7) as a motivating force behind her descriptions of women of the West. In *More Than Petticoats: Remarkable Montana Women,* she described several women who would be considered old-timers.

Most old-timers were seen as mysterious, unusual, and fiercely independent. They usually had characteristics that set them apart from the average member of the community. These characteristics might include dress, language, posture, size, unusual habits, or living arrangements. One such old-timer is described in the following way:

> *Larpenteur was a small, wiry man who never got over his French characteristics. He was highly intelligent, vivacious, well-informed and in the main a kindly person. Handsome, careful of his clothes and vain concerning his appearance and ability, he was to suffer greatly over these points of personality. Although Larpenteur was one of the most capable and trusted men on the upper river, he went from one company to another, with frequent intervals of freelancing on his own account, and he left the fur business*

without having enough to keep him comfortably in his old age. (Burlingame, 1942, p .62)

Books detailing memories of the past frequently provided descriptions of old-timers by occupation. One author described northwestern Montana loggers in this way:

Colorful human beings, all of them good workers, free-spenders, hard drinkers and independent as a hog on ice yet they were a friendly class of men, always there when a neighbor was in need. This independence seemed to stem from their always working alone, at their dangerous trade . . . They were the elite of the timber camps, for the skilled work brought them twice the wages paid other help. They always worked as piece workers and were called "Gyppos." (Green, 1969, p. 15)

Comments similar to this when describing the work done by old-timers were often made. Whether trappers, ranchers, prospectors, or cowpunchers, their work was usually described as dangerous and involved working alone.

Many old-timers were described as having a strong sense of personal privacy. They did not talk about their past and in this way seemed very mysterious. When asked about their past, old-timers would say that this portion of their life was not anyone's business. Green (1969) described a man who lived in northwest Montana in this manner:

Slim was a man of about forty, tall, slender, with bushy, black hair, friendly with his few distant neighbors, but extremely reluctant to discuss his personal history. No one knew him by any other name, nor where he came from. Many such men roamed the country in the early days. The name they went by, where they were from or where they went was no one's business but their own. (p. 85)

Green (1969) described another old-timer this way: "Buckskin Louie Bowman was a bachelor, half Indian and one of the first men to homestead in the valley, for he had been here for 20 years or more when I showed on the scene" (p. 29). Old-timers remained in an area but did not always remain in the same home. Frequent changes in residences within a region/area were common (Anderson, 1973; Burlingame, 1942; Green, 1969; Guernsey, 1936; Lee, 1968; Shirley, 1995; Stewart, 1913).

ATTRIBUTES OF OLD-TIMERS

From the dictionary definitions and the use of old-timer in the literature these defining attributes emerged:

(a) *age,*
(b) *length of time spend in a community,* and
(c) *establishment of a relationship within the community.*

Old-timer residents are usually of an older age, having lived in an area for a certain length of time. The length of time needed to attain old-timer status appears to be defined by the community involved. Also, old-timers have established a relationship within the community.

MODEL CASES

In concept development, a model case is one in which all of the attributes are exemplified. For the purposes of this concept analysis, two model cases were developed. The first model case that follows is one that illustrates the more historical folklore perspectives of an old-timer. The second model case represents a more present day version of an old-timer.

Model Case 1

This case is of a client for whom the author cared in an isolated, rural Montana community. The name has been changed to protect the privacy of the individual. Ole Johannesen was an 84–year-old man who had lived in this community for as "long as anyone can remember." He was married once, but "she up and left, without no warning." They had no children. He was usually reluctant to talk about himself or his past. He did have several cousins living in the area, and they kept an eye on him from a distance. Other members of the community would check on him. If he wasn't seen during the usual times, someone would notice and stop by to "see how he was doing." They stated that he did not appreciate anyone getting involved in his personal life or his business. He lived in a small cabin about seven miles from town. His relatives and neighbors frequently mentioned his "cantankerous behavior" when they would come to the clinic. They also were concerned that he was not taking care of himself. His response to these concerns was "they just want my land and house for themselves." He had been known to chase off strangers with a shotgun. The neighbors stated that during bad weather he was always willing to help dig a car out of the snow. He also chopped wood and brought it in for families or the elderly in the community who needed wood for heat. He had been a logger by trade. Mr. Johannesen was present at most community meetings and made his opinions known. Many other long-time residents would listen to him, and many newcomers would describe him as "that crazy old coot who lived up the mountain."

Ole was seen every Thursday at one o'clock in the clinic for treatment of his "dog bites." The "dog bites" were stasis ulcers. He would keep the appointment only if it were Thursday at one o'clock because that was when he was free. He also had arthritis, which he treated with Percodan. All efforts to change his arthritis treatment met with failure. His response was "Old Doc Smith told me this was the best treatment. He really knew how to treat people." The treatment for his stasis ulcers was application of Una Boots to both legs once a week. He refused to elevate his feet or to take any medications to treat the ulcers. He usually declined any interventions that would make any change in his lifestyle or usual routine. He said, "I am going to die the way I have lived."

This client displays the attributes of an old-timer. He is 84 years of age and a long-time resident of the area. He is recognized as an old-timer by other long-time residents and accorded a place of respect in community discussions. However, newcomers identified him as strange, unusual, and not very credible. He has definitely established a relationship within his community.

Model Case 2

Mary Michaelson, age 66, is a resident of a small town in a rural Western state. Mary's parents settled on a ranch outside this community. Mary and her brothers and sisters were raised in the community, and they all continue to live in areas surrounding the community. They all are involved in ranching, the dominant occupation in this area. The community is facing a declining population to support their hospital. The hospital board is exploring their two primary options—closing the hospital or becoming a medical assistance facility

(MAF). An MAF has most of the services of a hospital but fewer requirements for in-house staff, has limits on the length of stay, and can use the services of nurse practitioners and/or physician assistants to provide the care. Mary is opposed to either option. She feels that these changes are being proposed by the newcomer residents on the board of the hospital. She is very vocal at board meetings and has often been interviewed by the local paper. Her family members have begun to appear at public meetings to support her perspective.

Mary illustrates the attributes of an old-timer. Her age of 66 and her lifelong residency in the community bring her into the world of old-timers. She is very vocal about change in her community and has a support system of other long-time residents who view her as very credible.

Summary of Cases

These two real life cases reflect differing perspectives on the concept of old-timer. For both cases, age, length of time in the community, and the establishment of a relationship within the community are present.

CONSEQUENCES

The consequences of old-timer status involve the individual's identification as an old-timer. Other residents must recognize the individual as an old-timer. This process of identification as an old-timer serves to set the individual apart from the rest of the community. Recognition of the individual as an old-timer establishes a relationship within the community. The relationship may be viewed as positive or negative depending on the role of the viewer.

SUMMARY

The use of the term old-timer requires further evaluation. Old-timers may be a subgroup of long-time residents. No evidence appeared in the literature about whether persons who are native to the area and have resided in one area for a long time look at themselves as old-timers. In describing their role in a community, natives and long-time residents could view the label old-timer as an insult if they view the term in the Western folklore sense. Questions that must be answered before this concept can be used in research and further rural theory development include

(a) To what degree do communities of today use the concept of old-timer as it was understood in western folklore?
(b) How are old-timers identified in a community and how do they view themselves?
(c) What roles do old-timers serve in a community organization and social order?
(d) Are the attributes of old-timer the same today as they were in the past?

As pointed out by Weinert and Long (1987), "Rural dwellers used the concepts of 'old-timer' and 'newcomer' as a framework to organize their social interactions, their relationships within the community and were important to their 'view of the social environment'" (p. 453).

Until the above questions are explored, misunderstandings and miscommunication by rural dwellers, health care providers who are newcomers, and individuals who look at the social order in rural areas will occur. Terms used by rural dwellers to designate these individuals who play the important role of old-timers in rural communities must reflect both the role itself and the function of the individual in community organization.

REFERENCES

Adams, R. F. (1968). *Western words: A dictionary of the American west.* Norman, OK: University of Oklahoma Press.

Anderson, J. G. (1973). *Golden reflections of by-gone days.* Tumwater, WA: Quality Printing.

Anonymous. (1992). My dream practice had everything except patients. *Medical Economics, 69* (19), 115–121.

Barnhart, R. K. (Ed.). (1988). *The Barnhart dictionary of etymology.* Bronx, NY: Wilson.

Berliner, A. K. (1987). Group counseling with alcohol offenders: An analysis and typology of DWI probationers. *Journal of Offender Counseling, Services & Rehabilitation 11*(2), 33–51.

Burlingame, M. G. (1942). *The Montana frontier.* Helena, MT: State Publishing.

Chapman, R. L. (Ed.). (1986). *New dictionary of American slang.* New York: Harper & Row.

Edwards, B. (Host). (1994). The American culture wars, part 6. [Radio]. On *Morning Edition.* New York: National Public Radio.

Flexner, S. B. (Ed. in chief). (1987). *Random House dictionary of the English language* (2nd ed.). New York: Random House.

Green, C. (1969). *Montana memories, volume 1.* Kalispell, MT: Charles Green.

Guernsey, C. A. (1936). *Wyoming cowboy days.* New York: Putnam.

Johnson, Peter. (1996, February 5). Most Montanans see newcomers as threat to jobs. *The Great Falls Tribune,* pp. 1B-2B.

Klein, E. (1967). *A comprehensive etymological dictionary of the English language.* New York: Elsevier.

Lee, M. B. (1968). *Back in Cripple Creek.* New York: Doubleday.

Long, K. A., & Weinert, C. (1989). Rural nursing: Developing the theory base. *Scholarly Inquiry for Nursing Practice, 3,* 113–127.

Partridge, E. (1970). *A dictionary of slang and unconventional English,* 7th ed. New York: Macmillan.

Shirley, G. (1995). *More than petticoats: Remarkable Montana women.* Helena, MT: Falcon Press.

Stewart, E.P. (1913). *Letters of a woman homesteader.* Boston: Houghton Mifflin.

Walker, L. O., & Avant, K. C. (1995). *Strategies for theory construction in nursing* (3rd ed.). Norwalk, CT: Appleton & Lange.

Weinert, C., & Long, K. A. (1987). Understanding the health care needs of rural families. *Family Relations, 36*(10), 450–455.

Wertheimer, L. (Host). (1994). Santa Fe fighting loss of old way of life. [Radio]. On *All Things Considered.* New York: National Public Radio.

Wilson, J. (1963). *Thinking with concepts.* New York: Cambridge University Press.

Winning public support for education. (1983, April). *Here's How, 1* (5).

9

Newcomer

Dena J. Sutermaster

O blithe new-comer! I have heard,
I hear thee and rejoice.
O Cuckoo! Shall I call thee bird,
Or but a wandering voice?
Wordsworth (1807) in
To the Cuckoo (Partington, 1992)

The purpose of this concept analysis is to define the meaning of "newcomer." The concept analysis process used was Walker and Avant's (1995) model. Along with how the concept is used in various disciplines, attributes, antecedents, and consequences were identified. Cases using the attributes are presented.

In investigating the concept of newcomer, most of the literature addressed how established residents or employees viewed the newcomer. Little was written on how newcomers viewed themselves.

DEFINITIONS

The noun newcomer is defined as "one that has recently arrived: as a: immigrant b: novice c: something that is advancing toward a position of greater prominence or eminence" (Gove, 1986, p. 1523). There are several spellings of the word. These include newcomer, new comer, and new-comer. Newcomer is selected for use in this chapter.

Synonyms for newcomer found in *Roget's 21st Century Thesaurus* (Kipfer, 1986) include arrival, beginner, greenhorn, immigrant, incomer, neophyte, new kid on the block, novice, outsider, rookie, settler, stranger, and tenderfoot. The synonym greenhorn means "a beginner or novice, but willing to learn the cowboy way; pleasant to be around" (Yeo, 1995, p. 28). The *Barnhart Dictionary of Etymology* (1988) lists newcomer as a noun originating about 1450.

USES OF THE CONCEPT

The concept newcomer is used commonly to describe people and things or ideas. References about newcomer were found in the disciplines of nursing, sociology, education, management, literature (fiction and nonfiction), and the media (movies, television, radio, and writing)

Nursing

Long and Weinert (1987) introduced the concept of newcomer in relation to old-timer when discussing rural nursing theory. They thought the concepts of old-timer and newcomer were related and opposing. Of three descriptions of a newcomer, all dealt with the time lived in the area: three months to four years and more than ten years but less than twenty. The third description added the element of integration. Full integration into the community could not occur until the newcomer lived in the area longer than ten years. A newcomer's acceptance into the community was determined by family history, such as grandparents settling in the area and amount of time lived in the state.

Rural residents use an informal support system to help them care for ill family members and to deal with other problems (Long & Weinert, 1987). Therefore, newcomers who are professionals would not be relied upon by the community until they were accepted. Established residents need to accept the newcomer before they will allow the newcomer to care for them.

According to Long (1993), rural people are more likely to be independent and self-reliant and rely on informal networks, consisting of family, neighbors, and friends, which are affordable, accessible, and can be trusted for health problems. Therefore, for health care providers to be used, they must be accepted.

Informal social networks play a larger role in rural than urban areas (Blau, 1956). There are activities and outcomes in an organization that are not explained by official structures. Therefore, newcomers, including nurses, need to know how to work within informal networks (Weinert & Long, 1991).

Bushy (1993) notes that local residents in rural communities "often have a shared history and usually are well-acquainted" (p. 190). The history comes from the fact that many are decedents of homesteaders and have a sense of belonging to the community. Rural residents "prefer to interact with people similar to themselves" (p. 190). The concept of newcomer "implies that long-time residents are reluctant to establish close ties with new persons entering their community" (p. 190). Bushy describes a woman who moved to a rural town after marrying a resident of that town. After being married for decades, the woman continued to have feelings of being an outsider and of not being accepted by the extended family or the community.

Management

Within formal organizations, the term newcomer is used to describe someone who is new in an organization. Much of the research focuses on aiding the newcomer in his or her adjustment to the organization. Newcomers move from being outsiders to becoming insiders through a process of organizational socialization, a process of learning the ropes (Schein as cited in Bauer & Green, 1994).

Informal organizations occur spontaneously from the activities and interactions of people working together but have a structure different from a formal structure (Rakich, Longest, & Darr, 1985). The informal organization contains four different status positions: group leader, primary group member, fringe group member, and out of the group. The roles of each member are linked to communication. The group leader receives and distributes information to the members. Group structure arises from how often members associate with each other. Members at the fringe are most likely newcomers. Newcomers are evaluated by the primary group and can, in time, become full members. Members who are not accepted by the primary group will move to "out of the group" status. Out-casted persons who want to be members of the group may be unhappy with their status. These persons may continue to try to join the group or may resign.

Informal organizations are governed by convention, custom, and culture. They will attempt to maintain stability by resisting change, especially when it is perceived as a threat by its members. Employees who are part of any informal organization achieve a sense of belonging and security through group membership (Rakich *et al.*, 1985).

Morrison (1993) studied the effect of information seeking on newcomer socialization of new staff accountants. Her findings suggest that information seeking is important in socialization. Newcomers taking an active role in seeking information had an easier adjustment to their new environment.

Bauer and Green (1994) studied socialization by examining the effect of involvement in work-related activities. Their sample was newly enrolled science and technology Ph.D. students. Students actively involved in the program were better accommodated and had greater productivity as compared to those who were less involved. Accommodation was defined as a process by which newcomers discover their expected role in the organization and how to participate in work groups. Being accepted by the work group is an important part of the process. Greater productivity involved participation in research activities. Activities were measured on a 5–point scale; the items included working alone and with other students or faculty on research and writing projects. The active individuals reported less role ambiguity and felt an increase in perceived acceptance.

Sociology

According to Stinner and Kan (1984), migrants who arrive in a community include both newcomers and returnees. Newcomers have never lived in the community. Returnees had lived in the community before, departed for a time, and subsequently returned. Stinner and Kan studied the differences between newcomers and returnees in nonmetropolitan Utah communities. Returnees possessed some degree of familiarity with the social structure and cultural milieu of the community to which they returned. The study findings suggested that newcomers and returnees do not feel fully accepted by the community.

Education

Experienced teachers moving to a new school become newcomer teachers. This can present problems because they have prior knowledge of teaching but not of the school to which they have moved (Schram,

1992). When trying to maintain a previous level of standards, they may be seen as inflexible or assertive. This can threaten the other teachers, alienate the newcomers, and interfere with the development of colleageal relationships between the other teachers and the newcomers. In addition, newcomer teachers may be identified with their previous schools' academic records, thus influencing other teachers' perceptions of them. These perceptions, for better or worse, will affect how the newcomer teacher is accepted. Also, unwritten rules exist in schools; even an experienced teacher would not be familiar with the rules of a new school.

Newly arrived students from non-English speaking countries come to the United States with very limited experience of the language and the American school system (Constantino & Lavedenz, 1993). Instead of using a sink-or-swim approach, newcomer schools have been developed to aid these students. These schools emphasize integration by orienting students to American schools and society. Such schools provide an environment that allows newcomer students to adjust to their new language and environment by reducing cultural and educational shock.

Literature

In A. B. Guthrie's (1947) book, *The Big Sky,* about mountain men in Montana, his character Uncle Zeb states "She's gone, goddam it! Gone!" (p. 150). Uncle Zeb was upset because of the influx of people that were spoiling the once open, unpopulated area. He says,

> *Forts all up and down the river, and folk everywhere a man might think to lay a trap. And greenhorns comin' in and sp'ilin' the fun. Christ sake! Why'nt' they stay home? Why'nt' they leave it to us as found it? By God, she's ours by rights. God, she was purty onc't. Purty and new, and not a man tract, savin' Injuns,' on the whole scoop of her. (p. 150)*

In *Dakota: A Spiritual Geography,* Kathleen Norris (1993) discusses her experiences as a newcomer to a small town in South Dakota. Several times throughout the book, she discusses the newcomer's difficulty, and even inability, in being accepted by the community. She attributed the community's nonacceptance to the established residents' difficulty with change. Change, a contaminant brought in by outsider elements, can lead to instability in the community and potentially can mean failure of its way of life. A newcomer, someone who has made a major change in his or her life by moving, represents change and, like everything from the outside world, is suspect.

Norris (1993) also speaks to the local, unwritten history or story of the community. The newcomer is not knowledgeable of the history that dictates behavior in communities and families. One may need to go back fifty years or so to understand it. Because the history is not understood by newcomers, they are likely to break unwritten rules, further distancing themselves from the community. The newcomer can threaten the social order of the community, and "they have to be discouraged, put down, or even cast out" (p. 56).

The Media

Movies. An interesting use of the term newcomer comes from the motion picture *Alien Nation* (Hurd, Kobritz, & Baker, 1988). In the movie, extraterrestrials were marooned on Earth because of a problem with their ship. The aliens have no choice but to live on Earth and are called Newcomers. The Newcomers are not accepted by many Earthlings. Therefore, they experience discrimination.

Newspapers. A poll conducted by the *Great Falls Tribune,* a Montana newspaper, revealed a negative view of newcomers (Johnson, 1996). Sixty percent of the respondents thought that people moving into the state negatively affect the quality of life for residents. Complaints included increased real estate prices and property taxes; the negative impact on the state's environment; and the taking of jobs from Montana workers. One resident stated that it was all right for newcomers to come to Montana if there were not too many. Residents more likely to be critical of newcomers had lived in the state for more than ten years. Residents who reported living in the state less than ten years and having a college education were more likely to be in favor of newcomers. Conversely, 51% of the sample said that people moving into the state would bring new ideas and stimulate innovation.

Magazines. In a *Newsweek* article, Elliot, McGuire, Murr, and Glick (1995) reported on a culture clash in the mountain states. The West has become the chic place for new settlers. The reasons newcomers give for moving to the area are to get away from the crime and gang activities in California and to take advantage of the open spaces.

Established residents of several mountain states are not happy about the influx of new residents and blame the newcomers for their areas' problems. Residents complained about the loss of a town's uniqueness, urban development putting a strain on available resources, and rising housing costs. Verbal responses such as, "You must be a Californian," and the appearance of bumper stickers stating, "Welcome to Silver City. Now please go home," are examples of negative feelings of established residents toward newcomers.

Television. On November 14, 1995, *Good Morning America* (Reichblum) broadcast their program from Montana. One topic addressed was the migration of new people to Montana; it was called a range war: natives versus newcomers. The natives disliked newcomers because of increases in land values and taxes and newcomers bringing the problems they left with them. One man simply stated, "I wish they wouldn't come here." Another said "[they] come for something, once they get here it's gone." Reasons why newcomers came to Montana included improvement of their lives through better schools, no gangs, a better environment to raise their children in, and the wide-open spaces. Rock Ringling, Director of the Montana Land Reliance, commented that the wide-open spaces are being lost due to newcomers' building.

Radio. In May and December of 1994, National Public Radio (NPR) aired two programs about the problems of people moving into an area. The first, *The American Culture Wars* (Hoyt, 1994), specifically addressed people moving to Idaho. The old-timers were dismayed because the newcomers were making changes which dealt with their way of life; an example was the difficulty of moving large farm equipment on the road. Newcomers did not know they needed to respect the equipment; often they were rude to the farmers. Newcomers more accommodating to the residents' way of life had similar educational and political backgrounds. Many residents feared being crowded out by newcomers not wanting to live close to barns because of the smell. A retired school teacher called newcomers a "different class." They made her feel inferior because many have money, and she did not. In addition, she drove an old truck and lived in a house that "isn't really great."

City leaders tried to make the newcomers feel more at home by building new recreational facilities. Old-timers expressed no plans to visit the new facilities because they felt the newcomers "wouldn't want to meet poor farmers." Idaho writer Clay Morgan voiced the fear that "newcomers may be bringing with them the things they sought to escape" (Hoyt, 1984).

The NPR second broadcast from New Mexico was titled, *Santa Fe Fighting Loss of Old Way of Life* (Berkes, 1994). Hispanics, previously the majority group, were unhappy about becoming the minority group due to wealthy whites moving into the area. One man remembered as a child that whites moving to the area assimilated to the Hispanic's way of life. Now, the newcomers did not want to get to know the natives. Therefore, the Santa Fe the Hispanics had always known was changing. Many places the locals frequented no longer existed; an example was neighborhood stores. Rising taxes, more expensive housing, and low salaries of some locals created a need to move elsewhere. Conversely, some natives were happy to sell their adobe homes at inflated prices and move to more modern areas. The mayor of Santa Fe, Debbie Jaramillo, promised to control growth because she wanted the newcomers to live together with the natives, not separate themselves. While some newcomers said they were coming for the diversity of culture, many live in gated communities.

ESSENTIAL ATTRIBUTES

Three essential attributes were identified for the concept of newcomer from an examination of the literature. They are (a) *newly arrived,* (b) *unaware of the history of the area/institution,* and (c) *their existence may result in change* that can lead to insecurity among the established residents.

- A new arrival means that an individual or family has moved to a new place to live or work.
- Unaware of the social history of the area refers to the individual/family not being aware of the social structure that is in place and the whys of the communities'/organizations' decisions to do things a certain way. This is different from the actual historical beginnings of the area/organization. Unwritten rules dictate the culture of a community. Often individuals have difficulty in being accepted by the community because they break these unwritten rules.
- Their existence may result in change that can lead to insecurity

among the established residents—means that the established residents/employees may believe the newcomers are creating the likelihood that change will take place. Changes, caused by the presence of the newcomers, could be perceived by the community as threatening its security.

ANTECEDENTS AND CONSEQUENCES

To become a newcomer, individuals or families would have had a need or desire to move from their previous place of residence. The reasons they wanted to move would vary. The consequence of the actions of people moving to a new area would be that there is a new individual or family living in the community. These individuals would affect the community in some way.

CASES USING IDENTIFIED ATTRIBUTES

Two cases are presented. The first contains all the attributes, while the second, a borderline case, contains most, though not all, of the attributes.

Model Case

Sally Macleod is a nurse practitioner who recently moved to a rural Montana town from a large city in another state. She is the first nurse practitioner to practice in this area. Sally has never lived in this town before nor does she have any relatives who live in the area. After seeing Sally Macleod once, Mrs. Simpson now chooses to see the local pharmacist for her arthritic pain. Mrs. Simpson tells the pharmacist that "the new lady just doesn't know what we need. She tried to get me to wear braces on my hands. How am I supposed to work with them on?" The pharmacist replies by stating, "I don't know what's wrong with just going to the doctor. Why do people need to change things anyway?"

This case study meets all three of the attributes. Sally is a new arrival to the town and did not have any previous affiliation with the area. Her lack of knowledge of the social history of the area was pointed out by a woman who chose to use a pharmacist who has always lived in the area instead of the nurse practitioner who was not aware that being able to work is very important for rural people. By starting a new practice, Sally created change in the community through introduction of a new method of health care delivery.

Borderline Case

Joe Brook has moved back to the town where he lived with his family until he went to college. Through the years Joe has been home frequently and kept in close contact with his parents. His parents have been ill, and he and his wife will be helping in their care. Joe has been a bank loan officer for twenty years in a large city and will be working at the town's bank. In the coffee shop one morning, several long-term residents of the town were discussing Joe starting at the bank and how, "You can never trust those city bankers, and I'm not sure that I want one looking after my money."

This second case study only partially meets the attributes. Though Joe has newly arrived back in town, he is a returnee and not a true newcomer. The town's people are concerned about his ability to do his job at the bank because he has lived in a big city. They have expressed their wariness of him and of possible changes he could bring. Joe is familiar with the history of the community from growing up there, from frequent visits, and from his parents.

SUMMARY

The concept of newcomer was analyzed using information found in many disciplines. The concept of newcomer is one that cannot exist alone and is connected to the other concepts of rural nursing theory. Many references speak of newcomers and how they are treated by insiders and old-timers. Some references define a newcomer as an outsider trying to become an insider. Because newcomers are much more visible in a smaller town, they have less anonymity; their difficulty of integration into the community is a problem commonly seen in rural areas.

REFERENCES

Barnhart, R. K. (Ed.) (1988). *The Barnhart Dictionary of Etymology.* New York: Wilson.

Bauer, T. N. & Green, S. G. (1994). Effect of newcomer involvement in work-related activities; A longitudinal study of socialization. *Journal of Applied Psychology, 79* (2), 211–223.

Berkes, H. (Producer & Reporter). (1994, December 8). *All things considered: Santa Fe fighting loss of old way of life.* National Public Radio.

Blau, P. (1956). *Bureacracy in modern society.* New York: Random House.

Bushy, A. (1993). Rural Women: Lifestyle and health status. *Nursing Clinics of North America, 28* (1), 187–197.

Constantino, R., & Lavedenz, M. (1993). Newcomer schools: First Impressions. *Peabody Journal of Education, 69* (1), 82–101.

Elliot, M., McGuire, S., Murr, A., & Glick, D. (1995). The west at war. *Newsweek, 126* (3), 24–28.

Gove, P. B. (Ed. in Chief) (1986). *Webster's third new international dictionary of the English language, unabridged* (3rd ed.). Springfield, MA: Merriam-Webster.

Guthrie, A. B. (1947). *The big sky.* New York: William Sloan.

Hoyt, J. (Producer & Reporter). (1994, May 12). *Morning edition: The American culture wars—Part 5.* National Public Radio.

Hurd, G. A., Kobritz, R. (Producers), & Baker, G. (Director). (1988). *Alien Nation* [Film].

Johnson, P. (1996, February 5). Most Montanans see newcomers as a threat to jobs. *Great Falls Tribune,* pp. 1B-2B.

Kipfer, B. A. (1992). *Roget's 21st century thesaurus in dictionary form.* New York, NY: Dell.

Long, K. A. (1993). The concept of health: Rural perspectives. *Nursing Clinics of North America, 28* (1), 123–130.

Long, K. A., & Weinert, C. (1987). Understanding the health care needs of rural families. *Family Relations, 36,* 450–455.

Morrison, E. W. (1993). Newcomer information seeking: Exploring types, modes, sources, and outcomes. *Academy of Management Journal, 36* (3), 557–589.

Norris, K. (1989). *Dakota: A spiritual geography.* New York: Ticknor & Fields.

Partington, A. (ed). (1992). *The oxford Dictionary of quotations* (4th ed.). New York: Oxford University Press.

Rakich, J. S., Longest, B. B. & Darr, K. (1995, 2nd ed.). *Managing health services organizations.* Philadelphia, PA: Saunders.

Reichblum, B. (Executive Producer). (1995, November 14). *Good Morning America.* New York: American Broadcasting Company.

Schram, T. (1992). When a veteran teacher changes schools. *Principal, 72* (1), 20–21.

Stinner, W. F & Kan, S. H. (1984). Newcomer-returnee differences in non-metropolitan Utah communities. *The Social Science Journal, 21* (2), 136–148.

Walker, L. O., & Avant, K. C. (1995). *Strategies for theory construction in nursing* (2nd ed.). Norwalk, CT: Appleton & Lange.

Weinert, C., & Long, K. A. (1991). The theory and research base rural nursing practice. In Bushy, A. (Ed.). *Rural nursing* (Vol. 1) (pp. 21–38). Newbury Park, CA, Sage.

Yeo, B. (1995). *Montana outback.* Butte, Montana: Author.

10

Insider

Deborah D. Myers

In a discussion of the theory and research base for the practice of rural nursing, Long and Weinert (1989) identified the term "insider" as a key concept in understanding rural health care needs and nursing practice. The authors posit that the concept of insider relates to how rural populations view relationships and organize their view of the community. Moreover, Long and Weinert maintain that an understanding of the concept is essential for rural health care providers attempting to gain acceptance and, therefore, provide health care for a rural community.

AIM OF THE ANALYSIS

The aim of this paper is to clarify the meaning of the concept of insider and to facilitate the simultaneous analysis of the concepts of insider, outsider, newcomer, and old-timer. An appreciation of these concepts is essential for rural health care providers. Furthermore, the current movement from hospital-based to community-based health care compels nurses to understand the importance of gaining acceptance into any community in order to provide effective care.

Walker and Avant (1995) provide guidelines to be used for this concept analysis. Dictionary definitions and synonyms will be presented, and uses of the concept in various areas of literature will be identified. From these definitions and uses, defining attributes will be determined. Construction of model, borderline, and contrary cases will enhance the understanding of the concept. Finally, antecedents and consequences will be identified.

DICTIONARY ETYMOLOGY AND DEFINITIONS

According to Barnhart (1988), the term insider is derived from the English word inside and the suffix er. The term inside originated in Middle English, a compound of the adverbs, inne and side. Inside and its opposite, outside, first appeared in the English language after 1504 and referred to the interior of the body. The first recording of the term insider is in 1846. Insider was a noun, in American English, that referred to a book carried in an outside coat pocket. Two years later, the term appeared as someone who is a member of a group.

The term inside is currently defined by Webster (Merriam-Webster, 1986a) as

> *1 a: an interior or internal part: the part within b: inward nature, thoughts, or feeling c: viscera, entrails 2: an inner side or surface 3 a: a position of power or confidence (only someone on the inside could have told) b: confidential information (has the inside on what happened at the convention) 4: the area nearest a specified or implied point of reference: as a: the side of home plate nearest the batter b: the middle portion of a playing area c: the area near or underneath the basket in basketball. (p.625)*

Webster's Dictionary (Merriam-Webster 1986b) defines insider as:

> *n. A person recognized or accepted as a member of some group, category or organization: as a: a person having access to confidential information because of his position b: an officer or director of a company or a beneficial owner of 10 percent or more of an equity security registered on an exchange (laws regulating the manipulation of a company's securities by changes) (p. 1169).*

The *Oxford English Dictionary* (Simpson & Weiner, 1989) defines insider as "One who is inside; a person who is within the limits of some place, society, organization, etc.; hence, one in possession of special information, one who is 'in the secret.' Opposed to outsider" (p.1026). *Roget's Thesaurus* (Kipfer 1992) describes insider as in the middle; interior, central, inner, innermost, internal, inward, surrounded, secret, classified, confidential, esoteric, exclusive, hushed, internal, limited, private, restricted.

The dictionary definitions and etymology provide a basis for the understanding of the concept insider. An initial definition of insider is someone who is a member of a group and has access to special or privileged information.

USE IN NON-NURSING DISCIPLINES

The use of the concept insider is found in several disciplines including business, anthropology, philosophy, sociology, and organizational studies. The meaning of insider as it is used in these disciplines is presented in the following discussion.

Business

In business, the term insider is used with the term trading, i.e., insider trading, and in describing persons employed in a particular organization. Osti (1990) defines insider trading as "... the buying or selling of securities by someone who has obtained non-public information that is likely to be important to a reasonable investor and who uses that information in breach of an obligation of trust or confidence" (p. 71). Osti goes on to identify common characteristics of insider traders: desire for money, competitiveness, enjoyment of risk behavior, sense of invulnerability, need to identify with those in power, and the rationalization that it is a victimless crime. Osti's discussion of insider is consistent with the dictionary definitions in that the insider possesses or has access to special or confidential information. However, insider characteristics as identified by Osti are not consistent with the use of the term in other disciplines; the characteristic that is a possible exception is the need to identify with those in power.

Another reference to insider in the business literature describes insiders as those people currently employed by an organization (Leslie, 1992). This use of the term insider is consistent with dictionary definitions in that the insider is a person recognized as a member of a group.

Organizational Studies

Bartunek, Lacey, and Wood (1992), in writing about organizational change, use the term insider in describing founders of a group. The authors also identify the term in the context of research; i.e., an inside researcher as opposed to an outside researcher. In a more recent study of collaborative advocacy, Bartunek, Foster-Fisherman, and Keys (1996) again use a joint insider–outsider approach. That is, two researchers were insiders, founders of the advisory board being examined, and one was an outsider. The outsider collected interview and archival data about the board. According to Schein (1984), an inside researcher can understand the members' implicit assumptions. This is contrasted with an outside researcher who probes, searches, and holds assumptions about what is observed, thereby uncovering unconscious assumptions.

Other organizational studies direct inquiry to different topics but use the term consistently. Callen and Falk (1992) studied the efficiency of nonprofit health organizations that had a larger proportion of outsider, rather than insider, trustees. Insider trustees were defined as employees of the organization. O'Leary-Kelly, Griffin, and Glew (1996) suggested a research framework for studying violence in organizations. They also used the term insider to describe employees of an organization and added that the group to which the insiders belonged, i.e., the organization, provided an important social system. Additionally, insiders had more frequent contact with the group, and the interactions were more substantive. Finally, in a study of wage discrimination and fairness, Fehr and Kirchsteiger (1994) use insider to describe people who are employed by an organization and bargain collectively for wages. The authors go on to describe insiders as powerful and selfish.

Anthropology

Anthropologist Ewing (1994) discusses "going native," as opposed to remaining an outsider, while studying a given culture. Since "going native" is in opposition to outsider, the antonym of insider, it is pertinent to this analysis. According to Ewing, one significant danger in "going native" is the inability to maintain neutrality and, therefore, believing in another's reality, such as witchcraft or magic. An insider or someone who has "gone native," therefore, believes in another's reality. This definition is consistent with views of the disciplines of nursing, philosophy, and sociology.

In an ethnographic study of cultural differences in the ways Zuni and Anglo teachers operate in Zuni classrooms, Osborne (1989) discusses insiders and outsiders. Although insider is not clearly defined in the study, Osborne identifies that "insiders and outsiders" are a mechanism that provides or maintains power and provides protection of cultural heritage by controlling information. The control or possession of information is consistent with dictionary definitions of insider.

Philosophy

Philosopher Kamm (1990) identifies insider with respect to serving as advisor to a government commission. This is as opposed to an outsider who comments on the work of the commissions. Kamm suggests that being an insider, a member of the group, changes the way one interacts with the group.

Sociology

Oromaner (1984) discussed the role of community colleges in relation to research universities. He uses the term insider as one who is affiliated with the institution.

Sociologist Elias (1994) studied a community in Great Britain for several years and identified two groups of people in the community. He named these groups "the established" and "the outsiders" and focused mainly on the characteristics of the group of established. Elias' observations of the established are pertinent to the concept of insider because the established are opposed to outsider, the antonym of insider. The established are described by Elias as old families, i.e., families who had lived in the community for two to three generations. They shared a common past that included memories, attachments, and dislikes. There were no observable differences between the two groups as to housing, color, race, occupation, level of income, or education.

However, some specific characteristics of the established or insiders were identified (Elias, 1994). First, they held reserved social positions and were a cohesive group. Members of the established group did not associate with outsiders for fear of loss of status or fear of pollution. Second, established members viewed themselves as disciplined, trustworthy, and obedient, maintaining the laws and norms of the community. Third, emotional intimacy and group charisma were important characteristics of the established group, which maintained its identity and power by remaining detached and distant from the group of outsiders. Within the group, a ranking order was maintained, and the criteria for the ranks were known to everyone who belonged to the group. This was privileged information, however, because the criteria were not known to outsiders. These characteristics are consistent with other uses of the concept.

In a discussion of the sociology of knowledge, Merton (1972) identifies insider and outsider doctrines. Insider doctrines claim monopolistic or privileged access to knowledge. Furthermore, Merton explains that according to the insider doctrine, only members of a group can truly understand that group. In other words, the insider has experiences and socialization that produce intuitive sensitivity that makes empathic understanding of other members of the group possible. One characteristic of insiders that Merton identifies is that insiders share the deepest concerns of the group.

Summary

Examination of the use of insider in non-nursing disciplines provides additional information about the term. Not only is an insider a member of a group with access to privileged information, the insider has an intimate relationship with the group characterized by a deeper understanding of the group's norms and assumptions.

USE IN THE NURSING DISCIPLINE

The term insider is found in three areas of nursing literature. Authors in nursing case management, nursing research, and rural nursing all use the term as discussed below.

Nursing Case Management

Lamb and Stempel (1994) identify insider as a distinct role of the nurse case manager. Although they do not clearly define insider, they describe an insider as a nurse who has developed an emotionally intimate relationship with the client. To describe the insider nurse, clients use the terms "knowing me," "caring about me," "someone I can count on to be with me," and "interested in all of me."

Nursing Research

In nursing research, the term insider is consistently used to describe the group being studied (Masters & Shontz, 1989; Titchen & Binnie, 1992; Kauffman, 1994). Using quantitative analyses of behavior yields an outsider's view (Liehr & Marcus, 1994). Qualitative research, however, employs the ethnographic method to understand the insiders' view of their world and requires that the researcher enter the world of the group being studied.

Rural Nursing

Rural nursing literature provides additional applications of the term. Long (1993) describes an insider as someone " . . . who can be trusted to understand the social context of the health care problem" (p. 124). Weinert and Long (1991) consistently link insider with informal systems of health care delivery, e.g., the local drug store owner whose family has been a member of the community for generations. Characteristics of insiders have also been identified in the rural nursing literature. A long-time occupant of an area is a characteristic of an insider according to Nichols (1989). Additionally, Weinert and Long (1987) identified length of residence, family history, and type of occupation as important variables in determining a person's insider status.

Summary

Although insider is not defined in the nursing literature, the uses of the term are congruent with those discussed in other fields. The aspect of intimacy is readily apparent in the nursing literature. Nursing literature also provides another important characteristic of insiders, the length of time one has lived in the community.

DEFINING ATTRIBUTES

Defining attributes or characteristics of insiders identified from the dictionary definitions, etymology, and common usage of the term are a) *member of a group,* b) *having access to privileged information,* c) *an awareness of implicit assumptions and social context,* and d) *a long-time occupant.* Each of these is descriptive of the concept of insider relative to rural communities.

CASES

The development of case examples facilitates the understanding of the concept and helps clarify meaning (Walker & Avant, 1995). Model, borderline, and contrary cases developed from the author's experiences in rural and frontier communities are discussed.

Model Case

A model case is a pure example of the concept and includes all of the attributes (Walker & Avant, 1995). A 50–year-old man, Joe Smith, has always lived and worked in a mountain community that has a year-round population of seventy. The man's father owns and still operates the only general store, an inheritance from *his* father who delivered mail by foot across the mountains to the community around the turn of the century. Joe is a member of the group (community) and has lived there for a long period of time. In fact, two generations of his family have lived in the community. Therefore, Joe is a long-time occupant.

When we began to build a summer home in the community, Joe shared information with us regarding who built the best quality home, was most reliable, and was most knowledgeable. Several weeks after we selected a contractor, Joe informed us that this man was planning to move away from the community. Apparently, this was common knowledge to members of the community, but we had not been told. Joe has access to privileged information in that he knew characteristics of all of the contractors and the personal plans of at least one contractor.

Recently, a new family moved to the community and bought a business. Joe confided to me one day that the family was not being well received because they were not "introducing themselves around" and because they kept sheep behind their business. Rather, the new man would approach community members and make requests without introducing himself or engaging in social conversation. Joe understands *why* the new family is not being accepted. They are violating the social norms of the community by keeping sheep and by not becoming involved in the community. An implicit assumption in this community is that several minutes of social conversation precede the actual matter to be discussed. To "get to the point" of a conversation immediately is considered rude. Joe is aware of the social context and implicit assumptions of the community.

Joe demonstrates all of the defining attributes of an insider. He is a member of the group (community) and is a long-time occupant. Joe has access to privileged information and, finally, he is aware of the social context and implicit assumptions of the community. Joe possesses all of the attributes of an insider.

Borderline Case

A borderline case is one that includes many attributes of the concept but is lacking at least one attribute (Walker & Avant, 1995). Therefore, at first glance, the borderline case may appear to be an example of the concept. It has many similarities to but is not exactly the same as the concept.

In the community described above, there are many summer residents. One such resident is a 72–year-old retired physician. He and his wife return to the community annually to spend summers in the home they had built twenty-five years ago. Although both were born and raised in the state, they have lived and worked in another state for the past fifty years. The man possesses a wealth of information about the community, its members, and their histories. When I shared with him the information Joe had given me regarding the new family, he was already aware of it. However, he did not seem to understand why community members were reluctant to form a friendship with the new people.

This gentleman possesses some defining attributes of an insider. He has access to special information; i.e., he knows about the community, its history, and its members. He is a member of the summer community and may be a member of the year-round community (group). Although he has lived there for twenty-five years, it has been on an interrupted basis. He does not have the defining attribute of a long-time occupant. Moreover, he does not have a complete understanding of the social norms and implicit assumptions of the group. Therefore, though he has access to some information and is a member of the summer community, he is not an insider.

Contrary Case

A contrary case is one that is clearly not an example of the concept (Walker & Avant, 1995). The community described in the other two cases is a mountain community supported largely by tourism. A tourist in this community provides a clear contrary case. I overheard a conversation between the general store owner and a tourist who had stopped for gasoline on her way to another town. The woman was quite angry and said, "You mean you don't even have an ATM? How am I supposed to eat lunch? What kind of place is this?" I had seen the store owner cash checks for community members often, yet he did not offer to cash a check for her.

This case possesses none of the critical attributes for an insider. The woman had been in the community for approximately 10 minutes and was certainly not a member of that community. She did not have access even to basic information such as how to obtain cash. Furthermore, she demonstrated absolutely no awareness of social context. The members of the community see no need for an automated teller machine, and, in fact, are opposed to the idea. Moreover, she was completely unaware of an implicit assumption; the person she was speaking to was a long-standing member of the community and was to be treated with respect. In this community, treating someone with respect includes engaging in social conversation. This woman possesses none of the defining attributes and is not an insider.

SUMMARY OF CASES

Model, borderline, and contrary cases have been presented. The model case includes all of the defining attributes of insider, and the borderline case includes some, but not all, of the attributes. None of the attributes are present in the contrary case. Related, invented, and illegitimate cases could be developed.

ANTECEDENTS AND CONSEQUENCES

Antecedents are those things that must occur prior to the occurrence of the concept (Walker & Avant, 1995). To be a member of a group, one must first be accepted by the group. A person may be either born or socialized into membership. Therefore, acceptance by the group is an antecedent to being an insider.

Consequences are those things that occur because of the occurrence of the concept. (Walker & Avant, 1995) There are several consequences to being an insider. The first consequence, power, is discussed in three of the literature fields (Osti, 1990; Osborne, 1989; & Elias Scotson, 1994). Power is an important aspect of the concept of insider and comes because of having information that others lack. The second consequence is apparent in the discussion by Elias and Scotson (1994), reserved social position. Insiders often hold social positions that are unavailable to others. Third, lack of objectivity is a consequence of being an insider as discussed by anthropologist Ewing (1994). Finally, being committed to the group is a consequence of being an insider as illustrated in the discussions by Elias and Scotson (1994), and Merton (1972).

CONCLUSION

The concept insider has been defined using dictionary definitions, etymology, and synonyms. These definitions in combination with the uses in many fields of literature have provided the critical attributes of the concept. Model, borderline, and contrary cases were developed based on the identified attributes. Finally, antecedents and consequences were identified.

Several implications for rural nursing become apparent from the analysis. First, critical attributes, antecedents, and consequences need to be tested. Rural community members should be given the opportunity to validate or refute them. Additionally, nurses coming to a rural community to provide health care need to be able to identify and form a relationship with an insider. This must be done to begin to understand the assumptions and social context of the community and to gain acceptance by the community members, thereby providing health care that is viewed as important, effective, and useful.

REFERENCES

Barnhart, R. K. (Ed.). (1988). *The Barnhart dictionary of etymology.* Bronx, NY: Wilson.

Bartunek, J. M., Foster-Fishman, P. G., & Keys, C. B. (1996). Using collaborative advocacy to foster intergroup cooperation: A joint insider-outsider investigation. *Human Relations, 49* (6), 701–733.

Bartunek, J. M., Lacey, C., & Wood, D. (1992). Social cognition in organizational change: An insider-outsider approach. *Journal of Applied Behavioral Science, 28* (2), 204–223.

Callen, J. L., & Falk, H. (1993). Agency and efficiency in nonprofit organizations: The case of "specific health focus" charities. *The Accounting Review, 68* (1), 48–65.

Elias, N., & Scotson, J. L. (1994). *The established and the outsiders* (2nd ed.). London: Sage.

Ewing, K. P. (1994). Dreams from a saint: Anthropological atheism and the temptation to believe. *American Anthropologist, 96* (3), 571–583.

Fehr, E. M., & Kirchsteiger, G. (1994). Insider power, wage discrimination and fairness. *The Economic Journal, 104,* 571–583.

Kamm, F. M. (1990). The philosopher as insider and outsider. *Journal of Medicine and Philosophy, 15,* 347–374.

Kauffman, K. S. (1994). The insider/outsider dilemma: Field experience of a white researcher "gettin' in" a poor black community. *Nursing Research, 43* (3), 179–183.

Kipfer, B. A. (Ed.). (1992). *Rogets 21st century thesaurus* (1992). New York, NY: Dell.

Lamb, G. S., & Stempel, J. E. (1994). Nurse case management from the client's view: Growing as insider-expert. *Nursing Outlook, 42* (1), 7–13.

Leslie, D. (1992). Insider-outsider theory and the case for implicit contracts. *Economic Journal, 102,* 37–48.

Liehr, P. R., & Marcus, M. T. (1994). Qualitative approaches to Research. In G. LoBiondo-Wood & J. Haber (Eds.), *Nursing research: Methods, critical appraisal, and utilization* (pp.253–268). St. Louis: Mosby.

Long, K. A. (1993). The concept of health: Rural perspectives. *Nursing Clinics of North America, 28* (1), 123–130.

Long, K. A., & Weinert, C. (1989). Rural Nursing: Developing the theory base. *Scholarly Inquiry for Nursing Practice, 3* (2), 113–127.

Masters, M., & Shontz, F. (1989). Identification of problems and strengths of the hospice client by clients, care givers, and nurses. *Cancer Nursing, 12* (4), 226–235.

Merriam-Webster, Inc. (1986a) *Webster's ninth new collegiate dictionary.* Springfield, MA: Merriam-Webster.

Merriam-Webster, Inc. (1986b). *Webster's third new international dictionary of the English language unabridged.* Springfield, MA: G & C Merriam.

Merton, R. K. (1972). Insiders and outsiders: A chapter in the sociology of knowledge. *American Journal of Sociology,77* (15), 9–47.

Nichols, E. (1989). Response to "rural nursing: Developing the theory base." *Scholarly Inquiry for Nursing Practice, 3* (2), 129–132.

O'Leary-Kelly, A. M., Griffin, R. W., & Glew, D. J. (1996). Organization-motivated aggression: A research framework. *Academy of Management Review 21* (1), 225–253.

Oromaner, M. (1984). Insiders, outsiders, and the community college: A sociology of knowledge perspective. *Research in Higher Education, 21* (2), 226–235.

Osborne, A.B. (1989). Insiders and outsiders: Cultural membership and the micropolitics of education among the Zuni. *Anthropology & Education Quarterly, 20* (3), 196–214.

Osti, L. A. (1990). Insider trading: The causes of a behavioral phenomenon as presented in the business and financial press. *Journal of American Culture, 13,* 7–8.

Schein, E.H. (1984). Coming to a new awareness of organizational culture. *Sloan Management Review,* 3–16.

Simpson, J. A., & Weiner, E. S. C. (Eds.). (1989). *The Oxford English dictionary* (2nd ed., Vol.VII). Oxford: Clarendon Press.

Titchen, A., & Binnie, A. (1993). Research partnerships: Collaborative action research in nursing. *Journal of Advanced Nursing, 18,* 858–865.

Walker, L. O., & Avant, K. C. (1995). Strategies for theory construction in nursing (3rd ed.). Norwalk, CT: Appleton & Lange.

Weinert, C., & Long, K. A. (1987). Understanding the health care needs of rural families. *Family Relations, 36,* 450–455.

Weinert, C., & Long, K. A. (1991). The theory and research base for rural nursing practice. In A. Bushy (Ed.), *Rural Nursing,* vol. 1 (pp. 21–37). Newbury Park, CA: Sage.

11

Outsider

Michelle C. Bailey

INTRODUCTION

According to Walker and Avant (1988), concept analysis is an exercise that allows us to examine and define the attributes of a concept. The process also allows us to differentiate between defining and irrelevant attributes of a concept. A concept is a "complex mental formulation of empiric experience. . . . Theories are structured from ideas expressed as concepts" (Chinn & Kramer, 1991, pp. 58, 108).

The development of rural nursing theory is in its initial stages. Further theory development is needed to help define rural nursing (Bigbee, 1993). The rural nursing theory base includes the following concepts: work beliefs/health beliefs, isolation and distance, self-reliance/independence, lack of anonymity, old-timer/newcomer, and outsider/insider (Long & Weinert, 1989). While the concepts have been identified, they lack clarification.

The aim of this analysis is to clarify the meaning and use of the concept "outsider" so that the term is understood and used similarly by all within nursing. The guidelines for concept analysis described in Walker and Avant (1988) will be used for this concept analysis. Dictionary definitions, synonyms, and etymology of the concept will be stated; use of the concept in other disciplines will be identified; essential attributes will be determined; and a model case and a borderline case will be developed using the determined essential attributes.

DEFINITIONS

The concept of outsider is defined by *Webster's Third New International Dictionary* (Gove, 1986) to be

> *1a. a person not recognized or accepted as a member of some group, category, or organization (has lived there for 20 years but is still regarded as an outsider; a political outsider); 1b. a person who isolates himself or is felt to be isolated from the world around him (the artist ought to be an outsider-E. M. Forster); 2 a contender in a sports event that is not favored to win; 3 outsiders (pl.): a pair of long-nosed nippers for grasping the point of a key in the keyhole from the outside; 4 jaunting car. (p. 1604)*

The Random House Dictionary of the English Language (Flexner, 1987) includes these definitions: "1 a person unconnected or unacquainted with the matter in question: Not being a parent, I was regarded as an outsider. 2 a person or thing not within an enclosure, boundary, etc." (p. 1377)

According to *The Barnhart Dictionary of Etymology* (Barnhart, 1988), the term outsider originated in 1800 in Jane Austen's letters. Synonyms for outsider are many and include stranger, foreigner, alien, nonmember, and outlander (Chapman, 1992). Other synonyms are newcomer, outcast, reject, castoff, encroacher, trespasser, unwelcome visitor, gate-crasher, intruder, and invader (Urdang, 1978a, 1978b). Antonyms of outsider include insider and intimate. The Afrikaans use the term *Uitlander*; the Chinese use the term *foreign devil*; and the Spanish-Americans use the term *gringo* to refer to an outsider (Chapman, 1992).

The concept of outsider has many synonyms and many diverse definitions. Many definitions involve the idea of being exterior to the group, matter, or boundary in question.

USES OF THE CONCEPT IN OTHER DISCIPLINES

The concept of outsider can be found in many articles and in many disciplines. This review of the literature will illuminate some uses of the concept.

Sociology

According to Merton (1968, as cited in Merton, 1972), "Insiders are the members of specified groups and collectivities or occupants of specified social statuses; Outsiders are the nonmembers" (p. 21). However, according to Merton (1972), all of us are both insiders and outsiders, members of some groups and not of others. The Doctrine of the Insider maintains that "the Outsider has a structurally imposed incapacity to comprehend alien groups, statuses, cultures, and societies" (p. 15). In addition, "the Outsider has neither been socialized in the group nor has engaged in the run of experience that makes up its life, and therefore cannot have the direct, intuitive sensitivity that alone makes empathic understanding possible" (p. 15). Conversely, the Outsider doctrine holds that knowledge about groups is accessible solely to outsiders since they are unbiased by membership.

Sociologist Daley and attorney Kobak (1990) discuss "familiar outsiders," a new type of reformer who came to the Appalachian Mountains to escape from the emphasis on material success and individualism in American society. This familiar outsider "does not have an overt and well thought-out agenda to change mountain society nor does he or she have a stereotypical preconception of mountain people" (p. 248). The familiar outsider avoids and denies power. She or he wants to be accepted as an ordinary citizen and hopes to aid the community in realizing its potential. The familiar outsiders both are a part of and not a part of Clinch town society, an Appalachian community.

Philosophy

In his book, *The Outsider,* philosopher Wilson (1956) states, "What can be said to characterize the Outsider is a sense of strangeness, of unreality" (p. 15). Wilson writes, "At first sight, the Outsider is a social problem. He is the hole-in-corner man" (p. 11). He further states that "the Outsider problem is essentially a living problem" (p. 70). "The Outsider is not sure who he is. He has found an 'I' but it is not his true 'I' " (p. 147). Wilson writes that the problem of the outsider has been discussed by many authors. For example, Sartre and Camus wrote about the outsider on a metaphysical level, Boehme and Kierkegaard wrote on a religious level, and Dostoevsky wrote on a criminal level.

Literature and Art

Poet Kathleen Norris (1993) says that "many teachers, doctors, lawyers, and ministers in rural towns are outsiders" (p. 55). According to Norris, some outsiders can pose a threat to the existing social order because they have different standards. Furthermore, outside elements bring in change that is seen as a contaminant. She also suggests that outsiders have a different background and lifestyle. "It is a truism that outsiders, often professional with no family ties, are never fully accepted into a rural or small-town community" (p. 83). In addition, outsiders are often turned into scapegoats by a group that cannot face its internal differences.

The word outsider also describes a certain kind of art including psychiatric, naive, and folk art. Those who produce Outsider Art are "eccentric and reclusive" (Outsider Artists, 1993, p. 85). Many are disturbed people, and some are inmates of mental hospitals. Outsider artists are obsessed with self-expression.

Organization (Business)

Business professor Nelson (1990) discusses the transition from outsider to insider in terms of newcomer socialization in a new organization. Organizational politics are often interpersonal stressors for the newcomer. "The new member is not often privy to the intricacies of power and influence that are part of organizations" (p. 72). Nelson also believes that the transition from outsider to insider occurs gradually over time.

Education/Cultural Studies

In an ethnographic study conducted in a Zuni, NM, school district, education lecturer Osborne (1989) discusses the insider–outsider relationships that exist between Zuni and Anglo teachers. The Anglo teachers feel like outsiders when it comes to understanding Zuni life, while the Zuni teachers feel like outsiders when it comes to particular educational issues. The insider–outsider phenomenon maintains ethnic borders between the two groups and power within groups.

Rural Health Care

Nurse researchers Titchen and Binnie (1993) identify two models of action research in the nursing literature, the insider and outsider models. In the outsider model, action researchers come from outside the setting and have no authority to introduce change. They serve in a diagnostic role by relaying observations back to the participants.

A key concept identified in rural qualitative and quantitative research discussed by nurse researchers Long and Weinert (1989) is the concept of outsider/insider. This concept and others are "used by rural dwellers in organizing their view of the social environment and in guiding their interactions and relationships" (p. 119). According to Long (1988), variables that seem important in determining if a person is an outsider include cultural orientation, family ties, occupation, and length of residence in the area. Nurse researcher Nichols (1989) defines outsiders as "those who have come in response to transient industries" and insiders to be rural people who are "long-time occupants of an area" (p. 130).

Health professionals may be distrusted initially and seen as outsiders (Long, 1993). Nurse researchers Long and Weinert (1987) concur, noting that professionals who are new to the community would be categorized as "outsiders" and "newcomers" (p. 454). Long and Weinert (1989) note that the concepts of outsider/insider are applicable to the acceptance of all health care providers in rural areas. "There often is a fierce pride among rural populations that inhibits acceptance of help from outsiders" (Turner & Gunn, 1991, p. 124).

ESSENTIAL ATTRIBUTES

After examination of the use of outsider in the literature, three essential attributes were identified and consist of the following: (1) *differentness,* (2) *unfamiliarity,* and (3) *unconnectedness.* These three attributes were then defined using *Webster's Third New International Dictionary* (Gove, 1986).

1. differentness (in terms of cultural orientation, standards, lifestyle, education, religion, occupation, social status, world view, interests, or experience): "the quality or state of being differ-

ent;" different: "partly or totally unlike in nature, form or quality; not the same" (p. 630).

2. unfamiliarity with the matter in question: "the quality or state of being unfamiliar;" unfamiliar: "not well known; unknown; not well acquainted" (p. 2495).
3. unconnectedness: "having no family or other personal ties" (p. 2486).

ANTECEDENTS AND CONSEQUENCES

Antecedents to being an outsider include lacking understanding or knowledge of the social context, beliefs, rituals, customs, and history of the community. A minimal length of time in the area may also contribute to one being an outsider.

Because of being an outsider, one may be excluded from access to knowledge and information, not be accepted, not be recognized, be isolated, and be distrusted.

MODEL CASE

According to Walker and Avant (1988), "a model case is a 'real life' example of the use of the concept that includes all the critical attributes and no attributes of any other concept" (p. 40). The following is a hypothetical model case. It was constructed to provide an example of outsider that includes all the essential attributes and therefore is a pure case of the concept.

Katie Goldblum was recently hired to work in Stanford, Montana, as the primary care provider for the community. Stanford has been without a primary care provider for five years. Although the small town community originally wanted a family nurse practitioner, they settled for a physician's assistant. No other provider was willing to relocate to Stanford.

Katie is an upper-class Jew who has spent all of her life in New York City. Since Katie graduated in 1990 from Long Island University in Brooklyn, New York, she has been working in an inner-city clinic, primarily in the treatment of sexually transmitted diseases. This is Katie's first visit to Montana, her first time west of the Mississippi, and the first time she has seen "real-life farmers," she says. Katie has no family or friends in Montana. The majority of her family lives on the East Coast. Her closest relative is a cousin in California.

Since Katie is the only primary care provider in Stanford, her practice is doing relatively well. She is knowledgeable about diagnosis and treatment of common illnesses. However, the people of Stanford do not fully trust her. She is different. Katie has attempted to integrate herself into the community by attending local sporting events and serving as a Sunday school teacher Sunday mornings at a local church. However, she continues to be unfamiliar with the farming/ranching way of life. She also has done little to understand the local perception of health and unique needs of the community. To make matters worse, the community of Stanford has remained closed to Katie and has made minimal effort to help Katie to become a part of the community. Thus, Katie remains an outsider.

This case includes all the essential attributes of outsider. Katie Goldblum is different in many respects from the rural population of Stanford, Montana. She is also unfamiliar with rural people, specifically farmers, and the state of Montana. Furthermore, Katie is unconnected; she has no family or other personal ties to the community.

Borderline Case

A borderline case contains some but not all of the essential attributes of the concept analyzed (Walker & Avant, 1988). The following is a hypothetical borderline case.

June Running Deer is a 46–year-old Crow Indian who was born and raised in St. Xavier, Montana, on the Crow Reservation. She is a masters-prepared certified nurse midwife and holds the only college degree in St. Xavier. Besides being a midwife, June is also on the tribal council. She lives with her husband who is a welder along with their 15–year-old daughter in a two-bedroom house, much like the homes of other families in St. Xavier. June's family is well-respected and has been in St. Xavier since the late 1800s. Through June's work as a midwife, her involvement on the tribal council, and her being born and raised in St. Xavier, June is well acquainted with everyone in the community.

June delivers most of the babies in St. Xavier and the surrounding area. She also provides routine well-woman care to the women of St. Xavier. For the most part, the women of St. Xavier confide in her. She is not only a Crow Indian but speaks the Crow language. However, some Crow women are hesitant to disclose themselves fully to June. They believe that June is different since returning from her midwife training. June uses words that the women cannot understand. Moreover, June is not supportive of the lay midwives who have attended to births since before she was born. Therefore, June is periodically an outsider.

This case contains two of the three essential attributes of outsider. June is clearly familiar with the people of St. Xavier both through her work as a midwife and being raised in the community. She is also connected to the people of St. Xavier due to her family ties in the area. However, June is an outsider by virtue of her different level of education and her occupation.

CONCLUSION

This concept analysis clarifies the meaning of outsider through delineation of essential attributes and description of model and borderline cases. It also describes the use of the concept of outsider among different disciplines. An outsider is different in some way from the group in question. Furthermore, the outsider is unfamiliar with the group or matter in question and unconnected to the group by virtue of family or personal ties.

The concept of outsider has particular relevance for rural nursing practice. As stated by Long and Weinert (1989), it has implications for the acceptance of nurses and other health care providers in rural areas. Joint effort by both the community and the outsider, the health care provider, is needed to bridge the gap between them. Health care providers need to be open to the community and to familiarize themselves with local perceptions of health and unique community needs. In addition, the community must reach out to the outsider health care provider and help the provider become part of the community.

According to Walker and Avant (1988), "Concept analysis alone will not provide useful theories for nursing education, research, or practice" (p. 46). Valuable theories will result only when concepts are connected with each other. Thus, this concept analysis of outsider is a preliminary step in theory formulation. The next step will be to link it to other concepts and create a theory.

REFERENCES

Barnhart. R. K. (Ed.). (1988). *The Barnhart dictionary of etymology*. Bronx, NY: Wilson.

Bigbee, J. L. (1993). The uniqueness of rural nursing. *Nursing Clinics of North America, 28*(1), 131–144.

Chapman, R. L. (Ed.). (1992). *Roget's international thesaurus* (5th ed.). New York: HarperCollins.

Chinn, P. L., & Kramer, M. K. (1991). *Theory and nursing: A systematic approach* (3rd ed.). St. Louis, MO: Mosby.

Daley, N. K., & Kobak, S. E. (1990). The paradox of the "familiar outsider." *Appalachian Journal, 17*(3), 248–260.

Flexner, S. B. (Ed.). (1987). *The Random House dictionary of the English language* (2nd ed.). New York: Random House.

Gove, P. B. (Ed.). (1986). *Webster's third new international dictionary*. Springfield, MA: Merriam-Webster.

Long, K. A. (1988). The concept of "outsider-insider" in rural mental health nursing practice. In C. Weinert (Moderator), *Rural nursing: Concepts and their application in practice.* WSRN Symposium.

Long, K. A. (1993). The concept of health. *Nursing Clinics of North America, 28*(1), 123–130.

Long, K. A., & Weinert, C. (1987). Understanding the health care needs of rural families. *Family Relations, 36,* 450–455.

Long, K. A., & Weinert, C. (1989). Rural nursing: Developing the theory base. *Scholarly Inquiry for Nursing Practice: An International Journal, 3*(2), 113–132.

Merton, R. K. (1972). Insiders and outsiders: A chapter in the sociology of knowledge. *American Journal of Sociology, 77*(15), 9–47.

Nelson, D. L. (1990). Adjusting to a new organization: Easing the transition from outsider to insider. *Prevention in Human Services, 8*(1), 61–86.

Nichols, E. (1989). Response to "rural nursing: Developing the theory base." *Scholarly Inquiry for Nursing Practice: An International Journal, 3*(2), 129–132.

Norris, K. (1993). *Dakota: A spiritual geography*. New York: Ticknor & Fields.

Osborne, A. B. (1989). Insiders and outsiders: Cultural membership and the micropolitics of education among the Zuni. *Anthropology & Education Quarterly, 20*(3), 196–215.

Outsider Artists. (1993). *The Economist, 326*(7796), 85.

Titchen, A., & Binnie, A. (1993). Research partnerships: Collaborative action research in nursing. *Journal of Advanced Nursing, 18*(6), 858–865.

Turner, T. A., & Gunn, I. P. (1991). Issues in rural health nursing. In A. Bushy (Ed.), *Rural nursing: Vol. 2* (pp. 105–127). Newbury Park, CA: Sage.

Urdang, L. (1978a). *A basic dictionary of synonyms and antonyms.* New York: Elsevier-Dutton.

Urdang, L. (Ed.). (1978b). *The synonym finder.* Emmaus, PA: Rodale Press.

Walker, L. O. & Avant, K. C. (1988). *Strategies for theory construction in nursing* (2nd ed.). Norwalk, CT: Appleton & Lange.

Wilson, C. (1956). *The outsider.* Cambridge, MA: Riverside Press.

12

Concept Comparison: Old-Timer/Newcomer/Insider/Outsider

Helen J. Lee

INTRODUCTION

The authors of the four preceding chapters on old-timer, newcomer, insider, and outsider (chapters 8, 9, 10, and 11) each used the concept analysis process to provide the Rural Nursing Theory Special Committee (RNTSC) with information for furthering the work on rural nursing theory. While these terms (old-timer, newcomer, insider, and outsider) are used frequently within rural literature, no one had analyzed them as concepts. Early work done by the Montana State University-Bozeman graduate nursing students provided the only know research base for these concepts. This base stimulated the inclusion of the concepts in an article by Long and Weinert (1989) about rural nursing theory development.

According to Chinn and Kramer (1991), the creation of conceptual meaning facilitates communication and avoids misunderstandings in addition to providing a stable base for extending theory development. Morse (1995) expanded the process of conceptual inquiry for exploring the theoretical basis of nursing and suggested that several outcomes may evolve from the process: (a) concept development [concept is nebulous, not well explicated], (b) concept delineation [concepts are merged, used interchangeable], (c) concept comparison [competing concepts, area not well understood], (d) concept correction [clinical experience or participant observation shows the concept is not a good fit], and (e) concept identification [new concept needed for data not described]. A working group within RNTSC combined processes of (a) concept development and (e) concept comparison to examine old-timer, newcomer, insider, and outsider.

INITIAL WORK

The theory development work reported in these chapters (chapters 8, 9, 10, 11, and 12) was initiated by a graduate student's concept analysis of an outsider (Bailey). Subsequently, commitments were made by three faculty persons to analyze the concepts of insider (Myers), old-timer (Caniparoli), and newcomer (Sutermaster). Periodic teleconference meetings connecting the four campuses (Bozeman, Billings, Great Falls, and Missoula) were held to review the concept analyses papers and then to make comparisons among the four concepts. The purpose of this chapter is to share the comparison activity of the RNTSC working group. The concepts were reviewed and compared, controversial issues were addressed, the overlap between concepts was noted, and future direction was discussed.

Initially, examination of the concepts of old-timer, newcomer, insider, and outsider was accomplished by critically reading each of the individual concept analysis papers. Figure 12.1 shows a compilation of the attributes plus the antecedents and the consequences for each concept. The group consensus was that while the four concepts are separate, they are connected and, within the rural context, usually go together. The knowledge base providing examples of uses for the concepts of old-timer and newcomer was scant as compared with that for insider and outsider. Within the research base developed by the Montana State University graduate nursing students, little information is available about insider.

CONTROVERSIAL ISSUES

The group activity then moved to comparing the four concepts to look specifically at the differences between the attributes. A matrix

Antecedents	Critical Attributes	Consequences
Old-timer (Caniparoli)	- age - length of time spent in the community - establishment of relationship within the community	- recognition as an old-timer
Newcomer (Sutermaster) - decision to move	- newly arrived - unaware of history of area/institution - existence may result in change	- new individual/family in community
Insider (Myers) - accepted by the group	- member of a group - has access to privileged information - an awareness of implicit assumptions and social context - a long-time occupant	- power - reserved social position - lack of objectivity - committed to the group
Outsider (Bailey)	- differentness - unfamiliarity - unconnectedness	

FIGURE 12.1 Comparison of attributes, antecedents, and consequences for old-timer, newcomer, insider, and outsider.

was developed to allow focus on the critical attributes alone (see Figure 12.2). Two major controversies arose from the discussion surrounding the matrix. The first controversy was the attribute, "a long-time occupant," for the concept of insider. Some thought it was similar to the attribute "length of time spent in residency" for old-timer. One

Old-timer	Insider
- age - length of time spent in the community - establishment of a relationship within the community	- member of a group - has access to privileged information - an awareness of implicit assumptions and social context - a long time occupant
Newcomer - newly arrived - unaware of history of area/institution - existence (presence) may result in change	**Outsider** - differentness - unfamiliarity - unconnectedness

FIGURE 12.2 Matrix comparison of attributes of old-timer, newcomer, insider, and outsider.

group member noted the potential differences in perception of a "long time occupant." She noted that "if one is living in a rural boom town where people are moving in and out weekly, some who have lived in a location for a year may be considered long-time occupants. Whereas, in the small farming communities where hardly anybody moves in and many people move out, being there for generations is required." The response to her statement was that "long" is essentially contextual. Another group member asked, "If we use the attribute, long-time occupant, what is the position of this person in the community? Sometimes, 'long time' is a matter of social class. One could be living in a place for a long time but not be considered in the same way as if one happened to be one of the more influential people in the community." Another group member responded, "Maybe acceptance is really the issue. Since the insiders define how long long is, how long a time is long enough? It really is being accepted by the insiders that is the issue. The insiders accept you when they have decided you have been there long enough."

The second controversy centered around the concept of old-timer. Early in the review of the concept analysis of old-timer, one member of the group said that if her deceased father had been called an old-timer, he would have been insulted. His perception of an old-timer was that of a derelict, a vagrant, a bum. This perception may have its roots in the history of the American West, although the expression itself was infrequently used in historical literature. The more current use of the term seems to have a different perspective. This discussion included recognizing the cognitive baggage that accompanies the term old-timer; it revealed divergency in the way people use the term in their thinking (Miller & Dzurec, 1993). Rodgers (1993) suggests that concepts in existence for many decades may have changed and are applied differently than when first developed.

OVERLAP BETWEEN CONCEPTS

Often, persons living in rural communities have attributes or characteristics that fit more than one concept. A second matrix depicting the overlap was developed by group member Janice Buehler (see Figure 12.3). The old-timer who is also an insider is a person with whom nurses need to work to make changes in the community. Old-

Old-timer/Insider	**Newcomer/Insider**
- persons who are community influentials with whom nurses need to work to make changes in the community	-a wife (newcomer) marries insider (husband), member of old-time family - grandchild of old-timer family raised somewhere else who comes to community
Old-timer/Outsider	**Newcomer/Outsider**
- hermit - a seasonal resident (comes and goes) - marginal people - return to community (old-timer) after education (outsider)	- newly graduated nurse practitioner

FIGURE 12.3 Examples of persons who fit the overlap between concepts of old-timer, newcomer, outsider, and insider.

timers who are outsiders include many persons: (a) the hermit who isolates himself from the rest of the townspeople, (b) the seasonal resident who is present for the agreeable seasons and heads south to escape the cold winters, (c) marginal people who live in the community but are not truly a part of the community, (d) persons who leave the community for educational purposes and find they have become outsiders when they attempt to return to the community; i.e., the concept "you can't go home again" (Wolfe, 1940).

Newcomers may be insiders automatically by their links with old-timer families. A wife who is a newcomer may become an insider by virtue of marrying a member of an old time family. The grandchild of an old time family raised somewhere else who returns to the community to run the family farm may become an automatic insider because of the family link.

Most health care professionals who choose to work in the rural environment are examples of newcomers and outsiders. Newly graduated nurse practitioners are an example of the overlap between these two categories unless, of course, they come from and return to the same rural community after their educational preparation.

There was group consensus on the persons who fit each overlap between concepts. Once these overlaps were noted and recorded, no further discussion took place.

FUTURE DIRECTION

The terms old-timer, newcomer, insider, and outsider evolved from the earlier work of the graduate nursing students who talked with individuals in rural communities about their perceptions of health. Through dictionary definitions and use of each term in rural nursing literature, we now have identified attributes for each concept. If we truly believe these concepts are important to rural theory development and testing, further work is needed. Rather than automatically supporting the current use of each concept, perceptions of them from the perspective of rural persons is needed. A logical next step would be to return to the rural communities to find out whether the attributes fit. In particular, further illumination for the concept of old-timer using qualitative methods is needed.

SUMMARY

The work reported above suggests that concept analysis work within theory development should be an ongoing process rather than a static entity, "set in stone" once an individual concept analysis is completed. If our primary interest is ultimately to help health care providers who are newcomers and outsiders adapt to working in rural communities, we must reassess the relevancy of the concepts analyzed above and then evaluate the applicability of the concepts in different rural community settings (Rodgers, 1993). Through this work we can develop effective strategies in working with old-timers and insiders, many of whom are the influential persons in the rural communities we serve.

REFERENCES

Chin, P. L., & Kramer, M. K. (1991). *Theory and nursing: A systematic approach.* St. Louis, MO: Mosby.

Long, K. A., & Weinert, C. (1989). Rural nursing: Developing the theory base. *Scholarly Inquiry for Nursing Practice: An International Journal* 3(2), 113–132.

Miller, M. E., & Dzurec, L. C. (1993). The power of a name. *Advances in Nursing Science, 15* (3), 15–22.

Morse, J. M. (1995). Exploring the theoretical basis of nursing using advanced techniques of concept analysis. *Advances in Nursing Science, 17* (3), 31–46.

Rodgers, B. L. (1993). Philosophical foundations of concept development. In B. L. Rodgers and K. A. Knafl, *Concept development in nursing: Foundations, techniques, and applications* (pp.7–33). Philadelphia: Saunders.

Wolfe, T. (1940). *You can't go home again.* New York: Harper & Bros.

13

Self-Reliance: Characterization of Their Own Autonomy by Elderly Rural Women

Kathleen Chafey, Therese Sullivan, and Anna Shannon

INTRODUCTION

In this chapter, the construct of autonomy, expressed as self-reliance, in a cohort of aging, rural women is explored. The purposes for doing so were twofold. First, ways were sought to describe how these women viewed their self-reliance, what the term meant to them, and how they related the concept to aging and health. Second, the nature and extent of variations in self-reliance within the cohort were explored. All the women were living independently, either alone or with a husband, and they shared certain common characteristics including life-course perspectives.

The importance of this investigation lies in the long-term goals of the study: (a) to develop nursing assessment and intervention strategies that promote the ability of rural elders to remain at home in ways that are responsive to individual variations along this central value dimension, and (b) for those who can no longer remain at home, to address ways to foster autonomy in nursing home life, even when cognition is impaired. The study was predicated on the assumptions that (a) loss of autonomy and resulting dependence are not necessary concomitants of aging; (b) both intraindividual and environmental influences on autonomy are malleable; and (c) even into advanced age, individual changes in various expressions of autonomy, including self-reliance, can be viewed from a life-span developmental perspective. That is, the development of self-reliance begins early; undergoes gains, losses, and changes during all phases of the life span; follows varied developmental pathways for different individuals; and becomes more diverse with age and the experience of life-course events.

The underlying construct of interest in this study, autonomy, has been a central value in Western bioethics since World War II. Concepts related to autonomy such as self-reliance, independence, self-determination, individuality, and privacy have also been used frequently in literature about rural nursing to characterize the cultural values and attitudes of rural people. In this study, preliminary informal contacts and interviews led the authors to believe that the word "autonomy" was not in general use as a way to describe the experience and attitude they sought to study. For these reasons, the term autonomy was not used by the interviewers and never did a research participant use the term. Terms and phrases such as "rely on self," "independence," "self-competence," "decision-making," "control," and "self-confidence" were used by them as synonyms to describe some aspect of self-reliance, but "autonomy" was never used.

BACKGROUND AND SIGNIFICANCE

For the elderly, the specter of losing one's autonomy (usually expressed as self-reliance, independence, or control) looms large as a well-founded fear associated with aging and, particularly, with the prospect of institutionalization (Kohler, 1990). A growing literature chronicles the harm, both physical and psychological, that accrues to the elderly through restrictions of their autonomy and control. Evidence exists that there is wide variation in the ability of individual elderly to cope with these restrictions. An adequate understanding of the problem of autonomy, particularly as it relates to the elderly and decisions affecting their care, directs attention to the notion that autonomy is not only a cultural ideal but a key feature of psychosocial development across the life span, as well. As such, in the development of autonomy or self-reliance, individuals proceed along different paths, experiencing gains, losses, and changes according to the makeup of their personalities, cultural milieu, and life-course events. While the drive and capacity for self-reliance do not necessarily decline with age, neither is it safe to assume that self-reliance is both desirable and desired by all people, in all stages of adulthood, regardless of emotional and physical impairments of age or health.

Agich (1993) defines the construct of autonomy to include three concepts of individual freedom: self-reliance (the capacity to care for oneself), personal preference (attention to choice and decision, and to one's wishes, desires, and impulses), and, finally, self-assertion, the pursuit and fulfillment of the latter. Personal preference and self-assertion have been characterized by Collopy (1988) in some importantly different ways. Collopy differentiated *decisional* from *executional* autonomy, a potentially useful distinction in thinking about long-term care or about the elderly living independently but experiencing restrictions on their ability to act on their decisions. Decisional autonomy means having preferences and being able to decide freely, without coercion. Executional autonomy, on the other hand, means the freedom to act on, to pursue, or to fulfill those preferences, choices, and decisions. The distinction between decisional and executional autonomy may become blurred when executional autonomy becomes diminished. Individuals can decide but be unable to act on their decisions. If autonomy (or competence for that matter) is thought of primarily as executional, elderly clients may be viewed as nonautonomous, merely because they are unable to act on their decisions, or are restricted in the complexity of decisions they can make, or have relinquished to others certain categories of decision-making. Collopy observed that "as the outward reach of autonomy shrinks, its inner decisional core becomes a last and therefore most crucial preserve of self-determination" (1988, p. 12).

Agich (1993) noted that the tendency of Americans to draw apart, to value independence and privacy, has long been observed. These same values have often been attributed to rural dwellers in literature on rural nursing. Long and Weinert (1989) reported that the concepts of self-reliance and independence, expressed as "the desire to do for oneself and care for oneself" (p. 119) are central to understanding the health care needs and practices of rural dwellers. Long and Weinert also documented three additional studies that validated their findings that rural people are "resistant to care from persons viewed as outsiders," "[seek] health care information and assistance from local, and often informal sources," and "view the individual as responsible for health knowledge and care" (p. 122). A compelling example was provided by Grossman (1997) who found in a focus group session with older rural women that the women depended primarily on family and friends for information about breast and cervical cancer.

Rural families tend to be more self-reliant, according to Bushy (1991), doing more services for themselves, and relying on family and rural community organizations for assistance and social support. Wagnild and Young (1990) also found self-reliance to be an emergent theme in their study of resilience among older women residing in a metropolitan area of another state. The authors defined self-reliance as a "belief in oneself and capabilities" (p. 254) and cited examples of social and functional losses experienced by women in their study along with changes (often profound) in sources of social support. Many women experienced a ". . . new sense of self-reliance and confidence. Some had never had the opportunity to test their resources and were somewhat surprised at the strength and abilities found within" (p. 254).

Often, however, for the rural elderly, cultural ideals and personal identity founded on the values of independence, self-competence, and mastery can lead to feelings of diminished self-worth when these are no longer achievable. According to Agich (1993),

> *Self-reliance refers to the capacity to provide for one's own needs. In the course of aging, however, dependence begins as the diminishment of one's powers of self-reliance . . . and disability can compromise one's sense of personal worth precisely through compromising self-reliance (p. 8).*

Secondary defenses against dependence, including "denial of need, hostility toward helpers, even in the face of disabilities and limitations that require assistance from others" (Agich, 1993, p. 8), reflect a concept of individual freedom virtually synonymous with noninterference of others in the life of the individual. Clark (in Agich, 1993) has written that the concept of individual freedom held by older Americans is one that creates a definition of personal identity based on the ideals of self-reliance and independence. This position on autonomy may be too extreme, linking one's concept of self with one's capacity to provide for one's own needs without interference of others. As Lidz (Lidz, Fischer, & Arnold, 1992) has written, "all human life takes place in a historical, social, and cultural context. One's values and actions are necessarily affected by one's past and environment" (p. 7).

The concept of self-reliance has been described as a value important in Western society, a concept that characterizes rural people in particular, and as an important quality to be considered in planning health care for rural people. The aim of this study was an exploration and description of self-reliance as one of a family of concepts that make up the construct of autonomy.

METHOD

A qualitative research approach was used to explore and delineate the characteristics of the concept of self-reliance. This method of concept development has been advocated as appropriate to concepts that are in common use but have not been well explicated. This is particularly true of the concept of self-reliance in literature on rural nursing. The method uses techniques of qualitative inquiry as the primary tool for concept analysis (Morse, 1995; Morse, Hupcey, Mitcham, & Lenz, 1996).

Participants were chosen from two small towns of less than 40,000 people in the rural western state of Montana. Montana is the fourth largest state in the country in land size and has a total population of about 850,000 people. Its two major cities are each less than 100,000 in population.

The cohort of participants was selected based on gender, independent living arrangements, their many years of residence in a rural area, and as members of an age category having a unique history. All participants were known to at least one interviewer.

A structured interview guide was developed to elicit participants' perceptions of self-reliance. Each participant was asked what self-reliance meant to her, how important it was to her, how she thought she developed an attitude of self-reliance, at what age she began to notice a change in her self-reliance, and whether there were any particular areas in her life in which being self-reliant was especially important for her. Information specific to self-reliance and health care behaviors was also sought: would changes in her health status affect her self-reliance? and when she thought about the places where she received health care, how would each place influence her self-reliance? A second interview was held a year later with two participants who had undergone major changes in their lives. One experienced a major health crisis and the other had a significant increase in caregiving responsibilities for her husband.

The responses were transcribed and analyzed using thematic content analysis to identify the characteristics of the concept of self-reliance. Each interviewer studied all transcripts and reached a consensus on interpretation to ensure inter-rater reliability.

FINDINGS

Cohort

An effort was made to select a group of participants for these interviews who would be similar in age, rural residence, expectations of autonomy, socioeconomic status, ability to live at home, and life course perspectives based on historical events. All interviewees were between 70 and 85 years of age, lived in small towns (rural), were viewed by others as able to care for themselves, were of sufficient financial means to care for basic needs, were living in an apartment or house alone or with a husband, and had lived through major life course events as a rural dweller.

Despite these efforts, there was much diversity within the group. Several were approached because they were known to be decedents of "pioneer" families. Being rural dwellers, all had relied on the automobile for transportation and saw its continued use as critical to their ability to remain self-sufficient. One, who had very recently relinquished the use of her car for reasons of health and infirmity, expressed her dismay at the problems of transport via friends or taxis. All had health insurance, were within a few (less than ten) miles of health care, and had lived in their current residence for more than 15 years. All but one had lived in the general area all their lives. One had moved to the West from an eastern urban state as a young adult and had spent the rest of her years in the rural area. All but one either were married or had been married, and all but one had had a career. All were high school graduates and five had some college education. Four had done graduate work.

Experiences during the Great Depression and World War II told much about how historical events lead to different experiences. For three of the women, the Depression afforded them the opportunity to teach in rural schools for salaries of about $60 a month or for pay warrants that could not be cashed. These teachers lived with families more financially distressed than themselves and ate what the family raised, or in teacherages (a part of the rural school) far from other inhabitants, cooking lunches for the pupils. On weekends, some women did target practice to discourage unwanted suitors. Other women in the cohort did not mention either the Depression or World War II when they spoke of childhood influences on their development of self-reliance.

Primary Characteristics

In the process of analyzing the interview data, several primary and secondary characteristics of self-reliance emerged. The primary characteristics included *self-reliance as learned, decisional choice,* and *independence.* Secondary characteristics embodied an aspect of the interviewee's experience of self-reliance. These were *self-confidence* and *self-competence.* These key concepts are described below.

Self-reliance as learned. Interviewees who described themselves as self-reliant saw this experience and self-perception as emanating from previous learning events. Typically, these learning events started in their youth and revolved around family chores and assumption of responsibilities. The learning continued into adulthood and was reinforced by later life events such as death of a parent, a spouse, or retirement. The nature of self-reliance as a skill was acknowledged by one participant who did not consider herself self-reliant. This skill was described by her in this statement:

> *I don't know if I'm good at self-reliance . . . I don't know if I do practice self-reliance. [T-3]**

Interviewees who defined themselves as self-reliant emphasized responsibility, necessity, training, and the acquisition of task-skills as components of their development of self-reliance. The following excerpts illustrate these points:

> *Well, I think the building of self-reliance was a gradual experience. When I think back even early as a teenager after my father died, I had to take a lot of responsibility to help my mother. And that was probably the beginning of that, recognizing that I was developing that kind of ability to take care of my self and to help her [T-1].*

> *It's something I was taught at the very beginning . . . I had to rely on myself for a lot of things . . . and that necessitated for me being self-reliant*

*Refers to the inteview from which the quote was derived.

... You had to get to school on time. I had to be responsible ... Then I'd have the afternoon after school was out until [mother] got home ... I had definite chores ... I can't imagine having to rely on anybody else. [K-1].

I can't imagine being any way except self-reliant. I think we were taught self-reliance as we grew up ... we (siblings) were always given the opportunity to make decisions even though they weren't always the decisions my parents thought ... given the privilege of expressing our views even as children. [K-2]

Women who described themselves as dependent, gave examples from childhood as the origins of their dependence. In two instances, the primary influence was the relationship with the mother. These examples follow.

I was very dependent on my parents at first. And then I got more and more confidence that I could do things on my own from ... childhood on up ... But at first I was very dependent on my mother ... I didn't want to go anywhere that she didn't go ... (through) high school. [K-6]

I was raised by my mother ... and she did everything her sister told her to do ... I'd get awfully mad because she didn't think for herself too much. [T-3]

These same two women described their relationships with their husbands as one of dependence. With the death of the husband, each woman had to handle areas of life in which she had little or no skill. This is best illustrated by one participant:

I was so dependent and relied on my husband so much ... I don't like it [having to rely on self] because I liked the way I lived before ... dependent on my husband ... He [husband] never really sat down and talked to me about it [finances] and maybe it was my fault because I didn't want him to. [T-3]

Although most participants experienced change in their self-reliance with death of a spouse or retirement, the two most dependent ones experienced the change in self-reliance most negatively but saw adaptation as possible. The following brief excerpt describes this well:

[Since husband died] I think I am learning. I think I am. It's nothing that I want to do, and so I sort of get mad at myself ... [T-3]

Learned self-reliance has its roots in early life experiences of responsibility, task mastery, and decision-making. The data also support the notion that self-reliance as a skill can be learned at later stages of life when circumstances make that necessary or desirable.

Self-reliance as decisional choice. Decisional choice emerged as a primary characteristic of self-reliance. Making one's own decisions and choices, as well as being involved in decisions that affected their lives, were considered important by all. A clear illustration was provided by one participant when asked what self-reliance meant to her. She stated

I would think it would mean the dependence on yourself for decision-making, you know, and trusting your decisions . . . I think I want to be a part of decisions that affect me. I don't want other people directing my life. [T1]

When interviewed a year later after experiencing a significant change in her life involving a major increase in caregiver responsibilities for her husband, this participant still emphasized the importance of decision-making in maintaining her self-reliance:

You rely on yourself for everything that happens in your life and again back to the basic philosophy, that is you create your own environment; that takes a lot of your own self-reliance, I guess is the word; that you depend on yourself, you are grateful for other people who support you and are there for you, but the bottom line is that you are the one who has to call the shots and make the decisions. [T1]

The following excerpts are typical of the responses of participants who described themselves as self-reliant:

I manage my decisions about most everything. [K2]

I've always been self-reliant. I've done my own thing, I've been my own boss, and I don't like to have other people boss me. [K5]

Well, I might consult someone, but I'm going to make the final decision. [She explained that it was very important to her.] Because I feel that's my job to do that, and I understand what my life has been, and I understand all of this myself. [K3]

The decision-making theme was also prominent in response to the interview questions about health care. Participants were asked to think about the places where they received health care and about how each influenced self-reliance. One participant had received most of her health care in doctors' offices. She shared

> *You take the information that they can give you, and you process it yourself, and then you apply it as best you can to your situation. [In relation to long term care, in particular being in a nursing home] Again, I think I'd want to be involved in the decisions about whatever kind of regime has been established. I would hope that I would be mentally able to be a part of discussions about what I want to do and what I don't want to do. [T1]*

Another participant was interviewed a second time. She had, by then, recently spent about two weeks in a nursing home, having decided that she required more care post-hospitalization than she could receive at home. She described her reaction to the experience:

> *I think you cease to be a person when you go into a nursing home. You become a patient and don't dictate any aspect of your life. You have to conform. That is difficult for me. [She felt there was very severe regimentation in the nursing home setting] You are at the mercy of their hours, you are just at their complete mercy with everything. [K1]*

Changes in life circumstances such as those related to health and disability or death of spouses and other relatives altered the nature and the extent of restrictions and limitations on some participants' decisions and choices. Some examples follow:

> *[Following a stay in a nursing home] At this point, [self-reliance] means being able to live in my own house and being able to live the best way that I can under the circumstances. I think it means a lot to me to be able to stay here and do as I please. If I want to take a nap in the middle of the morning, I take a nap in the middle of the morning. I read until 12 or 1 o'clock [a.m.], not bothering anybody. [K1]*

> *[A significant increase in caregiver responsibilities for a spouse] During the last year there was some change in terms of relationships . . . I have increasing responsibility for [husband], and accepting the fact that he needs more help has taken a while. That, in itself, is a learning experience because when you finally, really agree that you have to increase the kind of help you*

give him rather than him being able to do things himself, then it becomes easier, and you make that a part of your life . . . I have not been as free to travel, so I am unable to really leave [name] at night which makes it very difficult to be gone overnight, especially if arrangements have to be made if I am going to be gone over night. Of course, I haven't planned to do that very often. I just have to limit that . . . I think there are times when I would like a little more freedom; then I think 'you made a decision early in your life' and you don't know the outcome of it and you can't change any of that. You accept it now, and if you can't accept, it you can make your life miserable.' I keep looking for alternative ways of handling the problems, getting more help, hiring more people, maybe finding some back up system so that I could get away a little bit more. [T1]

[Recent death of a spouse] Well, before, I never stayed by myself. Never. I'd have to go some place and stay. And since, I never have stayed any place but in my house, and I think I am getting better. I am not nearly as frightened, and I'm doing things that I never did before. Bills, things like that, things around the house. I never did and I'm really learning. However, I have lots of problems still that aren't . . . and I'm not coping too well with . . . [T3]

Decision-making and the importance (or inevitability) of choice were prominent in all interviews. Whether seen as a positive aspect of self-reliance or as a burden, decision-making and choice were integral to the concept.

Self-reliance as independence/dependence. Independence was a primary characteristic of self-reliance that emerged from the interview data and included independence or dependence on self, dependence on others, self-assertion or freedom of action, and self-identity. For example, reliance on oneself for personal care, decision-making, and freedom of action were evident in the following interview segments:

[What does self-reliance mean to you?] Dependence on yourself for decision-making, you know and trusting your decisions. [When asked about the value she placed on self-reliance] I value the independence. [T-1]

[Another participant, retired and a widow answered the question of what self-reliance means to you in this way.] That you have some independence, that you can work, and you are not a dependent person. [K-6].

Another participant who lived alone most of her adult life thought self-reliance was synonymous with independence. Statements about independence or self-reliance were made by this interviewee about growing dependence on others, especially for personal care, because of disability or health-related concerns. Following her first interview, this participant was hospitalized and spent two weeks in a nursing home before returning home. During the second interview, her comments about independence were made in the context of dependence on others:

> *[Since we last talked about self-reliance] I have lost a lot of my independence which we talked about . . . Of course, I could feel it flittering away. I lost most of my independence. I think I probably still have a little, or I wouldn't be here by myself. I knew I needed help [following her illness]. I needed people around me, I didn't like to be alone. I knew that I couldn't completely take care of myself and . . . I am quite dependent on the people around me. [K-1]*

As with decisional choice, independence/dependence became a prominent theme when questions were related to health care needs or settings. Overall, participants perceived the need for health care to be a threat to their independence as evidenced by the following excerpts:

> *There was never a time . . . when I felt I would have to have someone come in and care for me. And there were other women who were experiencing similar problems who had to have people come in and help them. . . . Now, if I had broken a hip or [was] damaged physically, or was mentally in a much worse way, then that would have altered it and I would have had to depend on other people which would have been hard for me. [T-1]*

> *[How would changes in health care affect self-reliance?] If I couldn't take care of myself that would be . . . you know, to be dependent on someone else . . . just being able to take care of myself no matter how limited; I mean, I just can't imagine not being able to bathe yourself or something. I just can't. [K-4]*

> *[Recognizing that one's own self-limitations might affect one's self-reliance] I'm sure the more limited you are, the less reliance you have on yourself. That must be a terrible feeling for people if you've been an independent, self-reliant person. [T-1]*

> *[Limited health care knowledge] I think as you get older and you lose touch with some of the more current approaches to health care, you become more dependent on health care workers to give you information . . . I do feel more dependent on other health care workers because of the advances that are being made . . . which does then lessen self-reliance . . . but it depends on your own judgment . . . not total dependence, in other words, on the expert. [T-1]*

For one subgroup of participants independence was focused on freedom of actions. However, when limitations due to health problems intervened, the feeling of independence was also limited.

> *[Do you feel that you're dependent on yourself for particular things?] Oh yes . . . I guess you would call it when I do the things I want to do . . . still being able to drive the car . . . still volunteer . . . still go to the grocery store. That, to me, boy, is self-reliance. Cuz you just gotta . . . once you lose your independence, you're gone as far as I'm concerned. [T-2]*

This participant placed central importance on the ability to drive, cook her own meals, and have her grown children and grandchildren be able to drop in:

> *If I lost my ability to drive a car, I don't know what would happen to me; because there isn't a day goes by that I don't use it to get around, because you can't live out here and take a bus .. . I'm just self-reliant because I can pick up and drive to Denver, Colorado, by myself. And that's self-reliance, I think. It's just being independent. [T-2]*

The participant who had been in the nursing home included driving as part of the discussion about "taking care of oneself" in her first, pre-nursing home interview by saying

> *Well, of course if I get to the point where I can't drive, then I will be really dependent on something. I'm not sure what yet. [K-1]*

After she became housebound her freedom of action was expressed in more limited ways. She discussed being dependent on others but still being able to "do as I please" within the confines of her own home.

Two participants, in particular, related the importance of independence to one's identity. One considered herself always to have been a self-reliant person. She so characterized herself and went on to say:

> *If you can't take care of yourself, there's really not much to live for. You'd get to be pretty much of a vegetable, and you can't enjoy the things that you enjoyed. [K-1]*

When asked if going into a long-term care environment would be difficult for her, another participant said

> *I think that would be hard. But I suppose again it's a matter of accepting whatever the situation is . . . if it was a situation that you could have prevented and didn't, then I think that you would feel guilty and would be disappointed in yourself. But if there was a necessity for you to be in an institution like that, I think you have to learn to accept that and then try to fit into that environment. And I think that you bring into that environment a good sense of yourself, a sense of pride about yourself, a sense of satisfaction with some of the things you've done in your life. I think you'd be able to accept that kind of dependence. [T-1]*

This individual recognized that forced dependence is not only difficult for those who view themselves as self-reliant, but it may evoke feelings of anger and hostility toward helpers, as well:

> *I hope I'd have enough consideration not to take it out on other people, but I think that's what happens to people who get sick and have to be dependent, especially if they've been independent. I think anger comes through, and it appears, I think, that they resent you, when in fact, what they're resenting is the limitation on their own lifestyle. I think that would be my response. Anger, resentment. [T-1]*

Secondary Characteristics

Two other concepts were voiced by interviewees as embodying an aspect of their experience of self-reliance: self-confidence and self-competence. For a few, one or both concepts were synonymous with their understanding of self-reliance. For others, these terms were used when describing a negative change in their feeling of self-reliance or when anticipating a threat to it. Each is further discussed below.

Self-confidence. The following quotations illustrate the general definitional sense in which many used the concept of self-confidence:

> *Actually it's all a part, the self-image, the self-confidence, the self-reliance. . . . The confidence to do that (make choices) or the confidence to even try anything new. It depends on how you feel about yourself and self-reliance. [T-1]*

For some, self-confidence was altered by a change in life circumstances or, if not changed, threatened:

> *[Self-reliance] makes a lot of difference in terms of how you handle every day. If you are threatened by events in your life and feel overwhelmed by them, then you are unable to really handle a lot of situations that you face. And sometimes the situation isn't as extreme as it seems to you if you lack self-reliance or self-confidence . . . I think they're the same thing. [T-1]*

> *[Speaking of being hospitalized] I've only had a couple of hospitalizations, and I felt very dependent on the people that were there to help me. And yet, I did question and ask questions. I think I didn't feel quite as confident and self-reliant as I would have if I was up and around. [Adjusting to changes in life] You've got to learn to rely on your own resources, whatever they are. It is hard if you don't have any self-confidence. [T-1]*

Self-Competence. Self-competence seemed to be tied to doing things. Its loss, or loss as perceived by others, was very distressing to the first participant quoted below. Two others expressed similar themes, but their losses were either more transient or anticipated in the future:

> *other people deciding for me. . . . These people think I'm getting incompetent, and I don't like that one bit. [K-5]*

> *[The car was significant for many interviewees] If I lost my ability to drive a car, I don't know what would happen to me [T-2].*

Whether expressed as a learned, decisional choice or as independence/dependence, self-reliance was important to all interviewees, even if they did not consider themselves self-reliant. All but two women stated the importance of self-reliance without equivocation. They used brief, "of course" statements in making these declarations:

[How important?] Oh, everything. [T-2]

If you're not self-reliant, you kind of slump down into nothing ... I think it keeps you on the track [K-6].

[Areas of living where self-reliance is important] Oh, gee, almost any, isn't it [K-4]?

I guess if I'm going to exist, it's pretty important [K-3].

Well, I think it makes a lot of difference in terms of how you handle every day [T-1].

I can't imagine having to rely on anybody else. I can't imagine being any way except self-reliant. [K-2]

DISCUSSION

This study of self-reliance in a cohort of aging, rural women had as its purpose a description of the ways women viewed their self-reliance. We sought to fill gaps in literature related to what the concept of self-reliance means to rural people, how they relate the concept to aging and health, and, finally, the nature and extent of variation along the dimension of self-reliance found in a cohort that shares certain demographic characteristics and life-course perspectives.

From data analysis, three primary characteristics and two secondary characteristics emerged and constituted critical attributes of the women's experiences of self-reliance. Primary characteristics included self-reliance as (a) *learned,* (b) *decisional choice,* and (c) *independence/dependence.* Secondary characteristics included (a) *self-confidence* and (b) *self-competence.*

The results of this study supported Agich's (1993) definition of autonomy that included self-reliance (the capacity to care for oneself), personal preference (attention to choice and decision), and self-assertion (the pursuit and fulfillment of wishes, desires, and impulses). The findings were also consistent with the view from psychology that defines autonomy as "the capacity to make decisions independently, serve as one's own source of emotional strength and otherwise manage life tasks without being over-dependent on other people . . . " (Sigelman & Shaffer, 1991, p. 586).

The finding that there had been a change in the self-reliance of participants over time supports the developmental nature of the phenomenon. Many changes related to health, death, or disability of a spouse, retirement, or earlier life-course events (war or the Depression, for example). Unlike what the literature had suggested, this group of women did not attribute change in self-reliance to age. Age, rather than being seen as a threat to self-reliance itself, was viewed as a concomitance to other events that would affect one's self-reliance, particularly decisional execution and self-competence. The fear of loss of independence attributed to age in the literature was, instead, related to feelings of self-competence and self-confidence. Age, in other words, did not decrease one's self-reliance in this group but changed the manner in which it was expressed. Where one had previously been able to meet basic needs, one now directed others to execute those actions. There was a fear, however, that loss of control over one's environment might mean an environment in which one's wishes would not be honored. Such an environment would leave the desire for the experience of self-reliance and independence but remove the means to achieve that goal.

Additional support for a developmental view of self-reliance included wide variation in views among the cohort about their own self-reliance, its desirability, and their responses to threats to independence. Those who saw themselves as self-reliant tended to have had early experiences that helped them learn to be self-reliant. Those who were not particularly self-reliant identified themselves as dependent on others even into adolescence and beyond.

The women interviewed expressed the idea that self-reliance was not only important to them but was part of their self-identity (For example: "I can't imagine being any way except self-reliant."), and the threat of loss evoked sentiments that supported the notion that loss of independence can lead to feelings of diminished self-worth. One participant even gave voice to the claim in the literature that loss of self-reliance may evoke secondary defenses against dependence, including hostility toward helpers or denial of need.

Self reliance as learned. The finding that self-reliance is learned supported, in part, one of the study's assumptions that self-reliance can be viewed from a life-span developmental perspective. Participants who viewed themselves as self-reliant tended to have had experiences beginning in childhood that contributed to the development of skills of self-reliance. Often, for this cohort, the experiences were related to household responsibilities including house and garden chores or helping with the care of younger children. The development of self-reliance continued into adolescence and adulthood, and most informants experienced change (either losses or gains) in their self-reliance with significant life events. Those who viewed themselves as more dependent than others during their childhood also experienced gains or losses with life events, particularly the death of a spouse, but the direction was toward loss of self-reliance. This finding expands Wagnild and Young's (1990) findings for women who had experienced social and functional losses. Many women in their study found a new sense of self-reliance, as did the women in the present study who had learned self-reliance early in life. For the more dependent participants in the current study, however, loss of a spouse was not necessarily accompanied by a discovery of latent self-reliance.

Decisional choice. Findings related to decisional choice supported associations in the literature between decisional autonomy, on the one hand, and executional autonomy, on the other (Collopy, 1988). This tension is similar to Agich's (1993) definition of autonomy. The definition distinguishes between having, on the one hand, choices or preferences that reflect one's values, goals, expectations, and desires, and on the other hand, having self-assertion, the ability to pursue and fulfill those choices. Like Collopy (1988, 1995), participants expressed the sentiment that it is important to have and express personal preferences and values, even when one might not be able to act on them.

Participants in the study cohort represented the full range of decisional versus executional autonomy. All but one participant defined self-reliance in terms of decision-making. One made and carried out her decisions and could not imagine being any other way:

> *Nobody moved me [into her apartment]. I made up my mind that I was going to move from my house to this apartment, made the decision by myself, told my sons about it, and did it. I manage my financial affairs. I manage my decisions about most everything. [K-2]*

Another participant was limited in the choices available to her and limited in being able to pursue and fulfill choices because of caretaking responsibilities to her husband. Yet another had full executional autonomy but was recently widowed and had always relied on her husband to make decisions.

Having desires, preferences, or choices and expectations about being able to fulfill those preferences was clearly shown to be subject to change and adjustment as health problems (their own or their spouse's) intervened to limit their abilities to act on their choices:

> *But one makes adjustments. I used to love to ride horseback and had horses. But when I got to the point where I couldn't ride comfortably, I gave them up, and I readjusted some parts of my life without too much turmoil. [K-1]*

Independence/dependence. Informants also described self-reliance as independence or dependence on self. They described the lack or loss of self-reliance as dependence on others. Independence meant depending on themselves for decision-making, freedom of action, or self-assertion, for example. It meant being able to work and, most commonly, meant taking care of oneself. For some individuals, independence meant being able (or unable) to maintain their homes without having to depend on others for simple maintenance chores. Health problems were influential in determining how members of the cohort described their independence. For those not yet facing serious, debilitating illness, independence related more to freedom of action and mobility. Driving a car was a key determinant in assessment of their self-reliance. Those still able to come and go as they pleased regarded with dread the idea of not being able to drive their cars.

Even those whose health was compromised placed a high value on being able live in their own homes, or as one woman articulated: ". . . to be able to stay here and do as I please." In this case, the participant's physical movements were severely restricted; her idea of self-assertion or freedom of action was staying up late or taking naps whenever she pleased. This woman maintained her connection with the freedom provided by a car by driving to the road to get her mail each day the weather permitted.

Most dramatic in its effect on independence was the emphasis on the capacity to care for oneself, even among subjects who faced no immediate limitations in the personal care arena. The need to "have someone come in" to help with personal care, either real or envisioned, was accompanied by reactions such as "lost most of my independence," "must be a terrible feeling . . . if you've been an independent, self-reliant person," "would have been hard for me," and "I just can't image [it] . . . I just can't."

Self-confidence and Self-competence. The importance of self-confidence and self-competence that emerged from the interview data relates to the relationship of autonomy and the concept of self-efficacy. The self-efficacy theory of Albert Bandura (e.g., 1982, 1989, 1991) frames autonomy as self-influenced, just as it is influenced by the environment. Autonomous decision-making and behavior occur not in isolation but within the context of individual abilities and the environment in which the individual functions. For example, one's sense of one's abilities and the sense that the social environment will be hospitable to one's efforts affect self-confidence and self-competence which, in turn, affect autonomy and a sense of well-being. On the other hand, people who believe they are inefficacious or believe the social environment will somehow thwart their efforts to assert control are apt to experience a high degree of stress (Beck, 1976), a sense of futility and helplessness (Seligman, 1975), depression (Holahan & Holahan, 1987), and hopelessness (White & Janson, 1986). People can give up trying because they expect their efforts to produce no results due to the unresponsiveness, negative bias, or punitiveness of the environment (Bandura, 1982, p. 140).

The relationship of autonomy as self-reliance and self-efficacy, or confidence in one's competence, was stated by at least one participant:

> *If you are threatened by events in your life and feel overwhelmed by them, then you are unable to really handle a lot of situations you face [T-1].*

Maintaining one's self-reliance. One final, unexpected, finding of this study was the spontaneous description by participants of actions they had taken to help maintain their self-reliance in the face of perceived or anticipated threats to it. These descriptions reinforce the interrelationships of the major findings of self-reliance as learned, as decisional choice, and as independence. All but two participants identified people or services they had engaged to ensure a level of independence while living in their own homes. The assistive services or people they employed depended on the participants' perceptions of their lack of knowledge or skill and their recognition of services or objects available. The examples given in the interviews reinforce the idea that self-reliance is learned, and that, when circumstances change, the necessary skills can be learned to enable one to be independent to a greater degree than without those skills.

REFERENCES

Agich, G. J. (1993). *Autonomy and long term care.* New York: Oxford University Press.

Bandura, A. (1982). Self-efficacy in human agency. *The American Psychologist, 37,* (2) 122–147.

Bandura, A., (1989). Regulation of cognitive processes through perceived self-efficacy. *Developmental Psychology, 25, 5,* 729–735.

Bandura, A. (1991). Social cognitive theory of self-regulation. *Organizational Behavior and Human Decision Processes, 50,* 248–287.

Beck, A. (1976). *Cognitive therapy and the emotional disorders.* New York: International Universities Press.

Bushy, A. (1991). Rural determinants in family health: Considerations for community nurses. In A. Bushy (Ed.). *Rural Nursing* (Vol. 1). Newbury, CA: Sage.

Collopy, B. J. (1988). Autonomy in long term care: Some crucial distinctions. *The Gerontologist, 28, (suppl.),* 13–16.

Collopy, B. J. (1995). Power, paternalism, and the ambiguities of autonomy. In L. M. Gamroth, J. Semradek, & E. M. Tornquist (Eds.), *Enhancing autonomy in long term care.* New York: Springer.

Grossman, L. (1997). *Breast and cervical health awareness project: Dissemination of information to older rural women.* Unpublished master's project, Montana State University-Bozeman.

Holahan, C. K., & Holahan, C. J. (1987). Self-efficacy, social support and depression in aging: A longitudinal analysis. *Journal of Gerontology, 42* (1), 65–68.

Kohler, P. A. (1990). Nursing model of care promotes elderly independence. *Nursing Forum, 25* (4), 5–9.

Lidz, C. W., Fishcer, L., & Arnold, R. M. (1992). *The erosion of autonomy in long-term care.* New York: Oxford University Press.

Long, K. A., & Weinert, C. (1989). Rural nursing: Developing the theory base. *Scholarly Inquiry for Nursing Practice: An International Journal, 3* (2), 113–127.

Morse, M. J. (1995). Exploring the theoretical basis of nursing using advanced techniques of concept analysis. *Advances in Nursing Science, 17* (3), 31–46.

Morse, M. J., Hupcey, J. E., Mitcham, C., & Lenz, E. R. (1996). Concept analysis in nursing research: A critical appraisal. *Scholarly Inquiry for Nursing Practice: An International Journal, 10* (3), 253–277.

Seligman, M. E. P. (1975). *Helplessness: On depression, development and death.* San Francisco: Freeman.

Sigelman, C. K., & Shaffer, D. R. (1991). *Life-span human development.* Pacific Grove, CA: Brook/Cole.

Wagnild, G., & Young, H. M. (1990). Resilience among older women. *Image: Journal of Nursing Scholarship, 22* (4), 252–255.

White, C. B., & Janson, P. (1986). Helplessness in institutional settings: Adaptation or iatrogenic disease? In M. M. Baltes & P. B. Baltes (Eds.). *The psychology of control and aging.* Hillsdale, N J: Lawrence Erlbaum.

14

Health Resources and the Rural Client

Jean Ballantyne

INTRODUCTION

Health care resources are considered deficient in much of rural America (Rosenblatt & Moscovice, 1982). Through this statement, Rosenblatt and Moscovice are referring to resources at the local level of the rural community. They propose this deficiency to be due to a lack of health professionals and facilities. In contrast to this view, Hassinger (1982) concludes that this level of resources was not a factor in the use of services. It was his finding that primary groups and social networks are influential for rural dwellers in accessing resources. Depending on the motivation of the individual, coupled with the support of his or her primary group and social network, health care needs of the rural client may apparently be met at a level other than locally. In considering the rural client and resources to meet his or her needs, one must often look beyond the local level to the regional and national centers available.

To better understand the relationship of resources to the health of a rural client, the concept of "resource" was analyzed through dictionary definitions and exploration of the concept in the disciplines of agriculture and sociology. Subsequently, the concept was used to examine rural health resources with a specific focus on a rural client with cancer.

DEFINITION

The word resource (resources, plural) comes from the root word *resurgere* which in Latin means to rise again (Gove, 1981). The French word *resourdre* also means to rise again and expands the meaning to include "relieve." Webster's dictionary (Gove, 1981) further expands the definition as follows:

> *1. A new or reserve source of supply; a fresh or additional store available at need; something in reserve or ready if needed; computable wealth (i.e., money, property). 2. A means of resort in exigency; something to which one has resource in difficulty. 3. The possibility of relief or recovery. 4. A means of spending or utilizing one's leisure time. 5. Capability of meeting a situation; ability to rise to an occasion. 6. An accounting asset. (p. 1934)*

Synonyms for resource include resort, expedient, shift, makeshift, stopgap, substitute, and surrogate. The synonym resort relates to turning inward to one's own resources. Another synonym, expedient, may apply to any continuance or plan for solution of a particular immediate problem, especially to one that is not customarily used. A summary definition in Webster's dictionary is as follows: "Resource may refer to any asset or means benefiting or assisting one, often to an additional, new reserved asset" (Gove, 1981, p. 1934).

AGRICULTURAL PERSPECTIVE

The agricultural industry is charged with the responsibility of producing the resource, namely food, utilized by humans for satisfaction of their most basic need. To produce basic food commodities, farmers look to the environment for resources necessary for this production. An agricultural definition of resource is any portion of the environment such as soil, water, rangeland, livestock, or human populations that can be used to promote man's well-being through production (Owen, 1971). Harmony between man's resource requirements and the resource base depends on conservation principles. With the multiple use of a given resource, a cardinal conservation goal is to ensure the greatest good for the most people over the long run. Due to conflicting interests over resources, the government has enacted legislation as an expedient allocator, thereby regulating use in a way that serves the best interest of the future (Sampson, 1981).

Legislation, however, is not always successful as evidenced by recent farm programs (Sampson, 1981). In the face of growing economic strife, much of which is caused by resource shortages, attempts to conserve resources are not always palatable though they make good sense. Many farmers do not have the capacity to be flexible to changing circumstances. The nation's agriculture base and its productivity will be challenged by increased demands for the future. Getting more for less will be difficult. The farmer must resort to methodologies that will promote the most valued production of the time.

Sociological Perspective

In the discipline of sociology, resources refer to characteristics such as physical strength, intelligence, and wealth that may be used by one individual to mediate with another individual for his desired goals (Scott, 1970). Levinger (as cited in Scott, 1970) defines a resource as any property or resort of an individual that he makes available to persons in his environment for their positive or negative need satisfaction. An individual using his resources for another's behalf may impose conditions on the recipient so that he has influence or power over the other. Therefore, resources may be used as sanctions.

The concept of resource is further defined by Scott (1970) as the actualization of properties for consumption. Accordingly, a resource refers to some act, past or present, which has the effect of facilitating or hindering the locomotion of other persons. In other words, an individual's power is based on the resources (i.e., money, skills, knowledge, strength) that he can expedite to help or hinder another's goal attainment or need fulfillment. Power is further related to the allocation of resources. Allocation basically refers to "who gets what and where." The location or deliverance of a resource in any area is greatly influenced by political, social, and economic power. The rational use of that resource may be related to individual power, as in the health care system with consumer and provider.

From the individual's perspective, taking the life span as a frame of reference, that individual at early life stages might view as rational the preferences for health care service of the type and level of expenditure that would maximize chances of living a normal life span (Clark, 1985). At the later stages of life, the individual might opt for fewer costly services that enhance quality of life at the risk of a shortened life span. Therefore, claims upon a resource are directly related to the allocation of the resource by the powers that exist and the values and perceived needs of the individual accessing the resource.

CONCEPT ANALYSIS

Common attributes and meanings can be derived from the definitions provided by the disciplines of agriculture and sociology and the dictionary. These attributes include the element property, which is used in the context of "property for consumption." In other words, a resource is a property or an asset that has value for consumption by populations in need of that property.

Another common element is the synonym expedient. As a dictionary definition, this element is called a continuance or plan for solution of a particular problem. From an agricultural perspective, expedient would relate to legislation as a plan for regulating resource allocation. Sociology includes expedient in reference to one's ability to employ a resource for another's behalf.

The third common element is that of the synonym resort. This element relates to the turning inward to one's resources. The farmer "resorts" to measures in his farming methods that will be conducive to meet the best production possible. The sociologist relates an individual's resort as a property made available to others.

Through the process of synthesization, a definition of this concept is derived: Resources are properties, resorts, or assets that are finite by nature and are *made available for use* by populations through an *allocation* process. Resources are *accessed* and used in response to a population's or individual's motivation for need satisfaction. At the level of the individual, the allocation, accessibility, and use of resources can be visualized as weights balanced on a scale. If the scale becomes unbalanced through any process that impedes one of these weighted elements, a deficit occurs. Furthermore, these three elements can be visualized in a circle with a flow of energy between the allocated resource, accessibility of the resource, and use of the resource. This flow of energy is bidirectional (see Figure 14.1).

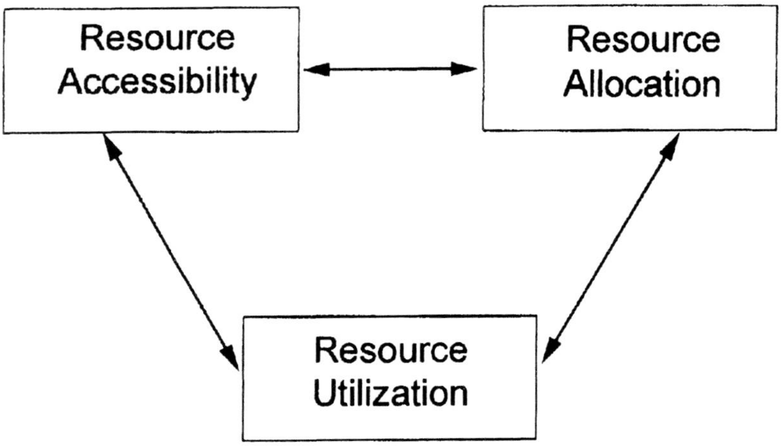

FIGURE 14.1 Circle of health care resource elements.

RURAL HEALTH CARE RESOURCES

For the rural client with acute health care needs, accessibility of an allocated resource and the use of the resource is dependent on several factors. The resources in the immediate community may not provide services that can adequately meet the client's needs. If the client is motivated to seek health care beyond the immediate boundaries of the community, factors such as transportation, distance, inclement weather, and finances become important issues. Another consideration is whether or not a health care provider such as a physician will make a referral to another level in the health care system.

Rural clients with serious health problems such as cancer are often motivated to seek help from local, regional, and national resources. Each level offers a different scope of services for the client. For example, the local level can provide initial diagnostic services and possibly more aggressive treatments such as surgery. Serving as tertiary and referral centers, regional centers offer chemotherapy and radiation. Most small towns in the region have rural hospitals served by physicians in general practice and nurses who are considered generalists. The rural hospitals and providers offer a variety of general services that are economically feasible and safe. For specialized services, however, referrals are made to the regional center.

A rural client with cancer who seeks access to a national resource is often at the point of desperation. Treatments have been unsuccessful at the local and regional levels and turning to a national resource such as a research center provides a shread of hope. The following case illustration is an assessment of the accessibility and use of resources at these three levels. Problems and barriers in this process are discussed as well as recommendations for improvement and implications for nursing. Health resources in relation to common attributes of the concept of resource are also included.

THE RURAL CLIENT

Mrs. Smith was a 35–year-old homemaker, mother, and registered nurse living in a town of 3,500 population in eastern Montana. The town lies in the heart of a large farm and ranch community and offers services as the main trading center for the county. Among the health care resources is the local hospital where Mrs. Smith was employed as a staff nurse. This facility is a 25–bed general hospital offering a broad repertoire of services including general surgery, medical surgical, obstetrical, pediatric, and emergency services. The hospital is modernly equipped and provides many educational offerings for the staff. Other community health resources include two physicians, twenty registered nurses, a mental health center, one public health nurse, and an EMS network.

A nurse-client relationship was established with Mrs. Smith to assess health resources she has accessed and used to meet her particular health problems. Mrs. Smith was diagnosed in March 1984 as having breast cancer with metastatic involvement of the axillary nodes.

Throughout her illness, Mrs. Smith used health resources at the local and regional levels. She was attempting to use a national resource at the time of her death in May 1987. In relation to the concept "resources," these three levels of resources were "properties that had value for consumption and expedients or plans for solutions for a problem." Mrs. Smith through her own "resort" searched for appropriate treatment at the national level. At all levels, these resources were allocated for use to provide need fulfillment for Mrs. Smith for diagnosis and treatment of the malignancy. This need fulfillment does not always have a successful outcome. However, the client was motivated to access and use these resources to fulfill the basic safety need

(Maslow, 1970). Cancer was life-threatening, and she sought resources that would prolong her life.

In the early stages of her illness in 1984, Mrs. Smith sought health care from her primary care physician for what she perceived to be mastitis. Having a palpable mass in the left breast with redness and swelling, she was convinced in her own mind that the problem was related to a "plugged milk duct." Her mother had had this problem when she was about Mrs. Smith's age, and Mrs. Smith was not alarmed over this lump that had been present for at least six months. After two weeks of antibiotic therapy that produced no appreciable improvement, a surgical biopsy was done at the local hospital. A tissue sample was sent to the regional medical center for examination by a pathologist. Within hours of the biopsy, results were telephoned by the pathologist to Mrs. Smith's primary physician showing that a malignancy was present.

Following diagnosis of the disease, Mrs. Smith, with the support of her husband, other family, and friends, decided to use the regional medical center for surgical intervention of a modified radical mastectomy. Although surgery could have been done at the local hospital, Mrs. Smith considered that at the regional medical center she would have access to an oncologist who would be able to expedite adjuvant treatment for the malignancy. The local physician facilitated the referral process in collaboration with Mrs. Smith's desire for the services of a surgeon whom she knew personally.

Considering how this client accessed these resources, one would have to concur with Hassinger's (1982) viewpoint about primary groups being influential in accessing resources. Also, according to Hassinger, this shows that even with rural resources in place, larger institutions are looked to for comprehensive care.

Following surgery, Mrs. Smith received chemotherapy followed by radiation treatment. For a total of six months, traveling the 85 miles to the regional medical center for treatment was necessary for Mrs. Smith. During radiation therapy, daily trips were required. Chemotherapy usually was given weekly. During this time, the client did not use local resources except for an occasional blood count at the hospital laboratory. By having this procedure done locally, she could prevent an unnecessary trip to the regional medical center should the cell count be too low to receive treatment. Although the many trips to the regional medical center were definitely an inconvenience and sometimes a hardship, the client was motivated to access the resource. At this point, her extensive social network became a resource to help with all the travel. Mrs. Smith was too ill to drive herself home after the treatments. Her social network of church friends and nursing peers helped by doing the driving or caring for her children at home.

Before starting chemotherapy and radiation, Mrs. Smith inquired about research center treatment. Her oncologist related that most research centers would not accept clients unless chemotherapy was unsuccessful. Knowing that she had advanced disease, she felt compelled to seek research therapy, expressing doubts about conventional chemotherapy. However, realizing she would probably not be accepted at a research center, she opted to continue with the conventional methods. At no point during the chemotherapy was consideration given to the option of providing any portion of this treatment at the local level. Such an arrangement was not explored by the oncologist and primary physician. The client had asked her oncologist if this would be a feasible option. His reply was that he needed to see her each week during therapy, thereby negating the possibility of this care being provided at the local level.

It is evident that barriers existed to accessing resources. Some of this phenonomen can be related to Rosenblatt and Moscovice's (1982) statement concerning the position of physicians in the health care system. They are viewed as the base of the system and also as the top in hierarchal power. In this client's case, physician power was evident in willingness to facilitate or not to facilitate accessing resources. Furthermore, this situation demonstrated that even though resources may be allocated for a given purpose, sanctions can be imposed on their use. This is not to say that physicians are totally responsible for these sanctions. Other constraints come into play as well. For example, experimental drug therapy is highly regulated, with strict criteria for the protection of human subjects. Varying degrees of financial constraints are an issue for many rural clients. Mrs. Smith had no serious financial concerns that would have been a barrier to accessing resources.

For two years, no disease recurrence was evident in Mrs. Smith. In September 1986, a palpable clavicular node was noticed. A biopsy performed at the regional center confirmed a malignancy. Subsequently, a second round of chemotherapy was initiated. Although the oncologist was approached again about referral to a research center, he convinced Mrs. Smith that chemotherapy should be started. This series of treatment lasted for six weeks. The process was identical to the first experience. She had severe nausea and vomiting with each treatment and alopecia. Again she was dependent on the social network as a resource for accessing treatment. Despite treatment, metastasis was subsequently discovered in the right femur and lungs.

When the 1986 Christmas season was over, Mrs. Smith began in earnest to identify and access a national research center for treatment. Looking to her own "resort," she contacted the National Cancer Institute in Bethesda, Maryland, by mail. She received information about various treatment locations and the modes of treatment. She presented her findings to the oncologist who did review the options with her. One possibility was immune therapy with Interlukin II, a therapy provided at the University of Wisconsin at Madison. Although this was not the only institution offering immune therapy, Mrs. Smith was interested in this site because of family located near that area.

Although her oncologist acknowledged the possibility of research center treatment, he convinced Mrs. Smith to undergo four weeks of a different drug regimen than the round of chemotherapy she had just finished. The third week into this treatment, Mrs. Smith's blood count was 1,200, and she was unable to receive treatment. At this time, she intensified her pressure on the oncologist to refer her to a research center. He agreed to pursue it for her and contacted the University of Wisconsin at Madison. However, he told Mrs. Smith that the most recent chest x-ray showed slight heart enlargement and criteria for admission included no evidence of cardiac involvement. He attributed the heart enlargement to the chemotherapy agent adriamycin and said that he expected her heart to return to normal.

During the last two weeks of April 1987, Mrs. Smith waited for a call for confirmation of acceptance to the program at Madison. Tentatively she received an appointment for May 5, 1987. However, on April 29, 1987, she was admitted to the local hospital with shortness of breath and congestive heart failure. X-rays confirmed a pleural effusion of the right lung and pericardial effusion as well. Despite aggressive medical treatment, Mrs. Smith died on May 2, 1987. She died without knowledge that she had not been accepted into the program at Madison.

RECOMMENDATIONS

Smooth access of resources is not always possible with barriers such as those discussed in the above case illustration. Although Rosenblatt and Moscovice (1982) relate that health care resources are deficient in much of rural America due to maldistribution of health professionals, deficiencies are also caused by barriers to accessing resources. Furthermore, barriers existed in the allocation of certain resources to a local rural area that could have been feasible as to economy and safety. Specifically, it was this author's recommendation that chemotherapy be offered as a service at the local level. This would have required a coordinated effort between the oncologist and the primary physician and also the local nurses. Nurses at the local hospital were willing and capable of learning chemotherapy administration.

NURSING RESOURCES

The case illustration clearly implies that nurses in rural areas need to increase the populations' awareness of local, regional, and national health resources. Following increased awareness, nurses need to encourage allocation, accessibility, and use of resources at appropriate levels. When considering appropriate resources, nurses need to remember that people are holistic beings with psychosocial needs as well as physical needs. Nurses should consider themselves a vital health resource for the rural client. Facilitating a client's access to appropriate resources is part of nursing's responsibility, that is, being a resource or "property for consumption."

CONCLUSION

Rural clients may access health resources at the local, regional, or national level for use of services to meet their health care needs. In any rural setting, a dichotomy exists between those services offered locally and those for which the client must travel (Moscovice & Rosenblatt, 1985). Appropriateness of services at each level needs to be periodically assessed. As previously discussed, accessing resources for the rural client is influenced by many factors including transportation and distance. The more services that can be provided in the local community, the less the client will have to deal with those issues. Also it is important to recognize that regional centers do not offer all the available sophisticated or research therapies, and, if the client so desires, a referral to a national resource is appropriate.

Meeting the acute care needs of the rural client can become a very complex issue. One should consider the three levels of resources as a framework. If appropriate services and referrals are offered at each level, the balance will be maintained between allocation, accessibility, and utilization of health resources for the rural client.

REFERENCES

Clark, P. G. (1985). The social allocation of health care resources: Ethical dilemmas in age-group competition. *The Forum, 25* (2), 119–125.

Gove, P. B. (Ed. in chief). (1981). *Webster's third new international distionary.* Springfield, MA: Merriam.

Hassinger, E. W. (1982). *Rural Health Organization.* Ames, Iowa: Iowa State University.

Maslow, A. (1970). *Motivation and personality,* (2nd ed.). New York: Harper & Row.

Moscovice, I., & Rosenblatt, R. A. (1985). A prognosis for the rural hospital, part 1: What is the role of the rural hospital? *Journal of Rural Health, 1* (1), 29–40.

Owen, O. S. (1971). *Natural Resource Conservation: An ecological approach.* London: MacMillan.

Rosenblatt, R. A., & Moscovice, I. S. (1982). *Rural Health Care.* New York: Wiley.

Sampson, R. N. (1981). *Farmland or wasteland.* Emmaur, Pa: Rodale Press.

Scott, R. W. (1970). *Social-Processes and social structures: An introduction to sociology.* New York: Holt, Rinehart & Winston.

15

Lay Care Network

Teresa S. Turnbull

> Language is a city to the building of which every human being brought a stone.
> Ralph Waldo Emerson, *Letters and Social Aims*

The ability to convey meaning based solely on the use of words is tricky business. Although words have a degree of universal meaning, in addition to the universality of meaning are interpretations colored by who we are, where we have been, and the context in which we have heard or used the word. "Speakers often make implicit assumptions about the real world, and the sense of an utterance may depend on those assumptions, which some linguists term presuppositions" (Fromkin & Rodman, 1988, p. 229). Subsequently, one can expect as many undercurrents of meaning for a word or phrase as there are human beings. The clarity of an idea can be clouded further by the inevitable clumping together of words to convey meaning. This is not to say communication is impossible but rather that it is more complex than it outwardly appears. Care must be taken to avoid the pitfalls caused by making assumptions or presuppositions regarding the universality of a phrase or word. That is the premise of concept analysis. "Concept analysis is ultimately a careful examination and description of a word and its uses . . . coupled with an explanation of how it is 'like' and 'not like' other related words" (Walker and Avant, 1988, p. 36). Careful definition of concepts develops a knowledge base that is prerequisite to a critical examination of their contribution to theory development and nursing research (Akinsanya, 1989, as cited in Fawcett, 1995).

Recurring themes in rural nursing theory are isolation, distance, and the resulting need for independence and lay care networks. Little, if any, reference is made to lay care in current literature, yet we have a "hunch" it exists as a health care resource, particularly in the underserved rural areas. We cannot base any kind of scholarly study, policy-making, or needs assessment simply on "hunches." To investigate lay care networks further, we must first define the concept, and that is the aim of this analysis. The rich, historical context of lay care networking will be explored to detect attributes specific to it. Additionally, model and other cases are developed in keeping with the Walker and Avant model (1988) for concept analysis.

DEFINITIONS

Grammatically, lay care network consists of two adjectives describing the noun "network." *Net* comes from the Latin word *nodus* meaning knot and Olde English *werc* similar to the present-day "work." The Oxford English Dictionary (1989) defines the noun network as

> *1. work in which threads, wires or similar materials, are arranged in the fashion of a net. 2. a complex collection or system of rivers, canals, railways or the like: the island, or network of islands, formed by the Danube. 3. A broadcasting system, consisting of a series of transmitters capable of being linked together to carry the same program: . . . broadcasting networks provide the people of the world with on-the-spot news reports, entertainment and educational programs through a billion radio and television receivers. (p. 345).*

Roget's II Thesaurus (1988) describes network as a "group of things that are linked or interconnected as if by weaving; WEB" (p.671). Synonyms include web, net, complex, interconnection, weave, and organization (Rodale, 1961, p. 791).

Lay is derived from the Greek word *laikos,* meaning of the people (Oxford, 1989). The noun lay has the following meaning: "weaving: The lay which carries the reed, is hung from a ba." (p. 724). As an adjective, lay carries the following meanings:

> *1. Of persons: Belonging to the 'people': . . . aid without confirmation from the Lay-Senate. 2. Characteristic of, connected or concerned with, occupied or performed by, laymen or the laity: A lay Sermon. 3. Uninstructed, un-*

> *learned: . . . they were unlearned and laye people. 4. Non-professional, not expert, esp. with reference to law and medicine: The prevention of disease, as well as the cure of it is too technical for lay inference. 5. Unhallowed, unsanctified; unspiritual, secular, worldly: Exchanging my lay-sword For that of the 'holy word.' (p. 724)*

Synonyms add to the explanation of the word lay: "Calm, unprofessional, wager, covert, and occupation" (Rodale, 1961, p. 662).

The Old English word *caru* translates into lament or trouble while *ga-karon* is the Proto-Germanic word for being concerned about (Barnhart, 1988, p. 144). "Care" in the *Oxford English Dictionary* (1989) includes the following meanings:

> *1. To feel concern, trouble oneself, feel interest: He cared only for his own interest. 2. Charge; oversight with a view to protection, preservation, or guidance: Under a doctor's care. 3. Mental suffering, sorrow, grief or trouble: The cares of the world could be seen in his eyes. (p. 893–894)*

Roget's Thesaurus (1984) states that other words for care included protection, control, custody, and ministration (p. 115). Synonyms equated with care were tribulation, load, concern, diligence, attention and discrimination (Rodale, p. 125).

USES OF THE CONCEPT

The phrase "lay care network" was not found in any literature per se. However, synonymous phrases, such as informal support network, lay consultants or lay referral network, and folk medicine were identified. This paper will examine their meaning to illuminate lay care network further. First, the rich historical context will be examined.

HISTORICALLY SPEAKING

> I was called in great haste to see Mrs. Hamlen who was in a fit . . . applied vinegar to her lips, temples, and hands, and onions to her feet, and she revived. Martha Ballard, October 14, 1790
>
> (Spriggs, 1984, p. 116)

When one refers to the lay care network throughout the centuries, one is typically referring to the woman of the house. Until recent times, women's access to education has been partially or completely restricted. Subsequently, the realm of "professional medicine" was completely dominated by men. In reading some of the cures used by physicians of their time, there was apparently less likelihood of iatrogenic consequences resulting from a nonprofessional's remedy than from a professional's. The following excerpt refers to Martha Ballard, a local lay midwife and nurse, who was practicing in a western frontier town in the late 1700s.

> *In contrast to the doctors, who relied heavily on bleeding and commercially available drugs, Martha treated her patients mostly with homemade remedies. Poultices, plasters, blisters, salves and 'decoctions,' and teas were her stock-in-trade. A list of her ingredients sounded like a grocery list. (Spriggs, 1984, p. 105)*

In Medieval days, all women were expected to have at least a basic knowledge of medicine that they practiced on their families. However, if they extended their practice outside the limits of their home, they could be prosecuted essentially for practicing medicine without a license. The following excerpt from 1322 describes a hearing for a 30–year-old lay care provider brought up for those very charges.

> *Various witnesses were called to testify to the skill of her diagnosis and treatment, and several of them said they had been given up by various doctors before being cured by her, and set forth names of these legitimate, but unsuccessful doctors. Her skill seems to have been generally accepted . . . She herself made an eloquent and sensible defense arguing that the statute under which she was arraigned was intended to restrain ignorant and foolish persons who knew not the art of medicine, whereas she was well instructed and skilled therein, as might be seen from her successful cures. She went on to speak of the need for women doctors in general, saying that many women were ashamed to reveal their infirmities to a man and that women had often died sooner than do so. Nevertheless she was prohibited from practicing; but as she had already*

disregarded a previous prohibition and fine, she probably went on as before. (Power, 1975, p. 88)

References from both the 14th and 18th centuries state that women's modesty was a serious hindrance in seeking medical care. Consequently, they either went without treatment or relied upon folk medicine and lay care networks (Power, 1975; Spriggs, 1984).

FOLK MEDICINE

> The young woman explained that Rosa was probably "hexed" and that she should seek help from "Aunt Pearlie," a voodoo woman.
>
> (See, 1991, p. 75)

One synonymous phrase for lay care network is folk medicine. Matthews (1987, as cited in See, 1991) refers to folk or *indigenous healers* as

community-based practitioners, known variously as spiritual counselors, religious store owners, priests, 'spiritual' ministers, 'root' doctors, evangelical counselors, witch doctors . . . shamans and voodoo doctors. Many people believe they provide counseling and supportive and therapeutic services, either free or paid. (p. 70)

Though folk medicine has existed for hundreds of years, its continued popularity has been attributed to a lack of available health care, limited understanding regarding anatomy and the disease process, and peer acceptance or promotion. Folk medicine relies on medicinal remedies that often have religious overtones and ritualistic behaviors. Religion and healing are inextricably bound, as it was considered that by the "grace of God" one could rid the body of bad spirits (Bushy, 1992). Without deference and humility toward one's higher power, the healer and her or his remedies would be rendered impotent (See, 1991). The remedies vary according to the cultural, ethnic, and regional context of the setting. Despite its origin, one consistent theme noted in all folk medicine practices is that of spirituality. "Folk healers recognize the existence of a spiritual dimension in the diagnosis, treatment, and prevention of illness" (See, 1991, p. 71).

LAY REFERRAL NETWORK OR LAY CONSULTANTS

> So when you think something is wrong and the man went through it, you can talk to him about it and he can tell you out of his experience what's what (referring to an "expert" consultant). (Furstenberg, 1985, p. 30)

The nonprofessional person being asked for health care advice is called the lay consultant.

> *It . . . [can] refer to everything from specific conversation about how to deal with an emergent health problem to diffuse and ostensibly purposeless discussions of symptoms and illness as a part of everyday conversation. Lay consultation is viewed as important in influencing the decision to seek medical care, the choice of practitioner, and compliance and continuation in care. (Twaddle, 1969; Friedson, 1961; & Suchman, 1965, all as cited in Furstenberg, 1985, p. 21)*

When examining the phenomenon of lay consultation, the traditional focus was an individual's decision to seek care and, later, comply with medical regimens for chronic illness. Furstenberg (1985) examined older people's pattern of consultation that revealed more about whom the key players are in a "lay referral network." Her study found that spouses were considered the primary consultants. More often than not, this population had lost spouses and, therefore, had to seek advice elsewhere. Age mates were often preferred over adult children as they interacted at the same cognitive level, within similar sets of circumstances and experiences.

A micro-ethnography about health care in a Montana Hutterite colony was done by a Montana State University nursing graduate student in 1982. In this study, she revealed some similar advice-seeking patterns as those found in Furstenberg's work. Colony members would "check aroun" the colony or have discussions at dinner regarding current health concerns, particularly those involving children. As with the elderly population, they would look for someone with a similar condition and compare symptoms and the results of various treatments. One home remedy after another was used until either the problem resolved or they ran out of remedies. "When there is a condition they can't collectively 'cure,' the decision would be made to see a doctor." Seeking outside help was viewed as a last resort (Johansen, 1982, p. 6).

INFORMAL SUPPORT NETWORKS

Informal support networks are similar to lay consultants except that their role entails more active involvement. This network is peopled by peers, adult children, intergenerational neighbors, and fellow church or club members. Whereas a lay consultant serves as a confidant and advisor, informal support networks' involvement could range from "keeping an eye on things" to bathing or colostomy care (Magilvry, Congdon, & Martinez, 1994; Ehrlich, 1985). Regarding the elderly, this group serves two functions: a) to maintain the elderly person's independence, and b) to maintain or promote health (Magilvry et al., 1994). Langlie (1977, as cited in Ehrlich, 1985) found a positive correlation between involvement of informal support networks with recovery from illness and appropriate health behavior. The network was also thought to act as a buffer for the stressors that cause one to be more susceptible to disease (Mitchell, 1969, in Ehrlich, 1985).

ESSENTIAL ATTRIBUTES

Reading through the meanings of lay care network, one can observe recurring definitions or words that characterize the concept. These are called essential or defining attributes (Walker & Avant, 1988). The characteristics noted were (a) *interconnection* or *net,* (b) *of the people,* and (c) *sense of concern.* An interconnection is the means by which one thing connects with another, whereas a net consists of fibers woven together for catching something. That which is "of the people" is belonging to, concerned with, or performed by the 'people' in a nonprofessional capacity. Lastly, a sense of concern refers to the idea that one develops or maintains an interest in the well-being of a person or object, to oversee with the intent to protect (Oxford, 1989).

CONSTRUCTED CASES

Constructed cases are another tool used in concept analysis to further illuminate meaning. For this analysis, a model, borderline, and contrary case have been presented. According to Walker and Avant (1988), a model case should be a pure representation containing all the essential attributes of the concept being defined with no attributes from other concepts. Borderline cases show only some critical attributes, and contrary cases contain none. Contrary cases strongly illustrate the concept by clearly stating what it is not.

Model Case

Janet Hedges is a 32–year-old mother of three children, ages 10, 9, and 7. Since all her children have been in school for the last two years, she found herself with more free time, part of which she spent getting to know her neighbors better. She was particularly drawn to one elderly woman, Lisha, who lived down the street. Lisha was 79 and had been living successfully by herself since the death of her husband 18 years ago. Janet spent hours talking with Lisha, as she found Lisha's life fascinating and occasionally similar to her own.

Recently, Lisha was hospitalized for an exacerbation of emphysema that she had been diagnosed with three years ago. She had to be taken to the nearest hospital forty-six miles away. Janet visited her two or three times a week during her three-week hospitalization. During her visits, she noticed Lisha becoming gradually more weakened and depressed. Before this episode, Lisha had managed her household quite well on her own. Now, Lisha was expressing her concern to Janet that she might never be able to return to the home she had known and loved for nearly 60 years. Janet also recognized this possibility, in that there were no local home-care agencies and affordability would be doubtful even if there were such agencies. Initially, Lisha would require round-the-clock care until she had an opportunity to gain her strength back. Someone would have to give her physical therapy twice a day, prepare her meals, clean the house, help with baths, and troubleshoot if problems arose with her oxygen equipment or new medicine regime. After contacting friends of both herself and Lisha, Janet arranged to provide care for Lisha in her own home once she was dismissed from the hospital. This proposal was welcomed by the hospital staff, because they had no beds in the long term facility which would have been Lisha's next stop after hospital discharge.

For the next two months, Janet coordinated the shifts and oversaw important details of Lisha's care. By the end of four months, Lisha could do most of her own daily living tasks again, except cleaning and shopping for which she hired a local woman.

This model situation meets all the attributes for lay care network. Janet Hedges has a nonprofessional background but because of her concern for her friend/neighbor, she learned the basic skills needed to care for her friend at home. She then wove a net between other people in the community in an effort to "catch" Lisha before she fell through the cracks. Due to effective networking, the network was able to give Lisha the opportunity to live in the manner and place that had significant meaning and importance for her.

Borderline Case

Ellen Johnson is a lay-midwife serving a community of 10,000 people in Eastern Montana. She trained with another lay-midwife for two years in the 1970s before establishing her own practice. She developed a commitment to providing safe and caring homebirths after encountering several women (herself included) who had very unpleasant birth experiences in the local hospital. Since she began providing services in the area, she has established herself as a competent midwife with a steady and satisfied client load. She has had 380 successful homebirths with good mother-baby outcomes and had to transport six women to the local hospital for problems she felt would be better handled in a hospital setting.

This exemplifies a borderline case for the concept of lay care network in that it meets only two of the three essential attributes. She has created an interconnection with the community by meeting a need not previously being met and doing it well. Her commitment to her work stems from and is fueled by a concern for women of childbearing age in the area. However, she did receive formal training, albeit not in a formal setting, and continues to advance her knowledge base. Some would argue that she is functioning in a professional capacity with an experiential background well beyond that of the average person which removes her from the category of the people.

CONTRARY CASE

Dr. Nadine Samuelson is a recent graduate of a prestigious medical school in California. Because of the debt she incurred in school, she signed a two-year contract to work in a rural community hospital in

Portent, Montana, sharing the practice with an older, established physician in town. She was appalled at what she viewed as the "backwoods" attitudes and ignorance of the townsfolk. Her disdain was apparent in many of her patient interactions, and she soon gained a widespread negative reputation. Because of her discomfort with small town living, she moved to the nearest "pseudo-metropolitan" area after arranging her schedule so that she could work three consecutive days at a time. This would enable her to spend as little time as possible in Portent while "serving [her] time" until her contract was up.

If Dr. Samuelson had concern for her patients, they would contend she never showed it. Rather, she was grudgingly and marginally fulfilling her contract. She did not develop any kind of interconnection with the community, nor was she regarded in any way as of the people.

CONCLUSION

The analysis of lay care network demonstrates a need not only for further refinement of the concept but also for a change in the wording of the concept itself. One suggestion would be to delineate lay providers from informal care networks. The review of the literature found they were clearly represented as two different concepts, but the wording lay care network combines them. Lay providers are viewed as people who have some special talents or training which makes people seek them out for their ability to heal. Since it is viewed as their "profession," lay providers often receive some kind of remuneration for their services, and it becomes their primary income. On the other hand, informal care networks represent caring friends, family, and neighbors who volunteer their time and energy to help an elderly and/or sick person at home. They fill the many gaps left by the formal care network, and their services range from advice-giving, to bathing, to acquiring skills needed to assist with routine medical procedures. Both groups seemed to be strongly represented in the culture of rural health care, so further clarification of the concepts and their roles are essential.

REFERENCES

Barnhart, R. K. (Ed.) (1988). *The Barnhart dictionary of etymology*. New York: Wilson.

Bushy, A. (1992). Cultural considerations for primary health care: Where do self-care and folk medicine fit? *Holistic Nursing Practice, 6*(3), 10–19.

Ehrlich, P. (1985). Informal support networks meet health needs of rural elderly. *Journal of Gerontological Social Work, 9*(1), 85–98.

Fawcett, J. (1995). *Analysis and Evaluation of Conceptual Models of Nursing* (3rd Ed.). Philadelphia: Davis.

Fromkin, V., & Rodman, R. (1988) *An introduction to language* (4th Ed.). New York: Holt, Rinehart, & Winston.

Furstenberg, A.L. (1985). Older People's Choices of Lay Consultants. *Journal of Gerontological Social Work, 9*(1), 21–35.

Johansen, S. (1982). An ethnographic interview: Health and healthcare at Fairhaven Colony. Unpublished manuscript, Montana State University-Bozeman.

Magilvry, J. K., Congdon, J. G., & Martinez, R. (1994). Circles of care: Home care and community support for rural older adults. *Advances in Nursing Science, 6*(3), 22–33.

Oxford English Dictionary (Vol. 2, 8, & 10, 2nd ed.). (1989). Oxford: Clarendon Press.

Power, E. (1975). *Medieval women*. Cambridge, MA: Cambridge University Press.

Random house thesaurus (college ed.). (1984). New York: Random House.

Rodale, J. I. (1961). *The synonym finder*. Emmaus, PA: Rodale.

Roget's II: *The new thesaurus* (expanded ed.) (1988). Boston: Houghton Mifflin.

See, L. A. (1991). Black Folk Healers and Folk Medicine in the Rural South. In A. Bushy, *Rural nursing* (Vol. 1). Newbury Park, CA: Sage.

Spriggs, J. (1984). *Domestick beings*. New York: Knopf.

Walker, L. O., & Avant, L.C. (1988). *Strategies for theory construction in nursing* (2nd ed.). Norwalk, CT: Appleton & Lange.

16

Informal Networks

Linda L. Grossman and Sarah McNerney

INTRODUCTION

Informal networks are ubiquitous in our society. We all interact with family, friends, and neighbors. Information, support, and guidance are received from colleagues or classmates. Because interpersonal interaction is essential for health, growth, and personal development, informal networks fulfill many needs.

Informal networks are an integral part of human existence. To create comprehensive services for rural populations, health care professionals must be aware of informal networks operating within a community. An understanding of informal networks is essential for holistic care of rural clients.

The steps used to conduct this concept analysis were patterned after Walker and Avant's (1995) procedure. These steps include (a) aim of analysis, (b) definitions, (c) use of concept in several disciplines, (d) defining attributes, (e) model case, (f) contrary case, and (g) antecedents and consequences.

AIM OF ANALYSIS

In this analysis, we will refine the uses of the concept "informal networks" in rural nursing practice. Relational statements in rural nursing theory are already in existence regarding the use of informal networks. "In rural areas help is usually sought through informal rather than formal systems" (Weinert & Long, 1991, p. 29) is one example of these statements. Informal networks is clearly a concept of significant value to rural nursing practice. However, ambiguity remains regarding a pragmatic definition.

Definitions

Many terms and definitions are used in relation to informal networks. Random House *Webster's college dictionary* (Costello, 1992) includes these definitions for informal:

> *1. without formality or ceremony; casual: an informal visit. 2. not according to the prescribed official or customary way or manner; irregular; unofficial: informal proceedings. 3. suitable to or characteristic of casual and familiar, but educated, speech or writing. (p. 691)*

Definitions for network include

> *1. any combination of interesting or interconnecting filaments, lines, passages, etc.: a network of caves. 2. any system or group of interrelated or interconnected elements especially over a large area. 3. a netting or net. 4. a computer or telecommunications system linked to permit exchange of information. 5. an association of individuals having a common interest and often providing mutual assistance, information, etc. 6. to place in or connect to a network. (p. 908)*

Informal is also defined as a gathering, discussion, or meeting (Carney & Nimmo, 1993). This is reminiscent of rural channels of informal communication such as town meetings, grange, and quilting circles.

Informal networks can be viewed as a safety net for rural clients "falling through the cracks" of formal health care. The concept of a safety net can be linked to the etymology of the word network; that is, a netlike structure (Barnhart & Steinmetz, 1988). The thesaurus (Lutz, 1994) provides the following synonyms for a network: weave, mesh, plexus, which aids in the visualization of a safety net. Another definition of network that alludes to this netlike structure is "networks are interconnected relationships, durable patterns of interactions, and interpersonal threads that comprise a social fabric" (Whittaker & Garbarino, 1983).

USE OF INFORMAL NETWORKS

Education

The school system benefits from the use of informal networks. Families are encouraged to take an active role in the education system. Families promote learning through educational instruction within the home. Parents, grandparents, and community volunteers all act as informal helpers in the schools. These roles may include playground monitors, teacher aids, and chaperones. Whittaker and Garbarino (1983) provided the following example:

> *Many times, the use of citizens as resources in the schools happens on an informal basis, as when a teacher invites a person from the community who has a particular skill to come to school and share that expertise with his or her students. For example, someone in the community may be knowledgeable about wildlife of the area, have a special collection of some kind, work in an unusual occupation, or be able to act as a living history text. (p. 279)*

Teachers informally network with one another for moral support. They share ideas, hopes and aspirations. This translates into improved interactions with students.

Sociology

Informal networks/groups are discussed extensively, under the umbrella of social networks, in the field of sociology. Hassinger (1982) discusses the relationship of informal groups and social networks to health behavior. He cites four functions of informal groups in matters of health. These functions are a) conduits of the health culture, b) instruments of social control in health behavior, c) sources of social support in illness, and d) channels of communication about health matters. Informal networks provide information about health and illness, routines for meeting problems of illness, and conditions for assuming the sick role.

An informal network is a series of channels through which people request support and make demands. The network becomes a series of communication links (Whittaker & Garbarino, 1983). A computer network is a perfect illustration of the essence of a network. By communicating via E-mail with friends, colleagues, and formal resources, we create linkages to others who may be in distant locations.

As instruments of social control, informal networks act as resources for providing information about the competency and characteristics of health care providers. Hassinger (1982) suggests that informal groups may require or deny members entry into the sick-role status, i.e., parents may judge the illness of a child to be malingering. Friends or neighbors may pressure a person to obtain professional services. However, Gottlieb (1981) noted that indigenous or natural helpers provide informal self-help or mutual aid activities within informal care networks.

Gerontology

Informal network is discussed in gerontology health care literature. Magilvry, Congdon, and Martinez (1994) refer to a "circle of informal care" consisting of family, friends, and neighbors providing meals, household tasks, shopping, personal care, health-related care, errands, transportation, and companionship. Many older adults could not live independently without the support of this "circle of informal care."

An "informal support network" is defined as an elder's spouse, living children, siblings, other relatives, friends, and neighbors—those significant others with whom the elder has close contact (Branch & Jette, 1983). A firmly established informal support network can be the first line of defense against institutionalization for many older adults (Soldo & Myllyluoma, 1983).

Psychology

Young, Giles, and Plantz (1982) refer to a "natural network" as an informal system of interpersonal linkages that exists for an individual because of family ties or friendships, personal accessibility (e.g., neighbors, co-workers), or a community role (e.g., minister, police, teacher). "Natural" is included as one synonym for the word informal (Lutz, 1994). According to Young et al., mental health professionals working with clients need to be aware of three important aspects of natural networks:

> *1. Even the most serious problems usually develop across time and are dealt with inside natural networks before being referred to the formal helping system. 2. The formal helping system may be unavailable, not readily accessible, or of limited assistance because of an overload. 3. A person's seeking expert help does not remove the need for continuing support from the natural network. (p. 467)*

DEFINING ATTRIBUTES

Attributes of informal networks identified were (a) volunteer, (b) information exchange, (c) support, and (d) guidance. These four attributes are described more fully:

- Volunteer is an individual who offers assistance free of charge. These volunteers are family members, friends, coworkers, and neighbors.
- Information exchange is the exchange of information among the members of the informal network.
- Support is the assistance given to members in the network. Support is further delineated into its emotional and physical components. The emotional component entails being a friend, listening, and "providing a shoulder to cry on." The physical component includes assistance with daily living, health promotion, and maintenance activities.
- Guidance can be given as advice, consultation, and information. Informal consultation is given regarding the availability of resources, referral to health care providers, and sources of alternative treatments.

Informal networks provide direction in conveying social norms of the wider community. Informal networks require information exchange, supportive assistance, and guidance provided by volunteers in a community.

MODEL CASE

This is a real life case. Bill is a 60–year-old male who lives in a small rural Montana community. He was admitted to the local hospital in

November of 1994 and was diagnosed with pneumonia. He spent the next five months in the intensive care unit on a ventilator. His medical insurance company was pushing to send Bill home on a ventilator with assistance from formal home health care. Bill was not strong enough to go home, so he was transferred to the inpatient rehabilitation unit. He spent the next four months trying to regain his strength but continued to be ventilator-dependent. His insurance company notified his wife that Bill had used his life time limit of health insurance.

Bill's main goal in life, at this time, was to go home and be with his family. He had a wife, four grown children, and many grandchildren. Before his hospitalization, he was very active with work, golf, family, and community activities. He and his wife had just bought a new home and were looking forward to their "golden years." He had spent the last nine months in the hospital; his body was emaciated, and he continued to be ventilator dependent.

Would Bill ever get his wish to go home? Now that his insurance had run out, he and his wife were short on hope and resources. His wife began to make calls, contacting members of her community and family for support and guidance. These contacts resulted in a chain of events that enabled Bill to go home. A strong bond existed between Bill, his family, and his friends. They wanted to fulfill his wish to go home. Neighbors and family members arranged their schedules to help with his care. He received care from a local home health agency eight hours per day, and the remainder of the day was covered by friends and family. The friends and family who cared for Bill at home provided physical and emotional support for both Bill and his wife.

Friends and co-workers organized a golf tournament and barbecue benefit to help with Bill's medical expenditures. The benefit, advertised widely throughout the community, was titled Giving a Helping Hand to your Neighbor. The benefit raised $145,000. There was now enough money to help with Bill's medical bills. Bill and his wife were also able to pay off their home mortgage. Bill lived at home for two weeks before he returned to the hospital with the diagnosis of sepsis. He died two days later.

Had it not been for the services volunteered by family, friends, co-workers, and community members, Bill would not have spent his last two weeks at home. This case includes all of the defining attributes of an informal network. It also includes the antecedent of a bond and a perceived need of support and guidance. The consequence was that Bill's needs were met.

CONTRARY CASE

Kay, a single mother of four children, has recently moved to a new community. She has no insurance and limited resources. One child has been complaining of an earache. He has been irritable and febrile. Kay decides she will need to take the boy to see the pediatrician. She is able to get an appointment later in the day. Upon arrival at the clinic, she is asked by the receptionist if she has medical insurance. Kay informs the receptionist that she does not have insurance. She is then informed that she must pay for her son's care before he is examined by the pediatrician. Kay replies, "I can't pay for it right now, but I could pay the bill later this month." The receptionist states, "If you can't pay for services, the physician will be unable to see your son." Kay is upset and disappointed. There is no one to offer support or guidance.

This is considered a contrary case. According to Walker and Avant (1995), contrary cases are those cases that contain none of the critical attributes. There are no attributes of an informal network associated with this case. Informal networks require volunteer supportive interaction and guidance among people who are linked by a bond.

ANTECEDENTS AND CONSEQUENCES

One antecedent noted in relation to informal networks is a bond. A bond refers to the tie that exists among family, friends, neighbors, and co-workers. These members are the core of an informal network. A bond is necessary to attach the links of a network. Another antecedent is that informal networks are generated in response to a perceived need. The consequence of an informal network is that the perceived need is met or not met.

SUMMARY

The concept of informal networks was analyzed using the procedures outlined by Walker and Avant (1995). Multiple definitions were provided and the use of the concept was explored. Essential attributes were determined and used in two cases. A model case and a contrary case showed a "pure" case of the concept and a clear example of "not the concept." Antecedents and consequences were included further to refine the critical attributes.

An informal network is a concept discussed extensively in the field of sociology but less frequently in the discipline of nursing. It is important that further analysis and research are pursued to increase understanding of how informal networks complement formal networks. Practical implications exist for informal networks within the formal system of rural nursing. Nurses practicing within a rural community need to recognize the value of informal networks as sources of support and guidance. Working within this framework is essential. Nurses can use informal networks to distribute and receive information regarding the health needs of the community. This in turn provides a foundation for the holistic care of rural clients.

REFERENCES

Barnhart, R. K., & Steinmetz, S. (Eds.) (1988). The *Barnhart dictionary of etymology*. Bronxville, NY: Wilson.

Branch, L. G., & Jette, A. M. (1983). Elder's use of informal long-term care assistance. *Gerontologist, 23* (1), 51–56.

Carney, F., & Nimmo, C. (Eds.). (1993). *French-English English-French dictionary* (unabridged ed.). Paris: Larousse.

Costello, R. B. (Ed.) (1992). *Random House Webster's college dictionary.* New York: Random House.

Gottlieb, B. (Ed.) (1981). *Social networks and social support* (Vol. 4). London: Sage.

Hassinger, E. (1982). *Rural health: Social networks and regionalization.* Ames, IA: Iowa State University Press.

Lutz, W. D. (Ed.) (1994). *The Cambridge thesaurus of American English.* Cambridge: Cambridge University Press.

Magilvry, J. K., Congdon, J. G., & Martinez, R. (1994). Circles of care: Home care and community support for rural older adults. *Advances in Nursing Science, 16* (3), 22–33.

Soldo, B., & Myllyluoma, J. (1983). Caregivers who live with dependent elderly. *Gerontologist, 23,* 605–611.

Walker, L. O., & Avant, K. C. (1995). *Strategies for theory construction in nursing.* Norwalk, CT: Appleton & Lange.

Weinert, C., & Long, K. A. (1991). The theory and research base for rural nursing practice. In A. Bushy, *Rural nursing,* Vol. 1 (pp. 21–38). Newbury Park, CA: Sage.

Whittaker, J., & Garbarino, J. (1983). *Social support networks: Informal helping in the human services.* New York: Aldine.

Young, C. E., Giles, D. E., Jr., & Plantz, M. C. (1982). Natural networks: Help-giving and help-seeking in two rural communities. *American Journal of Community Psychology, 10* (4), 457–468.

III

PERSPECTIVES OF RURAL PERSONS

The authors of the first four chapters of this part of the book used a variety of qualitative methods to gather information about the perspectives of persons living in rural areas. The first chapter (chapter 17) addresses the concept of health by using case examples. The second chapter (chapter 18) also addresses health; this phenomenological study reports the viewpoints of older persons living in North Dakota. The author of the third chapter (chapter 19) used grounded theory method to develop a substantive theory of protecting independence. The sample for this chapter was elderly women and men living in eastern Montana. The next chapter (chapter 20) reports the findings of two phenomenological studies exploring hardiness in samples of rural men and women over the age of 50 who live in middle and eastern Montana. This chapter also includes a commentary about the use of Parse's theory as an organizing framework for the two studies.

The last two chapters present analyses of two concepts pertinent to the perspectives of rural persons. Chapter 21 is about cultural isolation. Concerned about Mexican migrants in her practice, the author decided to address the isolation they felt after having migrated to work and live in Montana. The final chapter (chapter 22) focuses on ethnocentrism, a concept that must be recognized when all nurses, including rural nurses, work with persons from cultures different from their own.

Together these chapters form a framework for looking at health care through the eyes of rural residents.

17

The Concept of Health: Rural Perspectives*

Kathleen Ann Long

The concepts of health held by clients are known to significantly affect their health-promotion behaviors, health care seeking, and acceptance of preventive and treatment interventions. A considerable body of literature has addressed the importance of beliefs about illness susceptibility, illness seriousness, treatment availability, and treatment effectiveness in determining a variety of health-related behaviors.[1,5,13]

Smith[15] has identified four distinct sets of health beliefs, or "models of health" that affect how both consumers and providers behave in relation to health. Each model includes a definition of health, which is viewed as influencing the health goals set by individuals and the behaviors used to achieve those goals. For example, persons who conceptualize health within a clinical model focus on the absence of disease symptoms in defining health. Their health goals tend to be related to reducing or relieving symptoms, and they are likely to seek health care when a symptom is present. In contrast, those who conceptualize health using a role performance model are inclined to define health within the context of functional expectations and work requirements. Health goals are related to being able to work, meet family obligations, perform activities of daily living, and the like. Within this framework, health care is usually sought when one is unable to

Note: This work was supported in part by grant #1816001649A1 from the Division of Nursing, United States Public Health Service.

**Note.* From "The Concept of Health: Rural Perspectives," by K. A. Long, 1993, *Rural Nursing, 28,* pp. 123–130. Copyright 1993 by Nursing Clinics of North America. Reprinted with permission.

function based on self-expectations or the expectations of significant others.

Understanding an individual's, family's, or community's concept of health is critical to understanding that client's motivation for health promotion, health maintenance, and illness treatment. Knowledge of the client's concept of health is important for the development of assessment approaches and intervention strategies that are both relevant and acceptable to the client. Most health concept literature and research to date has not addressed place of residence as a relevant variable. There is increasing evidence, however, that place of residence and related environmental factors influence the way in which persons think about health. This article examines the health concepts of rural clients through consideration of global rural-urban differences, rural regional and subcultural variations, and unique client-specific factors.

RURAL VERSUS URBAN PERSPECTIVES

Early work in the field of rural health focused on what was unique and different in rural settings as opposed to urban settings. This was appropriate given a long history of health planning and research that neglected the rural perspective. More recent work,[12,18] however, has emphasized the diversity of rural areas. It is now generally accepted that there is no singular concept of health held by those in rural areas, just as there is no distinct and singular concept of health for all persons in urban areas.

A growing body of data indicate that certain definitions of and views regarding health are considerably more prevalent among rural dwellers than among urban dwellers. These general rural definitions and views have been found to hold true for rural populations across a variety of geographic locations and across age and gender differences.[3,14,18] Sound reasons exist for some general and basic differences in the way in which health is conceptualized by those in rural versus those in urban areas. As a result of their environment, rural dwellers are more frequently called on to be independent and self-reliant. Agencies and specialized services, related not only to health but to education, infrastructure and government as well, have been and continue to be less available in rural areas. Rural residents, whether by necessity or preference, tend to function as generalists. In many rural areas, geographic isolation requires the assumption of multiple roles. Those managing rural ranches, for example, often must also function as bookkeepers, veterinarians, market analysts, and carpenters. These diverse abilities are necessary to maintain homes and businesses in geographically isolated rural settings.

Of necessity and based on experience, rural dwellers learn to distinguish between those health impairments which, if untreated, will impede functioning, from those that can be tolerated for a period. Lack of health insurance, landbased work that does not permit "sick days," and long distances from formal health care providers influence the way health is viewed and illness is addressed. Informal networks of family members, neighbors, and friends are frequently used in diagnosing and treating health problems. This network is affordable and accessible. In addition, the help received comes from "insiders" who can be trusted to understand the social context of the health care problem.

Across different types of rural areas, several specific components appear to characterize the way in which health is conceptualized.[4,10,18] Health is often viewed within a role performance model. The ability to work, that is, to perform one's usual daily activities, is a major feature in the definitions of health provided by rural dwellers. Health as the ability to work has been reported by a variety of age groups and by both rural women and rural men. It has been mentioned by rural residents in such diverse locations as the northeast seacoast, the midwest plains, and the mountains of the west.[3,10,14] The "ability to work" aspect of health is, of course, also important to those who live in urban areas. The degree of importance or emphasis appears to be different, however. Urban dwellers more frequently and readily focus on the comfort, cosmetic, and life prolonging aspects of health. In contrast, rural dwellers tend to determine health needs *primarily* in relation to work activities.[4,10] For rural dwellers health needs are usually secondary to work needs. Rural residents, for example, have been found to tolerate pain for extended periods, so long as it does not interfere with the ability to work.[10]

This way of conceptualizing health, combined with the realities of the rural environment, have a significant effect on health-seeking behavior and the acceptance of both health care interventions and health care providers. The emphasis on work and self-reliance, coupled with inadequate health care resources, can place rural dwellers at special risk for premature death, long-term illness, and disability. Health care delivery systems have often failed to recognize and address the beliefs, preferences, and life-styles of rural dwellers. Certainly there is nothing inherently "unhealthy" about valuing work and relying primarily on self, family members, and close friends for initial health care and ongoing support. If these perspectives are overlooked in planning rural health care delivery, however, the result is health care programs that are inaccessible, irrelevant, or unacceptable to rural residents.

Although there appear to be general differences in the way health and health care are viewed by rural and urban dwellers, a knowledge of these general differences does not replace the need for comprehensive assessment of individuals and communities. The general differences do, however, provide a useful frame of reference for health care planning that can maximize the delivery of existing health care resources to rural residents.

Rural Variations

Differences within rural populations are substantial. Assuming that the general conceptualizations of health discussed earlier are applicable to all rural populations or that they represent a thorough explanation of health beliefs for any given rural population would be erroneous. Variations based on age, income, race, ethnicity, occupation, and health status are extremely important in understanding the concept of health among rural dwellers. Further research is needed to examine the interaction of these demographic variables with place of residence and the effect of these interactions on health status, beliefs, and practices. To date, little work has addressed health concepts among children or adolescents in rural areas. Work by Sorenson[16] has shown that rural children use coping and adaptive strategies that are quite similar to those of urban children. Rapidly rising rates of substance abuse and suicide among rural adolescents indicate that studies addressing the health beliefs and practices of this age group are particularly needed.

Rural minority groups, including blacks, Hispanics, and Native Americans, are known to have higher morbidity and mortality rates than white residents in the same or similar geographic areas. In addition, health care services, although limited for all rural dwellers, are often completely unavailable for these minority group members.[18] Barriers related to culture and belief systems, costs, and discrimination need to be better understood for specific minority groups within specific rural settings. Prejudice and poverty explain much in relation to health care access for all minority group members, but rural-urban differences in the health perspectives of minority group members should also be considered in the development of services and programs.

Health status is also an important feature of how persons conceptualize health. This appears to be a rather obvious notion; however, it has not always been considered in either health care planning or research. For example, the needs of terminally or chronically ill persons, regardless of place of residence, may be quite similar. A recent study of persons with multiple sclerosis has shown marked similarities in descriptions and perceptions of health, regardless of rural or urban residence.[9]

An understanding of the health concepts held by individual rural clients can be built on general rural-urban differences, but it must be tempered by careful consideration of the marked variations within rural settings and the characteristics of particular subgroups that reside in rural areas. This combination of knowledge is important for the timely and appropriate application of treatment and support services across diverse rural settings.

Specific Clients

The premise that client concept of health has a major affect on health and health-seeking behaviors is clearly conveyed in the following case examples drawn from rural nursing practice. These examples illustrate how aspects of the rural environment interact with belief systems and individual characteristics to determine health-related behaviors.

Michael T. is a 61–year-old wheat farmer. He maintains his large and profitable family farm with the help of his wife, three sons, and occasional hired help. He has managed and actively worked the same farm for almost 40 years. Mr. T. attended the state university for 2 years, studying agribusiness. By his state's standards he is well educated; he is in the middle-income bracket. During the harvesting season, he often works parts of his fields alone with the help of rented heavy farm equipment. Two years ago while working in this way, the middle finger of his right hand became caught in a moving part of his equipment while he was adjusting a machine component. He could not pull his finger free and the injury was quite painful. Mr. T. realized that it might be some time before anyone would come to his aid. The weather was changing, and there was need to complete the harvesting work in the field to avoid damage to the wheat crop and prevent additional equipment rental costs. He decided to pull his hand free, severing his finger at its base. He was able to control the bleeding with a tightly bound handkerchief, and he completed harvesting his field.

Once returning home his son drove him to the nearest town, 57 miles away, where he sought care in the hospital emergency room. The physician who saw him was very distressed that Mr. T. had not retrieved the digit and sought care immediately. While dressing Mr. T.'s wound, the physician explained that with prompt action and air ambulance transport to the state's major medical center, it might have been possible to reattach the finger.

Fortunately Mr. T. did not develop infection or other serious complications following his injury. He was able to manage his farm as usual after his injury. When he tells neighbors the story of this event, he often comments, "It simply goes to show you that if you go to those doctors too soon, you end up with lots of unnecessary treatment and bills."

The relationship between health and the ability to work are well illustrated. The cosmetic, and even the comfort, aspects of health were of little significance to Mr. T. For this lifelong rural resident, the time frame for treatment-seeking and the type of treatment sought were determined by his concept of health as the ability to continue work as a grain farmer.

A second case study depicts a rural community's definition of health and its effect.

Jamie C. is a 7–year-old girl, currently in foster care after 2 years of severe physical abuse by her alcoholic father. She has lived all of her life in a town of 1500 people that serves as the community center for surrounding ranches.

Jamie's teachers suspected that she was being physically abused from the time she entered school at age 5. Neighbors were aware of the abuse for several years, because they often witnessed beatings that occurred in the yard or on the porch. Almost everyone in the town knew that Jamie's father had a drinking problem, but alcohol abuse, especially weekend binging, was fairly common behavior for many of the men in the town.

Despite community knowledge about the abuse, it took more than 2 years for the Public Health Nurse and County Social Service Worker to gather sufficient data to arrange legal action and remove Jamie from her home. Even with existing child abuse laws, teachers were reticent to provide data, and the police and court systems were slow to act. At the hearing, the presiding official, a long-time town resident, commented to the nurse, I don't know why you're involved in this. Drinking and spanking your child don't have anything to do with staying healthy."

Certainly this narrow view of health and resistance to acknowledging and acting in domestic abuse cases are not unique to rural towns. What is somewhat unique is the power these views can wield in small, isolated communities and the implications this has for both abuse victims and health care providers. Similar cases of the impact of rural subculture on abuse situations have been documented.[8]

A final case example demonstrates the interplay of individual and group beliefs about health and a unique linkage between health and work.

Sylvester W. is a 39–year-old logger. He has worked in this dangerous and physically demanding occupation for more than 10 years. The pay is very good, although work periods are sporadic. One of the most demanding aspects of the job involves climbing high into trees to remove tops and branches.

Mr. W. presented himself at the First Aid Office complaining of "heartlock." The nurse practitioner at the office, a long-time resident of the area, readily permitted him to lie down and rest. She checked his pulse and found it to be rapid; his breathing was rapid and shallow. No further assessment was done, but Mr. W. was not sent back to work. The other loggers knew about and understood "heartlock."

The health care provider had come to learn the following about this ailment. "Heartlock" can best be explained as a type of anxiety attack. When it occurs, loggers often complain of tightness in their chests, a foreboding sense, and most importantly, a clear belief that they should not work. The development of occasional bouts of "heartlock" appears to provide loggers with a legitimate and acceptable way of seeking temporary respite from both the high levels of stress and the physical demands of their work. The episodes are accepted as legitimate health problems by logging contractors and by fellow loggers.

Clearly, the concept of health, determined by subculture and heavily influenced by the work environment, has been a major factor in determining the definition of this health problem by these rural residents. A health care professional unfamiliar with local definitions of health and the special care needs of this subgroup might recommend unnecessary procedures and exacerbate the client's anxiety state by refuting the existence of a health care problem.

Rural Nursing Practice

Client concepts of health have real and significant affects on health-related behaviors, and understanding these health concepts is relevant to nursing practice. There are implications for numerous aspects of rural nursing practice.

Assessment of both individual-and community-level health needs requires an understanding of person-specific and locale-specific health definitions. Although there are certain general, often physiologically, based parameters to guide assessment, these should be applied within the environmental context. For example, hypertension is determined by specific physiologic indicators, and these apply to all persons across location, culture, or subculture. The causes of hypertension, as well as client responses to this disorder, however, may vary widely, and can be heavily influenced by environment. Knowing how to assess the causes, significance of, and response to hypertension in rural settings requires an understanding of health as defined by rural persons. The data reported as a part of a health history depend on how the client perceives health. Client health definitions will affect willingness to use various diagnostic procedures and to accept the results thereof. These definitions will also influence the reporting or nonreporting of signs and symptoms. Substantial evidence exists that communities as well as individuals will not reveal information to health care providers if, based on the client's definition, that information is deemed irrelevant or unrelated to health. [4,8,17] Thus, hypertensive symptoms such as headaches or dizziness, which do not interfere substantially with the ability to work, may not be reported unless the client is thoroughly oriented to the importance of these symptoms and the long-term consequences of hypertension in relation to work. Likewise, community leaders are not likely to alter high-sodium drinking water unless clear connections between sodium intake, hypertension, and long-term disability can be elucidated.

Health care planning requires knowledge of and respect for the way in which rural dwellers conceptualize health. Ultimately the health goals that are set collaboratively by clients and nurses are circumscribed by the way in which clients view health. As discussed earlier, rural clients are often less likely to aspire to health goals that emphasize appearance, comfort, or longevity. An increasing body of theory and research is demonstrating that the health goals of rural dwellers may be better understood in relation to concepts such as "hardiness," "independence," and "ability to work."[2,4,7,10] Thus, rural health planning needs to focus on these goals. Planning efforts tied to the performance of work and functioning in various aspects of daily living are more likely to be endorsed and supported by rural families and communities. Exercise, for example, has become a major focus in health promotion plans nationally. Vast differences apply, however, in exercise plan regimens for sedentary office workers in urban areas and those for physically overburdened rural ranchers, miners, or loggers. Jenkins[6] emphasized the importance of considering the background, aspirations, and resources of each rural community in developing community health care initiatives. Mobilizing local resources for health programs is directly tied to the sense community residents have of understanding, endorsing, and ultimately "owning" the goals of those health programs.

Health promotion campaigns need to include implications related to work ability, or they will fail to tap key aspects of health-seeking motivation for rural persons. The planning of health screening and prevention services must consider rural work schedules, weather conditions, and the availability of transportation to large segments of the rural population. Another aspect of importance is the way in which rural residents may view professional providers who are new to the community. Health care providers and formal health care agencies may initially be seen as distrusted "outsiders." The provision of comprehensive health care, and mental health care specifically, can be adversely affected by programs that place providers in rural communities for short periods. Rapid staff turnover or the rotation of staff members to cover rural sites can inhibit the development of necessary provider-client interpersonal comfort and trust.

The effects of specific nursing interventions can be enhanced or limited based on their fit with the rural client's concept of health. Teaching, for example, as an intervention to address both preventative and restorative health care needs, has special relevance in rural areas. Rural residents are accustomed to "doing for themselves" because health agencies and formal systems are often unavailable. Teaching, done within a context that is sensitive to each client's motivation, learning style, and ability, allows rural residents to enhance on their own their ability to manage health care needs effectively.

Numerous opportunities exist for nurses to intervene in ways that strengthen existing, informal, and client-accepted health care resources. The degree to which these opportunities will be used is influenced by each nurse's ability to work with definitions of health and health care that may be quite different from the standards of professional providers. Working through a locally accepted "health expert," such as a drug store proprietor or a minister, may prove to be a more effective strategy for improving community health care than working separately from or in competition with such local resources. This does not mean that nurses in rural areas should endorse incompetent or unsafe providers, and it does not mean that rural dwellers should be expected to accept an "anything that's available" approach to health care. It does mean, however, that nurses and other professionals who are willing to appropriately enhance the knowledge base of indigenous care providers can do much to improve the informal systems that predominate in rural health care. In addition, through collaborative work, it is often possible to develop referral activities that ensure the appropriate use of both informal and formal health care resources. Understanding that health problems and health care needs are frequently addressed through family and neighbor systems in rural areas is a basis for integrating formal resources and professional providers into existing community networks. A clear and informative example of such integration is detailed by Memmot[11] in her description of the development of hospice programs in remote areas.

Nurses in rural areas can also use their knowledge about local concepts of health in developing relevant strategies for evaluating the outcomes of health care interventions and programs. Patient use, for example, needs to be applied cautiously as a measure of the value of a given health care service or professional in a rural area. Because informal networks predominate, a small number of individuals using a given health service or provider may actually result in a sizable number of clients who are affected, albeit indirectly. Changes in health practices or in health status also need to be evaluated in context. Health promotion and disease-prevention behaviors often change slowly and in subtle ways following the introduction of health promotion programs. Attitudinal changes among key local leaders regarding such things as alcohol abuse prevention or occupational safety can be important indicators of effectiveness, long before actual behavioral changes occur among rural residents in general.

SUMMARY

An understanding of the client's concept of health is necessary to conduct relevant and effective health assessment, planning, intervention, and evaluation. Client health concepts are affected by place of residence and further colored by specific community and individual level variations including occupation, education, subculture, age, gender, and health status. Rural nursing practice can be improved through knowledge of the health perceptions and definitions held by the rural clients to be served. Nursing, as a discipline, has traditionally emphasized the need to understand the client's perspective and to develop mutually agreed on health goals in collaboration with the client. Rural nursing practice offers unique opportunities to consider meanings of health within the environmental context. Further, it challenges nurses to work hand-in-hand with clients to develop strategies that fit the context, and thus effectively address rural health care needs.

REFERENCES

1. Becker MH: *Health Education Monographs.* San Francisco, Society for Public Health Education, 1974.

2. Bigbee JL: The concept of hardiness as applied to rural nursing. In Bushy A (Ed): *Rural Nursing,* vol 1. Newbury Park, Sage, 1991, p 39.

3. Brown K: Connected independence: A paradox of rural health? *Journal of Rural Community Psychology* 2:51, 1990.

4. Bushy A: Rural determinants in family health: Considerations for community nurses. In Bushy A (ed): *Rural Nursing,* vol 1. Newbury Park, Sage, 1991, p 133.

5. Green LW, Roberts BJ: The research literature on why women delay in seeking medical care for breast symptoms. *Health Educ Monogr* 2(2):129, 1974.

6. Jenkins S: The future of rural communities: Mobilizing local resources. In Bushy A (ed): *Rural Nursing,* vol 2. Newbury Park, Sage, 1991, p 16.

7. Lee, HJ: Hardiness: Its relevance for rural health and rural nursing. Paper presented at WSRN, Communicating Nursing Research Conference, Salt Lake City, 1988.

8. Long KA: Cultural considerations in the assessment and treatment of intrafamilial abuse. *Am J Orthopsychiatry* 56:131, 1986.

9. Long KA, Weinert C: Descriptions and perceptions of health among rural and urban chronically ill adults. Submitted for publication, 1991.

10. Long KA, Weinert C: Rural nursing: Developing the theory base. *Scholarly Inquiry for Nursing Practice 3*:113, 1989.

11. Memmott RJ; Developing hospice programs in frontier communities. In Bushy A (ed): *Rural Nursing,* vol 2. Newbury Park, Sage, 1991, p 63.

12. Miller MK, Stokes CS, Clifford WB: A comparison of the rural-urban mortality differential for deaths from all causes, cardiovascular disease and cancer. *The Journal of Rural Health 3*:23, 1987.

13. Rosenstock IM: *Why people use health services.* Milbank Mem Fund Q 44:94, 1966.

14. Ross H: Women and wellness: Defining, attaining, and maintaining health in eastern Canada. Dissertation Abstracts International 42:5175A-5176A, 1982.

15. Smith JA: *The Idea of Health: Implications for the Nursing Professional.* New York, Teachers College Press, 1983.

16. Sorenson ES: Daily stress-coping phenomena among rural American children. Paper presented at the ANA Council of Nurse Researchers 1991 International Nursing Research Conference, Los Angeles, 1991.

17. *Note:* This work was supported in part by grant #1816001649A1 from the Division of Nursing, United States Public Health Service. US Congress, Office of Technology Assessment: Health care in rural America. Washington, DC, US Government Printing Office, 1990.

18. Weinert C, Long KA: Rural families and health care: Refining the knowledge base. *Marriage and Family Review 15*:57, 1990.

18

Health Perceptions of Rural Elders: "Landscapes and Life"

Alice Running

INTRODUCTION

> I think of two landscapes, one outside the self, the other within. The interior landscape responds to the character and subtlety of an exterior landscape; the shape of the individual mind is as affected by land as it is by genes.
>
> (Lopez, 1988, p. 65)

Barry Lopez's (1988) description of landscape has great relevance for persons residing in rural areas. Nurse researchers have found that rural residents are private, independent, and self-sufficient (Lee, 1993). Additionally, rural dwellers are thought to be hardy (Bigbee, 1991), possess a sense of connected independence (Brown, 1990), and describe health in a functional way (Weinert & Burman, 1994), such as the ability to do work (Weinert & Long, 1987). These characteristics provide a way to envision and describe rural residents in general. However, each rural landscape brings with it its own characters. Therefore, the purpose of this research project was to describe the experience, and so the landscapes, of aging and health for a group of homesteaders in the Northwest Plains.

The lives, and so the minds, of these homesteaders were closely tied to the land. Without the ability to work, this group would not have survived. Because of the geographical distances to supplies, health care, and neighbors, these individuals developed a sense of independence, became very self-sufficient, and remained very private.

RESEARCH METHOD

In an attempt to uncover the meaning of the lived experience of aging and health for homesteaders in the Northwestern Plains, the phenomenological method was used. The phenomenological method is an inductive, descriptive research method. The goal is to understand everyday experiences and practices of health and illness. Phenomenology is holistic in that it seeks to study the person in the situation, rather than isolating person variables and then trying to put them back together.

Anthony Giddens (as cited in Morse, 1989) points out that "to speak of phenomenology is not to speak of a single, unified body of thought" (p. 15). Oiler (as cited in Munhall & Oiler, 1986) states that there is not one phenomenological methodology but a variety of methods that all hold to the primacy of the subjective experience. For the purposes of this research project, the first three of six steps in Giorgi's method—because of their somewhat directive nature—were combined with the Husserlian context for analysis of phenomenological themes.

The first three steps proposed by Giorgi (1970) are preparatory for moving into the thematic generation procedures consistent with the analysis of phenomenological themes. The last three steps in the Giorgi method require the transformation of concrete language or the language of the informant into the language of science and the communication of that language to other researchers for confirmation and/or criticism. However, it seems that the findings should be valued whether or not they can be confirmed by others. Therefore, the Husserlian field of consciousing the world also provides a context for analysis of phenomenological themes.

The Principle of Intentionality and the Multiple Modes of Awareness together are called the Husserlian Field of Consciousing the World (Reeder, 1991). "The Field of Consciousing the World is recognized as being the figure/ground context which makes attentive listening, constituting of meanings and synthesis of essential themes possible from the narratives shared by the participants" (Reeder, 1991,

p. 264). The skill of disciplined attention to the natural narratives of participants through first-hand, multiple-dimensional hearing is accompanied by reflection. Attitudes of reflexive listening, hearing, and reading lead to an appreciation of the rich data and to sensitive recognition of the meanings held by participants. From the analysis emerges a unifying grounding theme recognized in every narrative.

ENTREE AND PARTICIPANT SELECTION

Gaining entree into the sample chosen was not problematic. Entree as defined by Chenitz and Swanson (1986) deals with getting in, staying in, and getting what the researcher needs. Because my grandfather homesteaded in the area, my family was well known to this sample. While I had entree by virtue of my family, I did not at any time assume entree to persons and events simply because of family connections.

My first effort at entree was to attend a retired teachers' meeting with my mother, herself a retired teacher who had taught in rural North Dakota. After being introduced to all present at the meeting, I explained that I wanted to visit with people 80 years old and older about their lives in the Northwestern Plains. Before the meeting, I had discussed with my mother the possibility of establishing a "Committee of Experts" (people 80 years old and older). I explained that this committee would help me understand the perspective of aging and would, I hoped, guide my thoughts as I began to study that population. The committee of experts was established at the conclusion of the retired teachers' meeting, and a committee gathering was set for the following day at my parents' home. At the end of the committee meeting, the direction of my questioning was clearer. The committee was helpful in giving names of those people they thought would participate in the study.

SAMPLE

The sample was opportunistic because the "participants were selected according to their ability to articulate and provide explanations" (Agar, 1980, p. 20). In choosing participants, an effort was made to choose informants who represented different sectors of the population, to vary level of independence (and indirectly health), age, sex, and marital status. It is interesting to note that for this population, income was not a variable of concern. Neither my parents nor members of my committee could identify anyone who might be experiencing financial difficulty.

The nine participants ranged in age from 80 to 97, with a mean age of 89. One participant lived in a nursing home, one in a retirement center, and the remaining seven lived independently in their own homes. Of the nine participants, eight were women, and one was a man. One participant was Native American and French, two were English and Norwegian, and the remaining six were Norwegian. None of the participants were born outside the United States, but one had spent two years in Norway as a child. All of the participants spoke English.

The participants were contacted by telephone or in person and were asked to "visit" about their lives and their health. The term visit rather than interview was chosen to more fully describe the process used. As opposed to the word interview that implies one person asking questions of another, the word visit implies a discussion and best captures the attitude of this type of interaction.

PROTECTION OF PARTICIPANTS' RIGHTS

The participants were informed about the nature of the visit, the time required, and their involvement. They were told that the purpose of the visit was to obtain information for a research project and that their full names would not be used in a written report. Assured of confidentiality, each participant gave oral permission to be photographed and to a tape recording of what happened during each visit.

DATA COLLECTION

All visits began with a very general question asking about each participant's perceptions of his or her own life and health. As the process of exploration developed, the conversations were directed by the informant's responses. Questions that started at a superficial level increased in depth as the conversations progressed. Recognizing the potentially high "dross rate" (tendency to stray off the subject) (Field & Morse, 1985) with this age group, the participants were kept on the topic by reflective questions that guided the interview. "The interviews were closed when new questions ceased to be generated and the narratives were saturated with rich data" (Reeder, 1991, p. 264).

Because I personally knew the first participant, the one-hour-and-thirty-minute interview went smoothly. I was accompanied on the second interview by my mother because I did not know the participant. Thereafter, I included my 70–year-old mother in the interviews because of the comfort that she seemed to bring to the participants. All participants were aware that my mother would be accompanying me on the visit.

In keeping with the phenomenological methodology, the participants saw my mother as someone who could validate what they were saying because of similar life experiences, self-interpretations in the form of common meanings, personal concerns, and cultural practices shaped by a particular history. Unlike a positivistic paradigm that values distance and objectivity, the outcome of phenomenological inquiry depends on the researcher's ability to engage with the informants' reality (Swanson-Kauffman & Schonwald, 1988). After each interview, my mother and I critiqued what had happened and discussed whether the interviews should continue as they were or be altered in some manner. I explained the confidential nature of the visits to my mother, and we agreed that the visits would not be discussed with anyone else. The interviews lasted from one hour to one-hour-and-forty-five minutes. All interviews were audio-taped and transcribed verbatim. Field notes were written after each interview to portray the physical setting and the observed impressions of both verbal and nonverbal expressions.

TREATMENT OF DATA

The purpose of data analysis is twofold (Field & Morse, 1985). The first purpose is to code the data so that the themes may be recognized and analyzed and behaviors noted. The second is to develop a data filing system that will provide a flexible storage system with procedures for retrieving the data.

The first step required reading the entire description of the experience to get a sense of the whole, to dwell on the data. In this first step and throughout the process of data analysis, three operations were included which constituted the major processes of analysis in the phenomenological method. They are intuiting, analyzing, and describing (Parse , Cone, & Smith., 1985). The interviews were reread to relive the interview and the experience.

The second step, as outlined by Giorgi, was to read the description again more slowly, identifying transitions or units in the experience called constituents or themes. The Ethnograph computer program provided a convenient means of storing and sorting through the large amount of data. Codes or themes were developed from the transcripts.

Giorgi's third step called for the elimination of redundancies in the units, clarifying or elaborating the meaning of the remaining units by relating them to each other and the whole. Whereas steps one through three may have seemed reductionistic because of their step-by-step nature, the Husserlian thematic generation process used in conjunction with Giorgi was constructionistic in nature. The attitudes of listening, hearing, and reading reflexively during first and second level analysis of the natural narratives of the participants "lead to exceptional penetration of the rich data and to sensitive recognition of the conscious or unconscious meanings held by the participants" (Reeder, 1991, p. 267).

DESCRIBING THE FINDINGS

While the participants were asked specifically to talk about their health, the responses below reflect the intricate connection between health and perceptions of life in general. The underlying grounding theme recognized in every narrative of the study is described as follows: *The process of aging is a dynamic unity and harmony between internal and external landscapes that reflects lived values as individuals move forward with life.* Subthemes expressed in most of the interviews were (a) the value of hard work, (b) acceptance of life's uncertain challenges, (c) health, (d) faith in God, (e) the importance of independence and determination, and f) external landscapes. To understand the connections of the subthemes to the underlying grounding theme, "direct quotations are inserted as clarifying examples" (Reeder, 1991, p. 268). These quotations are listed for the reader so that the general tone of the entire sample can be appreciated.

Value of hard work:

I loved the homestead days—of course it was hard work, but then you done it for yourself, and things you do for yourself are never so heavy. Of course we worked hard; we were homesteaders, but what are we here for if we shouldn't do a little bit? You sure can't go around being dressed up all the time.

We had to work for things. I was brought up to work for things, and it didn't bother me. I worked hard all my life; I was just strong I guess; I just kept on a going. The harder I worked, the better I felt, and it made me strong. I suppose I wouldn't be here today if it wasn't for working hard and thinking hard, had to make the best of every day.

I think work keeps you young, so as long as you ain't sick keep it up, keep working. I went to work to make money for myself and to help the folks, it was pretty tough for the folks. It sure wasn't laziness that got me here.

Well, I'm almost 89, and the hard work didn't kill me. It was hard work, and sometimes you got real tired, but when the job was done, and you saw what happened, you could sit back and be glad that you had a part in making it a better place to live. There is no work now.

Well, it was some days work, and you never thought it was hard work because it was part of a day's work, and work never hurt anybody. We never thought about it being hard, that's the way everybody did. I'm glad I lived those days. They can talk about it, but we lived it, everyone of us, and we won't forget it. We Plains people are steadfast and have perseverence; we have an attitude for sticking and trying, a kind of sterlingness.

Acceptance of life's uncertain challenges:

Live each day to the fullest. If this is the last day, why then that's it. I don't want to think ahead, and I would hate to be a burden to anybody. Just keep an open mind.

You have to make the best of everything. When you get old you have to do it, that's all there is to it. I never dreamt I was going to be this old, but then we haven't got nothing with that to do, I guess. I go from day to day, and if something happens, it happens.

You lived and you worked and you kinda forgot about it. I guess we just lived and took it as it was, one day at a time. I am relaxed now like I say. You go from day to day, but if something happens, it happens. There are times when I feel really rotten, and I say I wonder if it is age, and I realize that I can't go on forever.

Health:

I'd think that if I had another go at this I'd try to take better care of myself, you know. Things are so easy now. You can just go to a dentist, and as far as education, I would try and better myself.

Well, my health isn't that good now because I can't walk very far now, walk or do much but I guess that I just go from day to day, and I don't worry like I used to. If something happens, it just happens, and you have to take things as they come.

I would have to say that I am content. I could be worse, I could be better, but I could be worse—you know we associate health with being absolutely disease free and having no kind of disability, and if you live long enough you are bound to get something, but you can still be content.

I think a lot of health is just your will power, you know what I mean, you just don't give up easy; I just don't fight it. I just live it and when the day is done, it is done. No use worrying about tomorrow because we really don't have any control anyway. You know, all at once we are gone, and so I live day-to-day and try not to worry and to see the funny side of things. That I suppose is my best feature. And I don't give up very easy either!

I say that I am healthy because I am not all crippled up; of course I walk with pain. You just get used to it and get on with life. Attitude is everything.

I feel like this—of course I have my aches and pains and a few problems but why bring it to somebody else who probably has enough of their own to worry about. You know, I was a homesteader, and I broke up most of my own land with a team of oxen. Now that was pain. So when I remember that pain I think heck, this is nothing.

I think that health means everything. You can have money, but money won't buy health, and health I think is being able to get around to do things that you like to do and do for yourself and not have to rely on somebody else.

I can remember when the family got that bad flu in 1918. We had to stay in the house, and the neighbors would come to do the chores, but they didn't come in the house. It was like being in jail, and now days you would just take a little pill. No pills in those days.

Faith in God:

I have a strong belief in God; it keeps me happy.

I think we (people who live in this town) have good values, moral values I mean.

Catholic, that is the only thing that really helps me is Catholic. If it weren't for my rosary and my holy water, I wouldn't be here today.

I have a lot of faith in people, that's what helps me is a lot of faith in people and God, and you are strong all over that way. I am a religious person and compassionate. I tried to live by the golden rule. I belong to the Methodist church, and I never miss a Sunday.

The importance of independence and determination:

I was nine when my mother died of pneumonia. In those days, they didn't have antibiotics, you know. I was the oldest of three children, so then I was in charge of things. I didn't get to finish up with school because there was too much work to be done at home.

I'm boss of myself. I have made 21 a couple of times, and nobody can tell me what to do, I'm free to do what I want to do.

I gotta come out of this cold cause nobody is gonna keep me down; I'm gonna get up and walk again. I try to get along on what I have, what I got is mine.

I loved it, even if it was hard work you done it for yourself, and things you do for yourself is never so heavy. If I worked for others, I should have thought I was a slave. We struggled and fought for a living like the rest of them. Well, I suppose it was because we wanted a home, it was our home we were working for, and that's the way it was for everybody. You hung on as long as you could.

Well, let's put it this way: we didn't want to give up. We worked and had to get along with little or nothing; we never thought about it, that's the way everybody had it. I can't remember that we ever complained or that we ever suffered any. I can't explain it; we had to do it you know, if we wanted to live, we had to do it and get it done.

I'm glad I lived those days, the hard days, because we got through with it, and everything went all right. It was hard, you know, but I still, it didn't hurt me, and we got to do many good things. I try not to depend on others too much and I try to take care of myself. What I have is mine—it isn't so fancy, but it is mine, but if I get sick I guess I have to depend on the insurance like everybody else.

External Landscapes:

Oh, I just love it out on the farm. I think of the freeness, the freshness of the air, the birds singing, and the open air is so beautiful, I can look out and see the Northern lights, see the sun rise, it's really neat.

Everybody grew up in the little three-room log cabins, Oh God, and I had them packed like sardines all over the floor, but they didn't mind. They had a roof over their heads, and that's all they cared.

Yes, they were hard, but even as old as I am now, I would go back again, over the same thing. I loved work, and I loved the Plains, too. I would go back to the farm anytime, anytime, anytime. It was hard, you know, because it seemed like the snow drifts always piled up around the barn, and hauling the water, that was hard too.

My dad and brother came out here, and they lived in a thrashing crew tent through the winter and built our house. You know, those old timers that come over here to homestead had a lot of guts to come out here; they didn't know what was out here or anything.

CONCLUSIONS

The different experiences of aging in the Northwestern Plains, as described by the participants in this study, are all closely connected to each other, and to the results of earlier research. While independence and self-care are very important qualities for the participants, their lives were so interdependent in the early years on the prairie that the stories all reflect the same underlying grounding theme. The process of aging for the participants of this study was and still is a dynamic, ever-changing unity and harmony between their internal landscapes and their external landscapes. Though they are no longer able to do the physical labor that was so important to them in their earlier lives, they are still very tied to the old values. The landscapes, both internal and external, have changed dramatically, yet they have managed to maintain their lived values and to move forward with life.

RESEARCH ISSUES

Results of this study can be generalized only to the participants in this study. The methodology chosen does not require a discussion of rigor, but to address that criteria, two factors discussed by Lincoln and Guba (1985) will be presented. These criteria are truth value and applicability.

Truth value is evaluated by how well threats to internal validity have been managed. In qualitative research, the truth value is an elusive goal but generally exists in the discovery of human phenomena as they are lived and perceived by the subjects. A qualitative study has truth value, or is credible, when it presents such faithful descriptions of a human experience that the people having the experience would immediately recognize it as their own.

A major threat to the truth value in a qualitative study lies in the closeness of the investigator-subject relationship or the threat of "going native." While the participants in this study were all acquainted with the researcher, the possibility of "going native" for the researcher was negligible because of the tremendous differences in life experiences between the participants and the researcher.

Applicability, or fittingness, is the second criterion for rigor. The aim of this naturalistic approach is not to generalize but to enable someone interested in making a transfer to reach a conclusion about whether transfer can be contemplated as a possibility (Lincoln & Guba, 1985). While the life experiences of these Northwesterners are unique to them, it may be that other homesteaders in other regions of the country experienced some, if not many, of the same hardships and triumphs. However, generalizing these findings to all homesteaders across the country is not appropriate.

NURSING PERSPECTIVE

Watson (1988) defines health as a unity and harmony within the mind, body, and soul associated with the degree of congruence between the self as perceived and the self as experienced. Roy (1989) states that human beings are dynamic, open systems that are continuously interacting with an ever-changing environment. Health, from Roy's perspective, is a dynamic process of being and becoming an integrated and whole person. Parse (1990) defines health as a complex process of living what is valued as one unfolds in an ever-increasing diversity. Human patterns reflect lived choices, as individuals move toward hopes and dreams in the process of becoming. My interest in discovering choices, hopes, and dreams of older persons living in the Northwest Plains led to my decision to explore their experiences of aging and health. The perceptions described within are a representation of the participants' internal and external environments, each perspective intricately spun from a combination of internal and external landscapes.

Nurses working in rural areas are reminded that rural residents are private, independent, and self-sufficient (Lee, 1993). Additionally, rural dwellers are usually thought to be hardy (Bigbee, 1991), possess a sense of connected independence (Brown, 1990), and describe health in a functional way (Weinert & Burman, 1994), such as the ability to do work (Weinert & Long, 1987). The stories provided here lend support to that research and provide nurses with an enhanced appreciation for the life-long experiences that have shaped each of their unique rural clients.

REFERENCES

Agar, M. H. (1980). *The professional stranger: An informal introduction to ethnography.* London: Academic Press.

Bigbee, J. (1991). The concept of hardiness as applied to rural nursing. In A. Bushy (Ed.), *Rural nursing* (Vol 1). Newbury Park, CA: Sage.

Brown, K. (1990). Connected independence: A paradox of rural health. *Journal of Rural Community Psychology, 11*(1), 51–64.

Chenitz, W. C., & Swanson, J. M. (1986). *From practice to grounded theory.* Menlo Park, CA: Addison-Wesley.

Field, P. A., & Morse, J. M. (1985) *Nursing research: The application of qualitative approaches.* Rockville, MD: Aspen.

Giorgi, A. (1970). *Psychology as a human science: A phenomenologically based approach.* New York: Harper & Row.

Lee, H. (1993). Health perceptions of middle, "new middle," and older rural adults. *Family and Community Health, 16,* 19–27.

Lincoln, Y. S., & Guba, E. G. (1985). *Naturalistic inquiry.* Newbury Park: Sage Publications.

Lopez, B. (1988). *Crossing open ground.* New York: Random House.

Morse, J. (1989). *Qualitative nursing research: A contemporary dialogue.* Rockville, Maryland: Aspen.

Munhall, P. L., & Oiler, C. J. (1986). *Nursing research: A qualitative perspective.* Norwalk, CT: Appleton-Century-Crafts.

Parse, R. R. (1990). Health: A personal commitment. *Nursing Science Quarterly, 3*(3), 136–140.

Parse, R. R., Cone, A. B., & Smith, M. J. (1985). *Nursing research: Qualitative methods.* Bowie, MD: Prentice-Hall.

Reeder, F. (1991). The importance of knowing what to care about: Phenomenological inquiry using laughing at oneself as a clue. In P. L. Chin (Ed.), *Anthology on caring.* New York: National League for Nursing.

Roy, C. (1989). An explication of the philosophical assumptions of the Roy adaptation model. *Nursing Science Quarterly, 2*(3), 26–34.

Swanson-Kauffman, K., & Schonwald, E. (1988). Phenomenology. In B. Sarter (Ed), *Paths to knowledge: Innovative research methods for nursing.* New York: National League for Nursing, p. 97.

Watson, J. (1988). *Nursing: Human science and human care.* New York: National League for Nursing.

Weinert, C., & Burman, M (1994). Rural health and health-seeking behaviors. In J. J. Fitzpatrick (Ed.), *Annual review of nursing research* (Vol. 12, pp. 65–92). New York: Springer.

Weinert, C., & Long, K. (1987). Understanding health care needs of rural families. *Family Relations, 36,* 450–455.

19

The Substantive Theory of Protecting Independence

Vonna Koehler

INTRODUCTION

As the end of the 20th century approaches, approximately 31 million people, constituting 13% of the U.S. population, are 65 years of age or older (Kapp & Bigot, 1985; Torres-Gil, 1992; U.S. Bureau of Census, 1989). U.S. Bureau of Census projections suggest that by the year 2050, the number of persons 65 years of age and older will number approximately 52 million and constitute 21.8% of the U.S. population (U.S. Bureau of Census, 1989).

RURAL ELDERS: A VULNERABLE POPULATION

The population of interest in this study was rural elders. Even though the majority of elderly persons reside in urban areas, there is a greater proportion of elderly living in rural areas (Cordes, 1989; Coward, McLaughlin, Duncan, & Bull, 1992; Glasgow, 1988). Recent data from the 1990 census revealed that 26% of the elderly population live in nonmetropolitan areas (U.S. Senate, Special Committee on Aging, 1992).

While the data are equivocal, the consensus still tends to be that, as a group, rural elders experience greater poverty, more chronic illness, poorer health, and substandard housing when compared to their urban counterparts (Bigbee, 1993; Bylund, 1985; Dwyer, Lee, & Coward, 1990; Glasgow, 1988; Krout, 1986; Lassey & Lassey, 1985; Palmore, 1983–84). Rural elders also tend to be more poorly educated, less adequately insured, and predominantly female (Bigbee, 1993).

Not all researchers agree that rural elders experience poorer health and more chronic illness than urban elders (Hassinger, 1982; Krout, 1989). Because of varying definitions of rural and the lack of sophisticated statistical analyses of data, Krout (1989) concluded that findings suggesting that rural elders are less healthy than urban elders are questionable. Krout and others (Dwyer et al., 1990) emphasized the need for further research to clarify differences between rural and urban elders on matters of health.

Rural America will continue to feel repercussions from the changing demographics of aging. This fact, along with spiraling health care costs, a huge federal budget deficit, resistance to revenue increases, and diminishing resources, leaves little doubt that the growing numbers of elders will have a major impact on the economic, political, social, and health care policies of urban and rural America well into the next century. Nurses working in rural areas will assume an even greater role in providing quality health care at reasonable cost in a variety of settings to increasing numbers of elders (Pickard, 1989).

RESEARCH QUESTIONS

A major research question guided this study: How do elders living in various locales of the sparsely populated, largely rural state of Montana manage their health care needs? Four subquestions derived from the major question were formulated to guide and focus the data collection.

(a) What behaviors do elders engage in to help them stay well and prevent illness?
(b) What actions do elders take to restore their health when they have an illness episode?
(c) Who are the persons elders rely upon when they require help managing their health care needs?
(d) What effect does geographic locale have on how elders manage their health care needs?

PLACING THE STUDY IN CONTEXT

The setting for this research project was the geographically large, sparsely populated, western state of Montana. The state, as a whole, has 5.5 persons per square mile. Twenty-four of the 56 counties in the state have fewer than 2.0 persons per square mile (U.S. Bureau of Census, 1992). Montana has at least three urban centers, Billings, Great Falls, and Missoula, which constitute the "big cities" of the state. However, 47% of the population of Montana live in communities of less than 2,500 inhabitants and are, therefore, considered rural by census definition (Cordes, 1989; Lee, 1991; Norton & McManus, 1989; U.S. Bureau of Census, 1992). Based on the population density of two to six persons per square mile, 45 of the 56 counties in Montana qualify for designation as the contemporary American frontier (Popper, 1986; U.S. Bureau of Census, 1992).

The very word frontier fosters an image, supported, in part, by Western folklore and history, of rugged individualism, independence, and self-reliance. This image, along with a low population density, more recent settlement patterns, and vast open spaces, are characteristics not shared by rural areas in other regions of the nation and may have contributed to attitudes and beliefs unique to the state of Montana.

Definition of Terms

For purposes of this study, the following definitions were used:

Urban. Urban was defined as a community with a population of 50,000 or greater. An urban community contains at least one hospital of 100 beds or more and has at least two medical clinics containing a variety of practicing physicians, including a full selection of medical specialists available for referral and consultation.

Rural. Rural was defined as a community with a population no larger than 10,000 located at least 15 miles away from a city with a population of 50,000 or greater. Rural communities have a local hospital of no more than 100 beds or a medical assistance facility. Rural communities have at least one practicing physician residing in the community. Small communities that do not have a local hospital, medical assistance facility, or resident physician but lie within a 15–to 39–mile radius of an adjacent urban community also were defined as rural.

Remote Rural. Remote rural was defined as a community with a population of 2,500 or less located 40 miles or further from a city with a population of 50,000 or greater. Remote rural communities do not have a hospital or a medical assistance facility. A practicing physician does not reside in a remote rural community.

Health Care Needs. Health care needs were broadly defined as any subjectively determined want, concern, issue, or condition arising within the context of promoting, maintaining, restoring, and managing one's own health or well-being.

METHOD

The design of the study was descriptive exploratory field research. Data were collected using semistructured interviews over a four-month time period. Data collection and analysis were guided by the grounded theory tenets of constant comparative analysis and theoretical sampling.

Working within a matrix in which data collection, analysis, and sampling were interactive and simultaneous, the investigator engaged in a labor intensive process of coding, categorizing, conceptualizing, and theorizing from the data with the aim of discovering the substantive theory that explicated most of the actions and processes found in the data. Memoing and diagramming were integrated into the analysis work and were helpful in identifying the core category and in relating the other categories to the core variable.

Sampling and Sampling Procedures

The number of participants included in the study were not specified a priori but were continuously selected to develop and saturate categories, a method which is consistent with the grounded theory tradition. Theoretical sampling, based on the emerging theory, directed sampling activities.

Inclusion criteria for study participants were (a) 65 years of age or older, (b) living in their own residence, (c) able to read, write, and speak English, and (d) cognitive alertness with no known history of disabling memory loss or confusion. Participants were recruited into the study from Senior Centers and networking or snowball sampling.

Participation in the study was voluntary, and all expected measures were taken to ensure protection of human rights. Participants were provided with a copy of the informed consent form, and, when possible, a second person witnessed the elder's signature on the consent form.

Demographic Characteristics of the Sample

A convenience sample of 30 elders participated in the study. All study participants were Anglo American. Minorities are under represented in this sample. Reasons for this include the convenience nature of the sample plus the generally small numbers of elder minority groups (other than Native Americans) in the state; this is particularly the case in rural and remote rural areas of Montana. Because of major cultural influences, Native American elders were not included in the sample.

The study participants ranged from 65 to 96 years of age, with a mean age of 75.4 years. The study participants included healthy (n = 18) and health-compromised elders (n = 12). The mean age of the healthy elders was 74.4 years and of the health-compromised elders was 77 years.

Healthy elders were those with no diagnosed illnesses, those who had experienced an illness from which they had fully recovered, or those who were living with a health condition that was well controlled (e.g., hypertension or diabetes). Healthy elders infrequently experienced illness episodes, saw themselves as healthy, and rated their health high on a scale of 0 to 10 ($M = 8.7$).

Health-compromised elders were those who had often experienced ongoing or multiple illness episodes within the past 5 to 10 years of their lives. On a scale of 0 to 10, health-compromised elders consistently rated their health lower ($M = 5.8$) than healthy elders and attributed the lower rating to ongoing or multiple illness episodes.

Rural elders had access to primary medical care in their communities but, depending on residence, might have to travel up to 200 or more miles to access any type of specialized medical care. Remote rural elders had no medical services in their communities and had to travel a minimum of 40 miles to receive any type of medical care. Again, depending on their residence, remote rural elders might have to travel up to 200 or more miles to receive any type of specialized medical care.

Urban elders had access to primary and specialized medical care in their communities and did not face traveling more than a few miles to access either. Not surprisingly, rural and remote rural elders in the study were more likely to be impacted by issues related to distance and resources than were urban elders in the study. Although the study sample was comprised of healthy and health-compromised elders, all elders in the study were currently capable of caring for themselves and considered themselves independent.

ISSUES OF CREDIBILITY

The appropriate way to judge the rigor of qualitative research is to use criteria that fit that naturalistic paradigm (Chenitz & Swanson, 1986; Lincoln & Guba, 1985; Sandelowski, 1986; Strauss & Corbin, 1990). The following measures were taken to ensure the rigor of the present study:

(a) Peer debriefing sessions—Throughout the study, the investigator sought out peers with and without experience or expertise in the method and exposed her thinking and writing for critique and feedback. This procedure provided an opportunity during which the working hypotheses, interpretations, biases, and feelings could be examined, challenged, and discussed.

(b) Triangulation of data sources through use of dictated field notes and transcribed interviews—Even though the primary source of data for the study was the semistructured interview, a conscious effort to be observant of the participants and their environment was made during the data collection experience. Observations deemed important or additive to the interview were dictated following the interviews and were preserved for referral during analysis.

(c) Informal and formal member checking—During the process of data collection and analysis, the investigator engaged in sharing key ideas gleaned from the data with subsequent study participants in an attempt to seek validation or to solicit variation. Once the substantive theory was written and the analytic diagram was finalized, the investigator met with selected participants to determine if the theory had fit, made sense, and seemed credible to the elders themselves.

(d) Creation of an audit trail by which dependability and confirmability could be assessed—Audit materials were preserved, including raw data, coding notes, lists detailing numerous categories developed from codes, numerous memos, working analytic schemes, and a personal journal reflecting thoughts, ideas, concerns, and feelings of the investigator during the experience.

THE SUBSTANTIVE THEORY OF PROTECTING INDEPENDENCE

Protecting independence is the core variable to emerge from the study. The analytic diagram that depicts the substantive theory of protecting independence is shown in Figure 19.1.

Protecting independence is defined as those health-related strategies and tactics taken by elders in the study for the ultimate purpose of guarding, sustaining, and supporting their autonomy, thereby reducing the possibility of losing independence and the potential changes associated with that eventuality. Elders in the study valued their independence and wished to protect it. The following comment from an elderly woman was typical of the thinking the elders expressed about independence:

> *Children sometimes mistakenly attempt to drag their parents into a protected situation. My son does that every once in a while. I tell him, "Back off. I'm getting in a corner, and I'm getting mad." But many times young people with the best intentions overprotect their parent and especially the men. A woman most of the time doesn't get overprotected so easily, but men are killed frequently just simply by being overprotected.*

The themes of independence and dependence are major issues for people across the entire age span. The literature on elders makes the assumption that independence is a universally held value and, therefore, a value of the elderly population as well. This assumption, along with assertions that declining health increases the likelihood for loss of independence, are prevalent themes in much of the literature on urban and rural elders (Davis et al., 1991; Ebersole & Hess, 1994; Hamdorf, Withers, Penhall, & Haslam, 1992; Kohler, 1990; Padula,

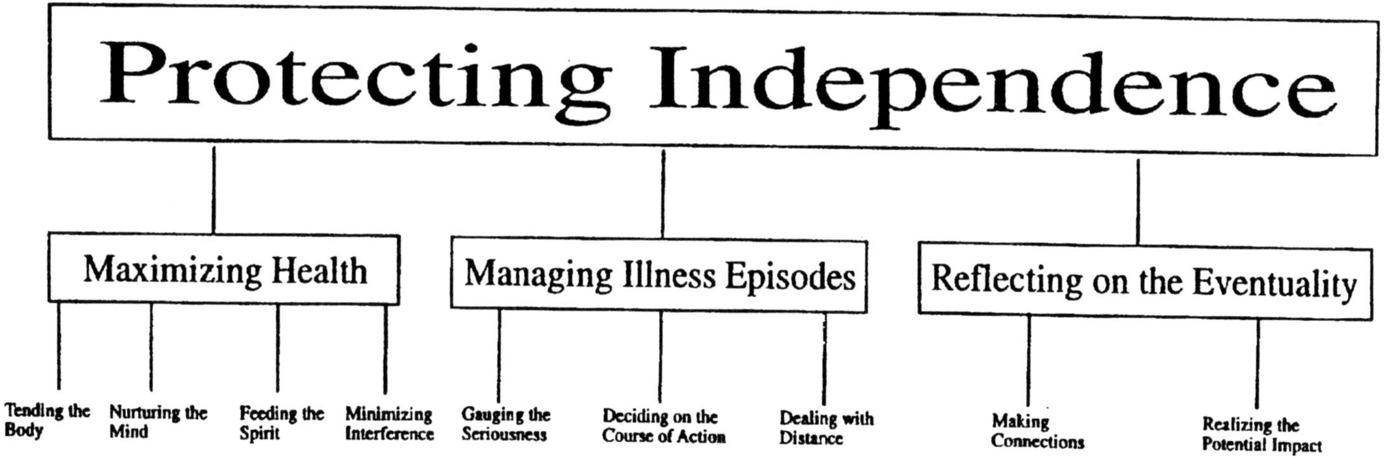

FIGURE 19.1 Substantive theory of protecting independence

1992; Schank & Lough, 1989, 1990; Shepard, 1993; Wold, 1993). The data from this study lend support to these ideas.

The three major properties of protecting independence are *maximizing health, managing illness episodes,* and *reflecting on the eventuality.* These properties of protecting independence, hereafter referred to as strategies, were influenced by and varied with health status, tolerance levels, and resources of healthy and health-compromised elders in the study. The following discussion explicates the strategies and tactics used by the elders in managing their health care needs.

Maximizing Health

Maximizing health is an holistic strategy comprised of the tactics of tending the body, nurturing the mind, feeding the spirit, and minimizing interference. Maximizing health is defined as actions taken by elders that were intended to augment and support their current health status. When discussing maximizing health, the elders acknowledged that all parts of a person's being affect health; therefore, the elders approached maximizing health from an holistic perspective as explicitly described by a 71–year-old man:

> *I think we're all one ball of wax, you might say. But I think we are composed of spirit, mind, and body. If the spiritual health is good, the odds are the mental health is going to be fine; in turn, if those two are in good shape, the body has no choice but to thrive and maintain its vitality and so on.*

Actions associated with the tactic of tending the body included obtaining exercise by being physically active, eating a well balanced and varied diet, being compliant with medical advice, and taking prescribed medications. None of the elders in the study, with the exception of one person, engaged in smoking. All but one elder reported seldom or never drinking alcohol.

Healthy and health-compromised elders in the study reported that being physically active and obtaining some type of exercise was important for staying well or preventing deterioration of current health status, thereby protecting independence. Variation was found in how elders tolerated physical activity or exercise, with the condition of tolerance being a deciding factor.

For healthy elders, tending the body through physical activity was easier to accomplish. Their activity levels were noticeably greater than those of health-compromised elders. Healthy elders were often quite vigorous physically and expressed pride in their physical prowess. When asked to what he attributed his health, a 79–year-old man who had been working cattle and riding horseback all day proudly stated:

> *Well, I think my eating habits, my exercise habits, and always being out as much as possible. I think that contributes to most of it. It's just like today, how many people do you know that are 79 years old and get up and ride a horse all day long? And come in like I am now. You don't see that I'm all in.*

Health-compromised elders in the study tended to have less tolerance and stamina for physical activity related to ongoing or multiple illness episodes. Health-compromised elders were generally older than healthy elders, but age in and of itself was not as important as health status in affecting the elders' tolerance levels for physical activity. Even though health-compromised elders experienced decreased tolerance to activity, they were still committed to engaging in some type of exercise as an important aspect of tending the body. For example, an 83–year-old retired rancher explained it this way:

> *My leg had been injured, my knee here [pointing to an area] one time, and that accounts for a lot of it. It makes me limp. . . . I can't go very far, but I did help with the branding and the vaccinating on the cattle here last month.*

Health-compromised elders in the study who had to ration their physical activity according to tolerance expressed varying degrees of dismay and frustration at the loss of stamina.

Fewer than five elders in the study engaged in a planned or regular exercise routine. In general, the study participants believed they were obtaining adequate amounts of exercise by doing housework, yard work, gardening, and staying physically busy.

In addition to physical activity, all elders in the study acknowledged the importance of eating a well balanced diet as part of tending the body. Most elders made a conscious effort to follow good dietary practices because they believed it was generally better for their health. Healthy and health-compromised elders reported eating reduced amounts of fat, meat, and salt, and increased amounts of fruits and vegetables as part of their dietary behavior as they grew older. However, the elders did not describe counting calories and fat grams or calculating food intake in any rigid manner, but described approaching diet using the guideline of moderation.

For many elders in the study, tending the body also involved being compliant with medical advice and taking prescribed medications. These actions were seen as ways for maximizing health and perhaps warding off an illness episode:

> *I have to take [pills] for my heart and then, of course, now one of those pills is a vitamin, and one is an aspirin. These three water pills and I take Minoxin. Oh, I hate it, but if I don't, I'm in trouble . . . but no, I wouldn't quit without the doctor saying I should.*

Actions associated with the tactic of nurturing the mind included staying mentally sharp by reading, working crossword puzzles, keeping abreast of social and political events, and maintaining a positive attitude:

> *I think that life is a great deal of attitude, and apparently I have the right attitude. I don't have the right habits altogether, but the body seems pleased with even my habits.*

Actions for the tactic of feeding the spirit included attending to emotional and spiritual needs by going to church, praying, helping others, and engaging in altruistic deeds.

In order to maximize health, some elders in the study also engaged in the tactic of minimizing interference. Elders who were minimizing interference generally were healthy and had experienced few illness episodes. These elders believed that, in addition to the tactics of tending the body, nurturing the mind, and feeding the spirit, their health status was augmented and sustained by avoiding unnecessary medical care or intervention:

> *Well, to me, I can have aches and pains, but that doesn't mean that I run to the doctor all the time. In fact, I haven't been to the doctor as such in several years now.*

Elders engaging in minimizing interference would see a physician only if it was deemed necessary. In general, elders engaged in minimizing interference did not have regular physician contact for common preventive care such as yearly physical examinations and flu or pneumonia shots. Elders who were minimizing interference displayed a high value for independence, wanted to maintain control over their health care, and reported trusting their ability to listen to and interpret body signals that would indicate dysfunction. While health status did not impact the elders' abilities to engage in nurturing the mind and feeding the spirit (both healthy and health-compromised elders engaged in these tactics equally), health status seemed to impact the practice of minimizing interference because this tactic most often was employed by healthy elders.

Overall, the data from the study participants suggested that, regardless of locale, the elders were knowledgeable about commonly advocated health behaviors such as obtaining exercise, eating a balanced and varied diet, not smoking or abusing alcohol, and attending to mental and spiritual needs. From the elders' perspective, however, this interest in, and commitment to, good health behaviors did not translate into adherence to a tightly controlled diet or a regularly scheduled exercise routine. The elders' tactics for maximizing health were implemented within what was realistic and achievable for them within the context of their life situations using moderation as their guideline. The elders in the study did not describe themselves as having any unhealthy habits and discussed the tactics of tending the body, nurturing the mind, feeding the spirit, and minimizing interference as augmenting and sustaining their health status, which, in turn, protected independence.

Managing Illness Episodes

The second major strategy of protecting independence is *managing illness episodes,* and it encompassed actions taken by elders for the purpose of assessing and controlling the episode, thereby preventing or reducing the threat to independence. For healthy and health-compromised elders in the study, managing illness episodes was comprised of the tactics *gauging the seriousness* of an episode, *deciding on the course of action* for an episode, and for rural and remote rural elders, *dealing with distance.* These tactics were often interactive and overlapping rather than sequential in timing.

Gauging the seriousness of an illness episode is influenced by the following conditions: how familiar or unfamiliar the elder is with the symptoms experienced; whether or not the elder believes the symptoms suggested progression, exacerbation, or reoccurrence of an illness; and whether or not the symptoms were acute, multiple, or unrelenting in nature. The dimension of time also was important in gauging the seriousness of an illness episode, with episodes of duration longer than five days more likely gauged as serious:

> *"I didn't think I was that sick, and I thought, Well, if I don't get over this in three days, then it would be time to call the doctor."*

Deciding on the course of action for an illness episode varied with the seriousness of an episode and the elder's health status. Illness episodes gauged as not serious were self-limiting in nature; were recognized as common ailments; and usually were managed by self-care practices such as rest, fluids, over-the-counter medications, self-monitoring, and, occasionally, use of home remedies. Only five elders reported even infrequent use of home remedies; these folks happened to be rural or remote rural elders. In view of the fact that two-thirds of the sample were comprised of rural and remote rural elders, the lack of familiarity with, or use of, home remedies was somewhat surprising. It may be that use of home remedies is more associated with rural elders living in different areas of the United States such as the South or Appalachia. Or perhaps the idea of use of home remedies is more of a stereotype than a reality about rural elders.

During gauging the serious of an illness episode and when deciding on the course of action, elders reported informally consulting with family members or, less often, friends or neighbors regarding the illness episode:

> *And my neighbor, I'm usually running over to her if I have something really, it seems like really major. . . . I don't know, she just has a gift of diagnosing, so if it's something really strange, I'll ask her about it.*

The role of informal consulting was one of discussion about the illness episode and did not involve direct caregiving activities, which may have been because the elders in the study were still capable of independent self-care. When asked, the majority of the elders in the study reported that should they became ill and need a caregiver, they preferred that the caregiver be a family member. Married elders, regardless of gender, expected their spouses to act in the caregiver role if needed. Participants living alone realized that family members might not be available to act as caregiver for them.

The elders in this study overwhelmingly preferred physicians for formal health care providers. This desire can be attributed to the elders' unwillingness to change (inexperience with alternative providers such as nurse practitioners or physician assistants), and a belief that physicians are the most prepared and knowledgeable health care providers.

When gauging and deciding, health-compromised elders were more likely to seek medical care earlier than healthy elders did. Reasons for this behavior were continued and ongoing contact with a physician, which made it convenient to seek physician care, plus a sense of heightened vulnerability related to ongoing or multiple illness episodes. All elders in the study, however, reported they would not hesitate to seek medical care early if they gauged their illness episode as serious.

With the exception of those elders who engaged in minimizing interference, the elders in this study did not express hesitancy about making physician visits. The health-compromised elders in this study reported a tendency to rely heavily on medical advice, care, and intervention in the event of an illness episode. In fact, when traveling, some of the health-compromised elders in the study preferred staying only in towns where they could quickly access medical care in the event of an illness episode. Further, healthy elders who were living with a controlled condition or who had fully recovered from a serious illness episode also tended to see physicians on a regular basis for preventive care and monitoring.

For rural and remote rural elders, managing an illness episode included the tactic of dealing with distance. In general, rural and remote rural elders discussed distance more as an inconvenience than a problem. Remote rural elders acknowledged that, for them, distance could be life threatening in an emergent situation, but remote rural elders did not worry about this unduly and accepted distance as a fact of rural life.

> *Well, I suppose a person could lose his life because he wasn't in town, if he had a heart attack or something, but it's just a way of life, and that's something you accept.*

The literature frequently reports transportation as a major problem for rural elders (Coward & Cutler, 1989; Helping the rural elderly, 1983; Krout, 1986; U.S. Congress, Office of Technology Assessment, 1990; Windley, 1983). The rural and remote elders in this study did not discuss transportation as a major problem and believed they could always find family or friends who would transport them for needed health care services. Rural and remote rural elders in this study were accustomed to living with distance and accepted it as a way of life associated with living in a geographically large, sparsely populated area such as Montana. However, it seemed reasonable to speculate that transportation problems for the study participants could potentially arise with deterioration in health status or advancing age.

Reflecting on the Eventuality

The final strategy for protecting independence is *reflecting on the eventuality. Reflecting on the eventuality* is defined as contemplating the relationship between health status and independence and is comprised of the tactics of *making connections* and *realizing the potential impact* that losing independence would have on one's lifestyle. Even though all the elders in the study currently were capable of and actively engaged in protecting independence, they identified losing independence as their major health-related concern.

Because of ongoing or multiple illness episodes, health-compromised elders in the study were more vulnerable to loss of independence than healthy elders. Health-compromised elders were aware of the relationship between their health status and the potential loss of independence. Healthy elders, although acknowledging that they were not invincible, did not feel the same degree of vulnerability for losing independence as health-compromised elders because they were in good health.

All elders in this study realized the potential impact that losing independence would have on their lives. Loss of independence might mean moving, selling the farm or ranch, entering a retirement home, or, even worse, a nursing home. The group at risk for greatest change related to losing independence was remote rural elders. Loss of independence for remote rural elders would have a significant impact on their lifestyles, owing to lack of accessible medical services or resources within rural areas:

> *Well, yeah, if something happened to us we'd have to either move to Laurel or Billings, get closer to our daughter down there or something, you know, to get by. . . . People that can't take care of themselves don't stay out in small communities.*

Even though there are no guarantees, urban elders and elders living in small rural communities with available services would be in a better position than remote rural elders to protect their independence and to delay the loss of it.

As the numbers of rural elders continue to increase and readily available resources for meeting their needs continue to decrease, it seems likely that protecting, sustaining, and supporting the independence of elderly citizens will become even more important. The reasons for protecting the independence of elderly persons should not be based solely on concerns about the costs or burden placed on society in providing services for dependent elders. Independence enhances not only the quality of life for the elder but for society as well. Prolonging and protecting independence will enable elders to make important contributions by sharing their wisdom, intelligence, experience, productivity, and stability in a time when the nation is in need of these contributions.

LIMITATIONS

The findings of the study are context bound and are not meant to be generalizable to other groups of rural elders. However, the substantive theory of protecting independence, while considered context bound to this sample of Montana elders, might be applicable in other settings with other elders, although future research is needed to determine if this is the case.

IMPLICATIONS

For Practice

The literature on health promotion and disease prevention behaviors of rural elders reports varying degrees of interest in, and practice of, health promotion and disease prevention behaviors. Evidence exists that rural elders are interested in health promotion and disease prevention behaviors (Bender & Hart, 1987; Holcomb, 1988; Riffle, Yoho, & Sams, 1989; Volden, Langemo, Adamson, & Oechsle, 1990). Data from the present study indicated that healthy and health-compromised elders were aware of, valued, and engaged in strategies and tactics for promoting and sustaining health with the goal of protecting their independence. While the development and implementation of health-promotion and disease-prevention programs for all elders, including rural elders, are recommended (Bender & Hart, 1987; Burnside, 1988; Ebersole & Hess, 1994; Johnson, 1991; Mockenhaupt & Muchow, 1994; Speake, Cowart, & Stephens, 1991; Wilson, Patterson, & Alford, 1989; Work, 1989), sensitivity to the views of rural elders and careful community planning can minimize and even overcome many of the barriers and challenges to developing healthy aging programs for elders in rural communities.

Rural elders do not understand the role or scope of services that nurses are capable of providing to them. Nurses need to work with other health care professionals and with rural elders themselves in order to create and establish acceptance and understanding of a nurse provider role in promoting healthy aging.

For Education

Nurse educators who live and work in largely rural states such as Montana have an interest in, and responsibility for, incorporating rural nursing into the learning experiences of students who will practice in rural hospitals and nursing homes. Theoretical and clinical learning experiences can be planned that allow undergraduate and graduate students the opportunity to focus on rural populations and rural elders, in particular.

Nurse educators could develop and present distance education programs for nurses working in small rural hospitals and nursing homes and, in conjunction with practicing rural nurses, can positively influence the knowledge and contribution that professional nurses can make in the quality of care available to all rural residents, including rural elders.

For Research

Further study is needed to uncover the impact that place of residence, health status, gender, age, values, attitudes, and health beliefs have on the strategies and tactics of protecting independence. It also would be useful to determine the quantity, quality, and types of services available to rural elders and what, if any, affect available services have on protecting independence? The data are scant and inadequate at this time.

Little, if any, information is known about the stressors and problems facing caregivers of rural and remote rural elders who need assistance or are dependent. Who are the caregivers for rural and remote rural elders? Is it predominantly wives and daughters as would typically be expected? What impact does lack of support services or, in many cases, of any type of service have on caregivers of rural and remote rural elders?

There is no doubt that the need for knowledge about the health care needs of rural elders will continue to grow. Nurse researchers living in areas with large proportions of rural elders can gear their work to the goals of promoting healthy aging, thereby assisting elders with sustaining and protecting their independence.

REFERENCES

Bender, C., & Hart, J. P. (1987). A model for health promotion for the rural elderly. *The Gerontologist, 27* (2), 139–142.

Bigbee, J. (1993). The uniqueness of rural nursing. *Nursing Clinics of North America, 28* (1), 131–144.

Burnside, I. M. (1988). Demography of the aged. In I. M. Burnside (Ed.), *Nursing and the aged: A self-care approach* (pp. 4–38). New York: McGraw-Hill.

Bylund, R. A. (1985). Rural housing: Perspectives for the aged. In R. T. Coward & G. R. Lee (Eds.), *The elderly in rural society: Every fourth elder* (pp.129–150). New York: Springer.

Chenitz, W. C., & Swanson, J. M. (1986). Qualitative research using grounded theory method. In W. C. Chenitz & J. M. Swanson (Eds.), *From practice to grounded theory: Qualitative research in nursing* (pp. 3–15). Menlo Park, CA: Addison-Wesley.

Cordes, S. M. (1989). The changing rural environment and the relationship between health services and rural development. *Health Services Research, 23* (6), 757–784.

Coward, R. T., & Cutler, S. J. (1989). Informal and formal health care systems for the rural elderly. *Health Services Research, 23* (6), 785–806.

Coward, R. T., McLaughlin, D. K., Duncan, R. P., & Bull, C. N. (1992, September 13–15). *An overview of health and aging in rural America.* Paper presented at Health and Aging in Rural America: A National Symposium, San Diego, CA.

Davis, D. C., Henderson, M. C., Boothe, A., Douglass, M., Faria, S., Kennedy, D., Kitchens, E., & Weaver, M. (1991). An interactive perspective on the health beliefs and practices of rural elders. *Journal of Gerontological Nursing, 17* (5), 11–16.

Dwyer, J. W., Lee, G. R., & Coward, R. T. (1990). The health status, health services utilization and support networks of the rural elderly: A decade review. *The Journal of Rural Health, 6* (4), 379–398.

Ebersole, P., & Hess, P. (1994). *Toward healthy aging: Human needs and nursing response.* St. Louis, MO: Mosby.

Glasgow, N. (1988). *The nonmetro elderly: Economic and demographic status.* Springfield, VA: National Technical Information Service. (ERIC Document Reproduction Service No. ED 303296)

Hamdorf, P. A., Withers, R. T., Penhall, R. K., & Haslam, M. V. (1992). Physical training effects on the fitness and habitual activity patterns of elderly women. *Archives of Physical Medicine and Rehabilitation, 73* (7), 603–608.

Hassinger, E. W. (1982). *Rural health organization: Social networks and regionalization.* Ames: Iowa State University Press.

Helping the rural elderly. (1983). *Journal of Gerontological Nursing, 10* (3), 105–109.

Holcomb, C. A. (1988). Age differences in personal health practices of rural women. *Psychological Reports, 62,* 794.

Johnson, J. E. (1991). Health care practices of the rural aged. *Journal of Gerontological Nursing, 17* (8), 15–19.

Kapp, M. B., & Bigot, A. (1985). *Geriatrics and the law: Patients' rights and professional responsibilities.* New York: Springer.

Kohler, P. A. (1990). Nursing model of care promotes elderly independence. *Nursing Forum, 25* (4), 5–9.

Krout, J. A. (1986). *The aged in rural America.* New York: Greenwood Press.

Krout, J. A. (1989). Rural versus urban differences in health dependence among the elderly populations. *International Journal of Aging and Human Development, 28* (2), 141–156.

Lassey, W. R., & Lassey, M. L. (1985). The physical health status of the rural elderly. In R. T. Coward & G. R. Lee (Eds.), *The elderly in rural society: Every fourth elder* (pp. 83–104). New York: Springer.

Lee, H. J. (1991). Definitions of rural: A review of the literature. In A. Bushy (Ed.), *Rural nursing* (Vol. 1, pp. 7–20). Newbury Park, CA: Sage.

Lincoln, Y. S., & Guba, E. G. (1985). *Naturalistic inquiry.* Newbury Park, CA: Sage.

Mockenhaupt, R. E., & Muchow, J. A. (1994). Disease and disability prevention and health promotion for rural elders. In J. A. Krout (Ed.),

Providing community based services to the rural elderly (pp. 183–201). Newbury Park, CA: Sage.

Norton, C. H., & McManus, M. A. (1989). Background tables on demographic characteristics, health status, and health services utilization. *Health Services Research, 23* (6), 725–756.

Padula, C. A. (1992). Self care and the elderly: Review and implications. *Public Health Nursing, 9* (1), 22–28.

Palmore, E. (1983–84). Health care needs of the rural elderly. *International Journal of Aging and Human Development, 18* (1), 39–45.

Pickard, M. R. (1989). Education of nurses for rural practice. *The Journal of Rural Health, 6* (4), 527–533.

Popper, F. J. (1986). The strange case of the contemporary American frontier. *Yale Review, 76* (1), 101–121.

Riffle, K. L., Yoho, J., & Sams, J. (1989). Health-promoting behaviors, perceived support, and self-reported health of Appalachian elderly. *Public Health Nursing, 6* (4), 204–211.

Sandelowski, M. (1986). The problem of rigor in qualitative research. *Advances in Nursing Science, 8* (3), 27–37.

Schank, M. J., & Lough, M. A. (1989). Maintaining health and independence. *Journal of Gerontological Nursing, 15* (6), 8–11.

Schank, M. J., & Lough, M. A. (1990). Profile: Frail elderly women, maintaining independence. *Journal of Advanced Nursing, 15* (6), 674–682.

Shepard, R. J. (1993). Exercise and aging: Extending independence in older adults. *Geriatrics, 48* (5), 61–64.

Speake, D. L., Cowart, M. E., & Stephens, R. (1991). Healthy lifestyle practices of rural and urban elderly. *Health Values, 15* (1), 45–51.

Strauss, A., & Corbin, J. (1990). *Basics of qualitative research: Grounded theory procedure and techniques.* Newbury Park, CA: Sage.

Torres-Gil, F. M. (1992). *The new aging: Politics and change in America.* New York: Auburn House.

U.S. Bureau of Census. (1989). *Current population reports, series P-25, No. 1022, United States population estimates by age, sex, and race 1988–2080.* Washington, DC: U.S. Department of Commerce.

U.S. Bureau of Census. (1992). *Montana 1990 census of population.* Washington, DC: U.S. Department of Commerce.

U.S. Congress, Office of Technology Assessment. (1990). *Health care in rural America* (OTA-H-434). Washington, DC: U.S. Government Printing Office.

U.S. Senate, Special Committee on Aging. (1992). *Common beliefs about the rural elderly: Myth or fact?* Washington, DC: U.S. Government Printing Office.

Volden, C., Langemo, D., Adamson, M., & Oechsle, L. (1990). The relationship of age, gender, and exercise practices to measures of health, lifestyle, and self-esteem. *Applied Nursing Research, 3* (1), 20–26.

Wilson, R. W., Patterson, M. A., & Alford, D. M. (1989). Services for maintaining independence. *Journal of Gerontological Nursing, 15* (6), 31–37.

Windley, P. G. (1983). Community services in small rural towns: Patterns of use by older residents. *The Gerontologist, 23* (2), 180–184.

Wold, G. (1993). *Basic geriatric nursing.* St. Louis, MO: Mosby.

Work, J. A. (1989). Strength training: A bridge to independence for the elderly. *Physician and Sportsmedicine, 17* (11), 134–136, 138, 140.

20

The Lived Experience of Hardiness in Rural Men and Women

Ellen F. Wirtz, Helen J. Lee, and Alice Running

INTRODUCTION

"Hardiness" was originally used in agriculture to describe plants and animals that survived despite adverse growing conditions (Lee, 1983). Occasionally, the term was used in frontier historical literature to depict rugged individuals who survived in challenging circumstances. In 1977, Kobasa, a social psychologist, used the term to identify study subjects who remained well despite experiencing life event stress equivalent to those who became ill. Her subjects were middle management executives in urban electrical companies. She detected the quality of hardiness using a large battery of instruments and determined the differences statistically between the two groups. She said that the hardy subjects possessed three qualities concerning their life circumstances: challenge, commitment, and control. These hardy individuals "view change as a challenge rather than a threat, . . . feel committed to the various areas in their lives, (and) . . . feel they have control over events in their lives" (Kobasa, 1979, p. 3).

The identification of hardiness and the availability of an instrument measuring the characteristic led to a plethora of quantitative studies measuring the variable and its relationship to an assortment of variables. Then, articles began appearing that urged caution about the measurement of hardiness and its relationship to theoretical models (Funk & Houston, 1987; Hull, Van Treuren, & Virnelli, 1987; Jennings & Staggers, 1994; Lambert & Lambert, 1987; Tartasky, 1993; Wagnild & Young, 1991). Jennings and Staggers (1994) voiced the opinion, "For such a enigmatic construct, it may be more beneficial to observe hardy subjects and allow their characteristics to drive scale selection" (p. 280). They recommended that "using qualitative approaches to conceptualize this elusive construct may be useful in differentiating hardiness from competing constructs" (p. 280).

RESEARCH QUESTION

About the same time that Jennings and Staggers (1994) were recommending the use of qualitative studies to study hardiness, the first author of this chapter (Wirtz), a graduate student enrolled in the rural nursing generalist program at Montana State University-Bozeman, was preparing to conduct a qualitative study focusing on hardiness with rural men. She selected this population because she pictured rural men as the embodiment of hardiness (Wirtz, 1996). She asked these men this question: What is the lived experience of being a hardy individual? One of her early findings was that these rural men described their wives and mothers as hardy individuals. Therefore, a second study using a sample of these rural women was conducted by the second author of this chapter (Lee). Reported in this chapter are the results of the two studies by each author followed by a commentary about the differing findings by the third author (Running).

NURSING PERSPECTIVE

Parse's (1981) nursing theory of human becoming was used as the framework for this study:

> *Theory creates a unity of meaning different from the individuals' words as they stand alone. . . . The combined words make it clear that human health is an ongoing process of participation with the world. The theory of human becoming is a unitary phenomenon that refers to the person's becoming through cocreating rhythmical patterns of relating as energy is exchanged*

> *with the environment, becoming an open process, experienced by the human, and becoming is human unfolding. (p. 11, 25)*

This theory supports the worth of the human experience as unique and invaluable to the understanding of humankind.

For this research, the meaning of hardiness is viewed as similar to Parse's (1981) phenomenon of health. The authors of this chapter believe that the characteristic of hardiness is developed through the process of human becoming. As with health, hardiness evolves in persons because of the rhythmic patterns created by connecting with and separating from the rural environment in their day-to-day lived experience. The development of hardiness is "as synthesis of values, a way of living" (Parse, 1981, p. 39).

Persons' definitions of a construct at any particular time are important to their perception of themselves and the world around them. Use of Parse's theory helps in

> *illuminating meaning; shedding light through the uncovering of the meaning of the past, present, and future . . . as clients talk about their meanings, the communicating of the impressions, thoughts, and feelings changes the meanings, making them more clear and explicit (Bunting, 1993, p. 25).*

This theoretical perspective enhances understanding of the lived experience; biological manifestations are not ignored but are subsumed within the experience of the person (Cody & Mitchell, 1992).

METHOD

A qualitative descriptive design, specifically phenomenology, was chosen to describe the essence of hardiness in rural-dwelling men. "Phenomenology attempts to understand the human experience through analysis of the participant's description . . . phenomenology attempts to understand the basic structures of phenomenon as humanly experienced" (Woods & Catanzaro, p. 134). Data analysis was accomplished by use of a series of steps: Colaizzi's (1978) process for Study One and Giorgi's (1985) method for Study Two. Both Colaizzi and Giorgi employ a similar series of steps: a) the original interviews are divided into units, b) the units are transformed into meanings expressed in psychological and phenomenological concepts, and c) the transformations are linked together to make a general description of the experience (Polkinghorne, 1989).

STUDY ONE-RURAL MEN

Sample

A purposive sample was used for Study One (N=6). Men identified as "hardy" by their family and friends and who lived in rural areas of Montana were contacted to participate in the study. Additional participants were solicited from these first men, creating a snowballing effect of gathering participants. The mean age of the participants was 66 years, and the mean years of education for the participants was 14 years. The nearest community to these men ranged from 0 to 28 miles; the size of the nearest community ranged from 23 to 25,000 residents.

Findings

Using Colaizzi's (1978) seven step reduction process, meaningful statements were extracted from the text of the interviews. These meaningful statements were clustered, and the result was five reoccurring themes in these men's experiences. These themes frequently overlapped and intertwined, but as the data were reduced, distinct themes did emerge. The themes were (a) **adaptability**, the ability to change and adjust to what life offered; (b) **positive attitude**, the ability to see opportunity and challenge in life circumstances rather than threat; (c) **endurance**, the ability to remain firm, steady, determined, or committed to something in life; (d) **learned experience** of being hardy, being mentored or observing others, primarily parents depicting hardiness; consequently leading to (e) **lived experience** of being hardy through individual life circumstances and experiences, of doing what needed to be done.

Each participant in this study equated **adaptability** or the ability with which to adjust to being hardy. Fred stated it this way:

In general, throughout their life, if people are hardy, they are going to be more flexible . . . adaptability makes them more hardy . . . it is a mind set of looking for how you can do something rather than making excuses for what you can't . . . it's an 'I can' sort of attitude, and I just haven't figured it out yet.

In another example, Carl did his own improvising:

You tend to do other things to try to help yourself. I converted some older buildings here because I didn't have the cash to build new ones . . . it's nothing fancy, it's strictly chain-saw carpentry, but it's functional.

A **positive attitude**, the ability to see opportunity in life situations, was another repetitive theme throughout each interview. This attitude was described in just a few words by Fred:

You can say that something looks tough to do, but then you look at it long enough and think about it long enough and decide, well I'm gonna try it, and generally you will get it done; it's all a matter of wanting to. You have to be positive all the time.

The attitude of each participant in this research study was vividly positive.

Another of the five emergent themes was **endurance** or the ability to remain firm, steady, or committed to something in one's life. These men primarily said that their commitment was to their family or their farm/ranch. Fred implied that he remained firm to the family and the farm:

When you have kids in college at the same time and you wonder, "How am I going to get through?" but we made it . . . if you don't believe in yourself, what do you believe in? Every time they (hardy people) get knocked down, they tend to get back up; not that they don't get knocked down, they keep on keeping on.

Learned experience, or learning by example, was a theme that emerged from the interviews. The men participating in this study identified one or both parents as mentoring or modeling hardiness as the men know and live it. Allan said,

Hardiness goes to my heritage . . . I am only two generations removed from the sod, the old country. I know a lot about the history of the family . . . I am a product of what I picked and chose from them . . . especially my

mother, she demonstrated the ability to do with very little material goods, demonstrated how to live with quality, a quality life. Others I used as examples overcame great hardship and adapted and kept on keeping on . . . I was trained in the skills . . . that older generation, they had to depend on things like taking care of themselves physically, a lot of home remedy type stuff, cooperation amongst themselves, working things out, survival things/skills. . . . If you have those skills in your background, it gives you a great sense of confidence and self-security. You are not helpless.

Carl also was mentored by his family:

There is a genetic factor there. My dad's dad was very hardy. I remember him very well and they rode horses until they were in their mid-eighties, in cold weather conditions and things not being fun type things; they just did it because there was a job that needed to be done out there . . . he would do whatever it took to tolerate bad weather or a bad horse.

Lived experience was that richness in life that people gathered from being a part of life circumstances. These men identified lived experiences as doing what needed to be done to live and taking what life had to offer. Allan stated,

Individual humans are adaptable to those conditions or environments that they are sufficiently motivated to adapt to . . . people are products of their environment. . . . It's the experience that comes with time . . . age seems to decrease your idealism and enables you to become more hardy, more flexible, more resilient.

Carl noted that his lived experience of hardiness was associated with the weather:

We've seen some very tough weather conditions, and we have to work outside in that weather. We are outside more when the weather is bad then when it is good . . . I suppose some of that is learned.

Don simply commented,

People probably become hardy because it is necessary . . . I guess we just adapted . . . so I think hardiness is taking life as it comes.

Discussion

Five themes were extracted from the rich descriptions of six rural men's perception of hardiness. These themes were (a) adaptability, (b) positive attitude, (c) endurance, (d) learned experience, and (e) lived experience. The themes seem to intertwine and overlap, but by using the participants' own rich descriptions of hardiness, clear and distinct themes were identified. They shed meaning about the lived experience of hardiness in rural men.

When comparing specific themes extracted from previous research studies to this work, similarities and differences were noted. The theme of *adaptability* seems similar to the control component identified in Kobasa's work (1979); however, her definition of control appeared to have an active, almost forceful component. Adaptability, as described by these six men, conveyed a more peaceful acceptance of life.

The theme of *positive attitude* appears to parallel and expand Kobasa's hardiness component of challenge. These men "felt the challenge of life's circumstances but also had the ability to see opportunity in situations. Challenge did not imply a foolhardy dare" (Wirtz, 1996, p. 35).

Endurance, remaining firm, was identified as a theme in these rural men's lived experience with hardiness. This theme seems related to Kobasa's component of commitment.

The two themes of *living and learning to be hardy* did not appear in other research about hardiness. These men spoke of learning how to deal with life through example and of mentors who modeled hardiness. Further, the environment, the severity of the weather, and the difficulty of farm life may have influenced their development into hardy individuals. These themes build on Parse's (1981) theory of human becoming "through cocreating rhythmical patterns of relating as energy is exchanged with the environment" (p. 25).

STUDY TWO-RURAL WOMEN

Life-Event Perspective

In addition to Parse's (1981) nursing perspective of human becoming, the Hultsch and Plemons (1979) life-event framework provided guidance for Study Two. Life's stage and the sociohistorical perspective form the context of this perspective. Life-event antecedents (marriage, new job, and birth or loss of a child) are mediated by variables such as physical health, intelligence, personality, family supports, and income. The hardiness characteristic (Lee, 1986) is considered a mediating variable. Appraisals of any threat coming into a person's life will elicit coping strategies. Subsequently, functional or dysfunctional outcomes will occur, dependent on the way the individual has managed the situation. Using the life event perspective to guide the interviews with the women, participants were asked to recall difficult times in their lives and to describe what helped them to manage the experiences.

Sample

Five women, the wives (n = 3) and mothers (n = 2) of Study One participants, were interviewed for Study Two. One mother is a widow; the other is divorced. The women ranged in age from 51 to 73. Interview time ranged from 45 minutes to one-and-one-half hours.

Emerging Themes

Using Giorgi's six-step method of data analysis (Polkinghorne, 1989), seven themes emerged. A key theme emerging from the data provided by these rural women is that of physical and mental **fortitude**. They each displayed patient courage in the face of difficult situations. They steadfastly hung on and continued with whatever was happening in their life situation. As each explained the situations she perceived as difficult in her life, she conveyed a **positive attitude** about the circumstances. These women **adapted** to differing circumstances by accepting what was and moving on with their life. Instead of viewing potentially difficult situations as threats, the rural women interviewed saw **challenge**.

Handling the trying times in their lives involved **spirituality**. This theme varied from the traditional beliefs involving participation in the formal structure of the church to the belief in the influence of a higher power. Also, these women took actions to **preserve self**. Four different ways of preserving self emerged from the interviews. First, they sought the help and advice of others in their lives. Secondly, they took specific steps to take care of themselves. Third, they sustained themselves through their commitment to others. Fourth, they made deliberate choices to accomplish the preservation of self.

The women said that they had learned to be hardy from their parents, principally their mothers. While their fathers had been very important in their lives, they thought that their mothers had been the principle **role model** for living and managing their lives. In the following paragraphs, excerpts from the interviews show the emerging themes.

Physical and mental fortitude. The participants described many difficult situations including the death of children, divorce, serious illness of self and of their children and husbands, and difficulty with finances. Bernice opened the interview by discussing the death of her two-year-old:

About the worst time was when we lost our little one . . . and I didn't handle it very well . . . I finally decided there was nothing I could do about it so I just, we just do the best you can. . . . finally ended up coming unglued over it before I could get myself . . . back on my feet. Took me about nine years to come unglued.

Later in the interview Bernice said:

I don't always think that I wanted to be (a hardy person), but actually I think it's kinda good for a person. You go through about anything, and you find out that if you can come through it, and you are either stronger or you curl up and quit. And I was never a curler-upper and quitter too easy, so you got to learn something by it.

Carrie shared her need to separate from the couple's business because of the differences between her and her husband's personalities:

. . . I came to the point, he's a very strong personality, and for me, it was a struggle to stay above the water . . . because my personality is much more mellow than his. And being around him 24 hours a day, I was just struggling to be who I was and I finally decided that it was time that I do something else, that I needed to get out get out on my own and do something of my own.

When asked how she managed the situation, Carrie continued by saying,

I looked for a job. It took two years 'til I found what I was looking for. And it was real difficult because I needed to say to my husband, "I have to do

> *something different, I cannot be here 24 hours a day." . . . But it was real hard. It changed the whole perspective of our business and our relationship. . . . I guess I tend to have a lot of fortitude. I guess, you just keep going. I knew that quitting wasn't an option for me. You just don't throw in the towel and say "I'm not going to do this" and sit back.*

While describing the circumstances of their difficult situations, the participants expressed them constructively and in a nonjudgmental way, displaying a **positive attitude**. Following a divorce from her husband Alice said:

> *. . . I never turned the kids against their dad; I don't believe in that kind of stuff. That was their dad.*

When asked how she managed the divorce and other difficult circumstances happening in her life, she said:

> *[by] having a good outlook on life, I mean, trying to think of the happy things of life rather than all the sad things, I think. Having more of a positive attitude.*

Evelyn and her husband were raising eight children; she returned to teaching to better the couple's financial situation. She said:

> *I enjoyed the high school kids. They were people, and when you felt like making an effort, you could talk to them as people.*

The third theme was **adaptable**, being able to accept what is and moving on. Alice said,

> *I was raising kids alone, and my pay was very small. . . . (Nevertheless) we always managed to eat; I always said the refrigerator didn't look very full but mama always came out with a decent meal.*

Carrie spoke of her being able to leave her family to be with her father in an urban coastal city for the last two weeks of his life. Her husband

> *. . . sent all the kids down to see their granddad. . . . It was really . . . a surprise. They all showed up at the house. Well, it was unsettling to me in that there was a lot of commotion . . . four extra people in the house. It was*

a big house but they didn't have any furniture in the bedrooms. And they slept on the floor. We got air mattresses and blankets, we scrounged up blankets. . . . And I didn't have food. . . . I was able to have them stay with their Grandpa while I ran to the store and got groceries, and so there were tradeoffs that worked out ok.

The next theme is **challenge**, the ability to view experiences as an adventure rather than a threat. Evelyn explained:

I was a city girl when I came there (to teach) . . . and I went to this (northeast Montana) farming community and felt like a pioneer. And continued to feel like one for about five years. And then (it) kind of lost its adventure and came a little more real, down to earth.

Bernice discussed experiences her family had during the summer months when they accompanied her husband to shear sheep:

I scrubbed my clothes and cooked on a little two-burner cook stove. I even cooked with a frying pan and Presto cooker. And, you know, we did fine. It didn't bother me any . . . it was always kind of a challenge to me.

The fifth theme was **spirituality**. Two forms of spirituality emerged, the more traditional form in which one participates in a formal religious structure, and the less informal form in which one verbalizes the belief in a higher power. Doris provided an example of a *traditional belief*:

I taught Sunday school, and I took my kids to Sunday school and church. But my husband would never go so when they all got through school, I kinda quit church. I listen on the radio every Sunday. . . . And a lot of time, I go in the third Thursday of every month and take communion with my mother in the nursing home.

Sharing a *belief in a higher power*, Bernice made this comment:

And you think you're the only one in the world that can take care of things, you know. That's a bunch of baloney. You aren't. There's something stronger that can tell you that you're wrong.

Preserving self was evident in these interviewees. This theme consists of four components. The first component is to *seek help/support.*

Evelyn shared that when she realized that she was having suicidal thoughts she

> *had sense to go to the doctor and (to) talk with my priest. . . . (I also) talked things out with my husband. . . . My mother-in-law who was the best friend I had at that time came out and stayed with me so I wouldn't be alone.*

Alice related the difficult circumstances that surrounded the unexpected recent death of her adult son:

> *I retired when (my son) died . . . I went over and seen Pastor Smith, I did. I was pretty down . . . and he helped me a lot. He had just lost a brother so he understood a lot. . . . And he gave me alternatives on what to do.*

The second component of preserving self is *taking care of self,* nurturing oneself. Alice nurtured herself by surrounding herself with young people:

> *. . . young people bring you lots of happiness . . . I like being around young people, young kids . . . because they have positive things they're thinking of, not negatives.*

Evelyn shared that after her experience with depression, she

> *. . . consciously tried to do more things I enjoyed. (Now), I give myself all kinds of treats. If the housework builds up (and) the sink stacks up, I go out on the porch and read. Sometimes then, after my brain is tired of reading, I can come back and do the work.*

The third component of preserving self is *commitment to others.* For these women, commitment to their children was particularly evident. An example of this component was shared by Doris:

> *Well, we had our other little boy, he'd have been about two then [at time of loss of second pregnancy] . . . you gotta think about him. . . . [and] you've got other people to think about too, you know.*

Evelyn related that people were really important to her, "particularly my children." She later added,

> *. . . I try to put people ahead of things so that when there's a people problem I try to solve it as much as I can.*

The fourth component of preservation of self is *making choices.* Alice related that she

> *. . . left nursing so I could be home weekends and evenings . . . it was less pay . . . I loved the patients . . . (but) when you're raising three kids alone, you gotta, they've to be it (the priority).*

Bernice said that she

> *didn't want an empty house so I just kind of filled it up. Boy, did I fill it up! Loren was disgusted with me, but I just told him, I said "I want another baby." I was 40 years old, for God's sake. I told him, "Well, if you won't accommodate me, you know, I'll get a neighbor." Well, I wouldn't have [laugh].*

The last theme in the concept of hardiness is the **presence of a role model**. The women discussed learning to be hardy from their parents but leaned toward their mothers as a principle role model. Bernice brought forth a picture of an older couple and said:

> *. . . let me show you. This lady right here, and my Daddy. . . . I think Mother was the main stay of the family. . . . calm . . . To tell you the truth, I really don't know how she could handle it, but she did.*

Evelyn indicated:

> *. . . my mother . . . believed in self control . . . that she should hold herself to high standards and that she shouldn't let up with the duties she thought were proper to her . . . right along with that she raised me and my brothers and sisters in a rather relaxed atmosphere, and . . . saw to it that we had lots of good things as children.*

Discussion

Five rural women were identified as hardy individuals by the husbands and sons participating in Study One. The women shared their lived experience of managing difficult life events. Themes emerging from the analysis of the interview data were fortitude, positive attitude, adaptability, challenge, spirituality, preserving self, and presence of a role model. Each theme is discussed in view of the many concepts linked with the hardiness characteristic in the literature.

Fortitude. This theme, specifically identified by one participant, is new to the multitude of concepts identified with hardiness. While the term has close association with endurance, "the physiological and/or psychological toughness to continue" (Lee, 1983, p. 33) and strength, "the ability to resist force, stress, hardship" (Lee, p. 33), the added dimension of patience makes use of the word, fortitude, a better choice. The patient courage exemplified by these women is similar to that described in the life history of an 85–year-old Australian woman (King, 1989). King suggested that her participant valued the characteristic of hardiness. She "made her life by relying on herself, working through life's events and stages" (p. 21). The perspective of the effect of life events on one's life course was evident in King's work and in this study.

Positive attitude. The finding of a positive attitude coincides with the same finding in Study One explicated above. Also, King (1989) noted that her life history subject "talked about the importance of having a positive attitude" (p.21).

Adaptability. While not previously identified in the qualitative work about hardiness, the concept is frequently seen in discussions by Pollock (1986). She has examined hardiness in the successful adaptation of persons to chronic illnesses.

Challenge. Challenge, originally identified as a component of hardiness by Kobasa (1979), was also a finding with these rural women. The finding could be equated with boldness, "the quality of being courageous, daring, adventurous" (Lee, 1983, p. 33). Challenge may also be related to robustness, curiosity, the tendency to find experiences interesting, and the expectation that change is the norm, four concepts identified by Lindsey and Hills in 1992.

Spirituality. The finding of this theme is new to the research findings for hardiness. The finding could be indirectly related to the second part of the concept, tendency to find experiences interesting and meaningful (Lindsey & Hills, 1992). While variations of this theme were found between participants, the need for the belief in a higher power or for the ongoing rituals associated with a religious institution was deemed a necessary component of hardiness.

Preserving self. The first component of this theme, seeking the help and advice of others, is supported by mediating variable of family support from the life-event perspective. This finding may be related to Consolvo, Brownewell, and Distefano's (1989) findings. They "conducted several semistructured question-and-answer sessions" (p. 335) to learn how Neonatal Intensive Care Unit (NICU) nurses handled stress. Using Kobasa's three components of hardiness—control, commitment, and challenge—as the framework for their discussion sessions, they added the component of "companionship" to their perception of the personality characteristic of hardiness. The NICU nurses saw "companions as an integral part of their ability to cope with stress" (p. 337).

The second component, taking care of self, does not appear related to other concepts already identified for hardiness. Taking care of self may be an attribute that women in general identify as a need in comparison to men.

The third component, commitment to others, is related to one of the three components identified by Kobasa (1979). Kobasa's definition encompasses commitment as "an ability to feel deeply involved in or committed to the activities of their lives" (p. 3) rather than specifically to other people.

The last component, making choices, is related to the control component of the original hardiness characteristic identified by Kobasa (1979), the power to control by Lee (1983), and the self-assertiveness identified by Lindsey and Hills (1992). Being able to make choices does give persons a sense of control over what happens in their lives.

Role models. This finding was similar to that of Study One with rural men. It is supported by the life-event perspective of family support, a mediating variable in dealing with life events. The presence of a role model to imitate can be stabilizing force in the presence of difficult situations.

SUMMARY

Many differences and similarities exist between the findings in these two studies and those in the literature. The findings of these two studies add to a beginning knowledge base of perceptions of hardiness from the perspective of hardy individuals themselves. The third author of this chapter comments on the findings of the first two authors.

COMMENTARY

Each researcher has referred to Parse's Human Becoming theory as their nursing framework of reference. A framework provides the researcher and the research project with a foundation, or an outline that gives support to the research process and so to the research results. The Human Becoming theory provides a filter or a kind of lens that focuses on some phenomenon of concern to the discipline. In nursing, the phenomenon of concern has been broadly defined as the human-health interrelationship (Mitchell & Cody, 1993). For the researchers, the phenomenon of concern was hardiness in the health-human interrelationship. What nurse researchers must remember is that as humans, each of us is in constant interaction with a world that is ever-changing. Because of this ever changing environment, our interpretations of experience (hardiness) will change. Each change will influence the next experience, and each experience will affect the next change. And while there may be different interpretations of any experience, there will also be similarities. So that while each person's life is uniquely his or her own, there are junctures of interface or inter-relatedness with others because all humans must coexist.

This is proven out in the results of these two research projects. Commonalities, or themes thought to be related to hardiness in both samples, were identified by the respective researchers. Both researchers identified the themes of positive attitude, adaptability, endurance, challenge and/or fortitude in their data. These themes have been identified by other nurse researchers as well and so could be common to the concept of hardiness. However, what can also be appreciated from these two studies are those themes that are not common or generalizeable in both studies; those themes that could be identified as having arisen out of each participant's unique process of participating in the world.

Guided by the belief that the human experience is unique and invaluable to the understanding of humankind (Parse, 1981), the two researchers actually both identified (by different names) themes that by their very definition attest to unique interpretations of similar circumstances. The themes of self preservation, the learned/lived experience, and spirituality speak to unique interpretations of, or interrelations with, an ever changing environment. These relations allow for the integration of unique life events (Hultsch & Plemons, 1979) into what Parse (1981) describes as an "unfolding" (p. 11,25).

Any time a researcher is required to interpret the meaning found in a participant's narrative, the researcher will use his or her personal experiences and understandings of hardiness to make sense, or science, of the individual descriptions. And because people interact with each other through language, we will at times choose the same language in our effort to explain ourselves to others. However, as rural nurses caring for unique individuals, we can also appreciate the different words or language chosen by different individuals to express meaning or understanding.

The findings presented here demonstrate the quality of uniqueness. The researchers have presented their interpretations of experiential descriptions provided by their participants and have seen that while there are common interpretations, there are also interpretations that provide for a glimpse of each of the participants as a unique individual. Rural nurses must remember that each person who requires care is a unique individual. That individual will have had his own life events and will have incorporated those life events into who he is as a person today. Having done that, he will naturally have unique dimensions and understandings of whatever has brought him into contact with a nurse. If rural nurses can understand those things that are common, and appreciate those things that are unique, they will not only utilize Parse's Human Becoming theory in research, but will live it out in their practice of the art of nursing.

REFERENCES

Bunting, S. (1993). *Rosemarie Parse: Theory of health as human becoming.* Newbury Park, CA: Sage

Cody, W. K., & Mitchell, G. J. (1992). Parse's theory as a model for practice: The cutting edge. *Journal of Advanced Nursing Science, 15* (2), 52–65.

Colaizzi, P. F. (1978). Psychological research as the phenomenologist views it. In R. Valle & M. King (Eds.), *Exestential phenomenological alternative for psychology.* New York: Oxford University Press.

Consolvo, C. A., Brownewell, V., & Distefano, S. M. (1989). Profile of the hardy nurse. *Journal of Perinatology, 9* (3), 334–337.

Funk, S. C., & Houston, B. K. (1987). A critical analysis of the hardiness scales's validity and utility. *Journal of Personality and Social Psychology, 53,* 572–578.

Giorgi, A. (1985). Sketch of a psychological phenomenological method. In A. Giorgi (Ed.), *Phenomenology and psychological research* (pp. 8–22). Pittsburg, PA: Duquesne University Press.

Hull, J. G., Van Treuren, R. R., & Virnelli, S. (1987). Hardiness and health: A critique and alternative approach. *Journal of Personality and Social Psychology, 53,* 518–530.

Hultsch, D. F., & Plemons, J. K. (1979). Life events and life-span development. In P. B. Baltes & O. G. Brim (Eds.), *Life-span development and behavior: Vol. 2* (pp. 1–36). New York: Academic Press.

Jennings, B. M., & Staggers, N. (1994). A critical analysis of hardiness. *Nursing Research, 43* (5), 274–281.

King, P. A. (1989). A woman of the land. *Image: Journal of Nursing,21* (1), 19–22.

Kobasa, S. C. (1979). Stressful life events, personality and health: An inquiry into hardiness. *Journal of Personality and Social Psychology, 37,* 1–11.

Kobasa, S. C. Q.(1977). Stress, personality, and health: A study of an overlooked possibility. (Doctoral dissertation, University of Chicago, Microfilm No. T26446).

Lambert, C. E., & Lambert, V. A. (1987). Hardiness: Its development and relevance to nursing. *Image: Journal of Nursing,19* (2), 92–95.

Lee, H. J. (1983). Analysis of a concept: Hardiness. *Oncology Nursing Forum, 10* (4), 32–35.

Lee, H. J. (1986). Relationship of hardiness and current life events to perceived health in rural adults. *Research in Nursing & Health, 14,* 351–359.

Lindsey, E., & Hills, M. 1992). An analysis of the concept of hardiness. *The Canadian Journal of Nursing Research, 24* (1), 39–50.

Mitchell, G. J., & Cody, W. K. (1993). The role of theory in qualitative research. *Nursing Science Quarterly, 6* (4), 170–178.

Parse, R. R. (1981). *Man-living-health.* New York: Wiley

Polkinghorne, D. E. (1989). Phenomenological research methods. In R. Valle & S. Halling (Eds.)., *Existential-phenomenological perspectives in psychology* (pp. 41.60). New York: Plenum.

Pollock, S. E. (1986). The hardiness characteristic: A motivating facor in adaptation. *Advances in Nursing Science, 11* (2), 53–62.

Tartasky, D. S. (1993). Hardiness: Conceptual and methodological issues. *Image: Journal of Nursing Scholarship, 25* (3), 225–229.

Wagnild, G., & Young, H. M. (1991). Another look at hardiness. *Image: Journal of Nursing Scholarship, 23* (4), 252–255.

Wirtz, E. F. (1996). Perception of hardiness in rural men. Unpublished master's thesis. Montana State University-Bozeman.

Woods, N. F., & Catanzaro, M. (1988). *Nursing research: Theory and practice.* St. Louis: Mosby.

21

Cultural Isolation

Patricia Carrick

INTRODUCTION

"It's so weird! *She has a sign on her door, and we're supposed to wear masks when we go into the room. We didn't wear masks yesterday,* before *we brought her to the hospital. Why do we have to now?"*

"We've got to isolate this viral strain conclusively; then we can develop an effective vaccine."

"Our patron helped my husband get a drivers license so he could run the tractors on the ranch, but he has to work every day, and I don't drive, so I can't get into town very easily."

"They just hang around together and talk among themselves. They never even try *to speak English. If they're going to live here, I think they ought to speak English!"*

"A Mexican family moved in next door to us, but I only know a couple of words of Spanish, and I feel stupid trying to say to them, so I haven't dared to speak to them yet."

"I have lived here for almost 18 years, and I recognize lots of the people I see, but only my Mexican friends talk to me in the grocery store. I know my English isn't very good, but . . ."

Despite differences among them, each of the statements above reflects an accepted interpretation of the concept of isolation. In fact, isolation is used in many disciplines to refer to a variety of conditions including physical separation, microscopic localization, geographic distance, ethnic segregation, and linguistic or cultural exclusion.

The potential for isolation in rural settings is readily acknowledged by rural residents who refer frequently to the importance of reliable transportation and communication services. The difficulties of negotiating remote roads in bad weather, the inconvenience and potential dangers of radio and telephone outages, and the crucial nature of informal social support networks are familiar themes threading the casual conversations of rural dwellers. Isolation in rural settings is referred to in the rural nursing literature, especially as related to geographic distances, access to care, social networks, and independence. In her discussion of the very definition of the word rural, Lee states, "Rural ecology is characterized by a geographic area containing a small and unconcentrated population that is relatively isolated from the influence of large metropolitan centers" (1991, p. 13). Geographic isolation is discussed by Dietz (1991) as both a stressor and a benefit to rural women. Bicknell (1991) identifies isolation with both social and geographic qualities as one of several obstacles to provision of services to rural Maine's mentally ill elderly. But the nature and intensity of the isolation experienced by culturally diverse minority populations in rural settings has not been thoroughly addressed. The aim of this chapter is to explore the characteristics of isolation particular to the circumstances of non-English-speaking, ethnically diverse, rural residents.

WHAT DOES IT MEAN?

The Oxford English Dictionary (Simpson & Weiner, 1989) defines the word isolation as

> *the action of . . . standing alone; separation from other things or persons; the separation of a person or thing from its normal environment or context . . . as a result of its being . . . set apart; the complete separation of patients suffering from a contagious or infectious disease, or of a place so infected, from contact with other persons; a defence mechanism whereby a particular wish or thought loses emotional significance by being isolated from its normal context; the obtaining of a chemical element or compound as a*

> *separate substance; the limitation or prevention of interbreeding between groups of plants or animal. (pp. 123–124)*

The Random House Dictionary (Flexner, 1987) adds, "the separation of a nation from other nations" (p. 1013).

The word isolation derives from the Latin *insula,* island or isle, and comes to us in English through the Romance Languages from the French word *isole* which also means, literally, island (Klein, 1966, p. 818). This derivation confirms the physical or geographic quality of isolation, a quality which in itself carries no emotional weight. However, when applied to humans, isolation develops a distinctly negative feeling tone. When John Donne wrote in 1657, "No man is an island, intire of it selfe; every man is a peece of the continent" (Evans, 1968, p. 352), his words carried implicit warning about the inability of humans to survive in an isolated state, separated from others, without social contact and support. Thomas Carlyle put it even more bluntly in 1843 when he wrote in *Past and Present*: "Isolation is the sum-total of wretchedness to man" (Evans, 1968, p. 352).

Thus far isolation has been referred to as both a word and a concept. But does a word differ from a concept? *Webster's New Collegiate Dictionary* (1979) defines a word as "a speech sound . . . that symbolizes and communicates a meaning" (p. 1340), while a concept is "an abstract or generic idea generalized from particular instances" (p. 231). Chinn and Kramer state that a concept ". . . is derived from perception and experience" (1987, p. 84). In order to develop a conceptual understanding of the word isolation, already observed to have varying meanings, its application in several disciplines or particular instances and in the personal experience of the author will be explored. Specific attributes will be identified and discussed and sample cases relevant to the experience of rural minorities will be described. The process delineated by Walker and Avant (1988), for the analysis of concepts provides a guideline for the following exploration.

A WORD OF MANY COLORS

Hospital Isolation: A Double-Edged Sword

In the field of hospital infection control, isolation is the practice of separating patients physically from other patients, from hospital staff, and from the public when actual or suspected infectious disease is present or when the patient is considered vulnerable to contracting an infectious disease because of compromised immunity. Such separation has a bidirectional character which confers protection to both the patient and those surrounding the patient. Physical and procedural elements are involved. An elaborate set of guidelines defines circumstances under which specific isolation policies are to be implemented (Bennett & Brachman, 1986; Garner & Simmons, 1983). A patient may be placed in a private room (physical separation). Access to the room and/or the patient may be limited (social isolation). "Personal protective equipment" such as gloves, gowns, and face masks may be worn to provide tangible physical barriers to infectious microbes. Although hospital isolation is still considered sound practice in regard to microbiologic containment, the concomitant inhibition of human contact is thought to have ramifications to patient well-being which are extremely serious and potentially detrimental. In her work on hospital isolation, Coleman (1987) describes its harsh impact:

> *Isolation is the bitterest pill some hospitalized patients are forced to swallow. . . . The patient in isolation may find himself confined to a strange room with practically nothing to distract him from the discomfort and uncertainty of his illness. Even the usually caring nurses seem to avoid him, partly because the inconvenience of donning gown and gloves before entering his room naturally motivates them to limit the number of their visits. . . . The mere fact that all of his nurses wear gowns, gloves, and masks while caring for him can affect his morale. Gowns and gloves make caregivers look cold and unfeeling. Masks hide the faces and smiles a patient longs to see. (p. 50)*

In recognition of the potential negative effect of isolation procedures, the original Centers for Disease Control's "Guideline for Isolation Precautions in Hospitals" (Garner & Simmons, 1983) contains an admonition that concerted efforts by caregivers are required in order to maintain a healthful level of human contact with patients placed in isolation.

Linguistic and Cultural Isolation: How We Know What We Know

Anyone who has traveled alone in a country whose language she did not speak or understand knows only too well how complete is the sense of isolation when verbal communication is inhibited. In these cases, physical separation is not the critical factor. Indeed, one may be surrounded by people, yet completely unable to express thoughts, questions, concerns, or emotions and equally unable to comprehend those of others. Under such circumstances, it becomes clear that verbal indicators act not only as tools for personal expression, but as crucial cues to appropriate cultural behaviors, to what is expected or acceptable, and to the significance of specific cultural signs and symbols.

In February, 1987 I found myself walking alone down a muddy track in the jungle highlands of Papua New Guinea. In an isolated spot, I rounded a corner in the path and suddenly encountered a group of Huli warriors carrying huge, machete-like knives; their bodies decorated with leaves, grasses, paintings, and little else; ears and noses punctured by wooden plugs, gesticulating wildly as they shouted angrily at one another. I was upon them before I could stop or turn back. There was no escape; I was too obvious—too white, too female, too alone. They all turned to me at once with the fiercest of looks and raised their machetes. With no options I could think of, I continued toward them, doing my best not to look scared to death. They made threatening faces while I forced leaden feet to step forward. As I drew abreast of them, with a violent gesture the warrior closest to me . . . broke into a huge smile and began to shake one hand up and down in mid-air just before he grasped my own and almost shook me over in greeting!

I came to understand that the Huli people are unremittingly expressive and energetic. The signs I took to be expressions of anger were typical of everyday conversation; they may have been discussing their gardens with just such frenetic tones and gesticulations. The threatening faces were a demonstration of masculinity presented for my appreciation and approval, and the machetes were essential for path-clearing on even the most casual amble to the neighbors' by any route but the busiest thoroughfare. Because I could not understand their language and the cultural symbols were unfamiliar to me, I could not interpret correctly what was happening around me until finally the extroversion and good humor of the Huli Highlanders transcended my fears.

An iconoclastic Hispanic-American scholar, Richard Rodriguez (1982), writes about language as the key to cultural assimilation, the antithesis of cultural isolation, in his autobiography, *A Hunger of Memory*. He speaks against bilingual education:

> *... proposed in the late 1960s by Hispanic-American social activists, later endorsed by a congressional vote. It is a program that seeks to permit non-English-speaking children, many from lower-class homes, to use their family language as the language of school. (pp. 11–12)*

Mr. Rodriguez argues that refusal to adopt the language of the dominant culture perpetuates, rather than alleviates, isolation and powerlessness in minority populations:

> *... bilingual educators say that children lose a degree of 'individuality' by becoming assimilated into public society ... [they] simplistically scorn the value and necessity of assimilation. They do not seem to realize that ... such assimilation makes possible the achievement of* public *individuality ... Those middle class ethnics who scorn assimilation seem to me filled with decadent self-pity, obsessed by the burden of public life. Dangerously, they romanticize public separateness and they trivialize the dilemma of the socially disadvantaged. (pp. 26–27)*

No stranger to the terrible loneliness, the "wretchedness" of true linguistic and cultural isolation, Rodriguez describes from personal experience how adoption of the language of the dominant society is fundamental to individual comprehension and acquisition of culture, to resolution of the pain of "public separateness." For him, it is language that provides the enabling tool with which to banish the pain of exclusion, the key to credibility and success for ethnically diverse people within a foreign culture.

Ethnic Isolation: The Fear and Stigmatization of Segregation

As Rodriguez describes, for minority residents in a dominant foreign society incomprehension of cultural symbols can be a persistent, daily experience rather than an occasional event. When the dominant society simultaneously misinterprets the verbal and behavioral symbols of a minority population distinguished by identifiable physical/racial characteristics, isolation can become multifaceted. The bidirectional nature of isolation previously referred to for its protective qualities in the discussion of hospital isolation may develop in far less constructive forms. The consequences of resultant racial, social, and cultural misunderstanding can be frightening and self-perpetuating.

A study by Moore (1985) of young Chicano men in East Los Angeles describes the gradual process of stigmatization and resultant isolation arising from conflicting ethnic identification and cultural interpretation. In an effort to retain cultural identity and to prevent an overwhelming sense of social isolation within a dominant foreign culture, Mexican immigrants of the early 1900s transposed a Mexican tradition of male youth groups into the context of U.S. society. As these groups developed in the 1920s and '30s, their cultural identity *was,* in fact, recognized by the dominant culture. But it was misinterpreted: the youth groups were called "gangs;" participants were assumed to be violent and delinquent, and Anglos gradually came to assume that *all* young Chicano men were included, a process Moore refers to as "ascribed deviance." The assumption of delinquency resulted in stigmatization and setting apart or segregation, a form of social isolation often related to racial and other visible identifiers (Flexner, 1987). Group or gang participants, experiencing the consequent frustrations and disappointments of being stigmatized and isolated, further solidified group boundaries over time, creating a self-isolation which, in combination with the suspicion and isolation imposed upon them from without, has effectively divorced them from the dominant culture.

DEFINING ATTRIBUTES

Certain characteristics have resurfaced repeatedly in this exploration of the literature on isolation. The identification of specific defining attributes may contribute to the effort to create a pure or concentrated description of the concept. Attribute definition is, in fact, an effort to isolate the essence of isolation!

In every case referred to thus far, isolation has included certain essential qualities. It involves *separation,* being cut off or set apart from a more inclusive context. When applied to humans, isolation entails a sense of *dissatisfaction or unhappiness*; it is (remember Thomas Carlyle) a "wretched" condition. Isolation is a distinctly *unnatural* state. Isolation may be endured temporarily but is *neither desirable nor healthful.* Isolation is, therefore, in most cases *involuntary* if it is sustained. In the sociocultural sense, isolation is a condition which happens to or is inflicted upon another by some entity powerful enough to effect or enforce it. There is, therefore, a condition of implicit power inequity in the state of isolation and a quality of *passivity and victimization* about one who is isolated.

ANTECEDENTS

There must be an existence "in relation to" before being "set apart from." Mere distance alone does not constitute a state of isolation. A rock lying on a remote mountainside could be said to be isolated from town, but there is no prerequisite relationship from which it is cut off or set apart, so it would be inaccurate to attribute to the rock a condition of isolation, although it is certainly distant.

An inequity of power or control must characterize a system in order for social or cultural isolation to persist. Since isolation is undesireable and unhealthful, an animate entity rarely moves naturally or willfully toward a state of isolation, except in the case of dysfunction or extreme eccentricity. Something or someone must have the ability to impose isolation upon another.

CONSEQUENCES

Brock, Smith, and Madigan (1984) report that absolute isolation results ultimately in the death of a strain or species. Replication of regressive genes and/or social characteristics, in the absence of all external biologic or social input, without opportunity to incorporate hybrid and adaptive traits, generates deformities and reduces survivability in a biologic system. Less extremely, various levels of social and cultural isolation appear to result in dysfunction and antisocial behaviors (again, see the discussion in Moore, 1985).

These defining attributes, antecedents, and consequences of the concept of isolation as developed in this discussion may be clarified by a few examples.

CASE EXAMPLES

Model Case

Luisa, a Hispanic child in the third grade, is seated quietly at her usual desk in the back of the classroom. She moved to the United

States when she was six years old. Although she understands a considerable amount of English, she speaks it poorly and has learned to read neither Spanish, which is not taught at her elementary school, nor English. As the reading lesson progresses, she becomes restless. She watches three rows ahead of her an Anglo girl she has admired and hoped all year to befriend. When the moment seems right, she passes her favorite barrett to the student seated immediately ahead of her and tries to explain in whispers that she wishes to have the gift passed forward to the girl who is the object of her admiration. She is not readily understood by her classmate, however, and the teacher notices the whispering, accuses her of disrupting the class, and angrily demands that she stand by the doorway with her face turned toward the wall for the rest of the reading lesson. She hides her tears until the end of the school day and sits alone on the bus, afraid someone from her class will make fun of her on the way home.

Discussion

This scenario demonstrates all the defining attributes of isolation. The child is set apart from her classmates literally by the teacher who removes her from her desk and stands her in a separate place. She is chagrined and shamed by the event, but in the face of the power inequity of the teacher-student relationship, she accepts a passive role and does not argue or attempt to defend herself. Her punishment is enforced by the teacher until the school bell rings at the end of the class period. The bidirectional nature of isolation is also reflected here when Luisa, overwhelmed by her sense of helplessness and shame, chooses to sit alone on the school bus in order to protect herself from the ridicule she fears.

Borderline Case

Paula is married to Antonio, a farmworker from her own home region of Jalisco in Mexico. Since the spring after their marriage three years ago, he has come to southwestern Montana to work for seven months every year. This year they agreed that Paula could join him in the United States, although Antonio warned her of the many difficulties she might encounter. She arrived in late May, one month after his arrival for work, to find the living quarters spare but manageable. Without her familiar things from home she felt odd but busied herself cleaning the small cabin to make this their home together for the next 5 months. She was, however, unprepared for the distance from town or neighbors. The ranch is 7 miles by road from the next ranch, 13 miles from the nearest (tiny) grocery and bar, 52 miles from the next town. Antonio drives and has a U.S. license which his patron helped him acquire so he could drive farm machinery on the county roads around the ranch, but Paula has never driven a car nor does she speak or read English. Paula is very lonely and often feels depressed while Antonio is at work. She is used to seeing her mother and other family and community members daily, but here the few people she has met are miles away. She has decided she *must* learn enough English to pass the driver's license written exam. On Sunday afternoons Antonio drives her to any one of several ranches in the same valley where they socialize with other Mexican ranchworkers. Paula particularly enjoys these outings and has borrowed two Spanish/English textbooks from her new friends in order to gain the language skills she will need for the exam.

Discussion

Paula is experiencing several aspects of isolation. She is geographically separated from the society of other Spanish-speakers and even from the casual, functional interactions of English-speaking shopkeepers in town. She finds her circumstances unsatisfactory and experiences an unhealthful state of dis-ease (depression) as a result. However, Paula does not feel disempowered. She participated in the decision to join Antonio in the U.S.—even in recognition of some of the difficulties she would have to face. Additionally she has found an active, constructive approach to her immediate problem (she is studying English to prepare for the driver's license test) and has refused the passivity that might threaten to keep her removed from others. Her active stance in these two regards provides an exception to the criteria of involuntariness and enforcement of isolation by others and makes this a borderline case.

Related Case

Rum Dum is a middle-aged Tibetan ascetic who has studied Buddhist philosophy for almost 40 years. Exiled from his own country by political circumstances, he has lived and worked in the United States throughout his adult life. During these years he has been recognized as a great teacher: he has taught spirituality, he has worked devotedly in many service organizations, he has given freely of himself, and he has meditated rigorously. Now he declares he is off to the mountains to spend the rest of his life as a hermit, in peaceful meditation in a simple hut in Colorado. He will welcome few visitors and will not have a phone or a car, although he will arrange for his sustenance and medical necessities to be provided for as needed.

Discussion

At first glance, this case might appear to be an example of isolation. Physical separation is certainly a significant factor. However, none of the other attributes essential to isolation as the concept has been defined in this chapter is present. This setting apart does not bring with it a sense of dissatisfaction or unhappiness but quite the contrary, a sense of peace, of retreat, perhaps even of relief. There is no effective power inequity operating. This is a voluntary separation and has about it an aspect of inner strength and healthfulness. What is described here is an example of solitude, a concept, indeed a tradition, held in high regard in the spiritual disciplines. This concept shares with the concept of isolation the quality of being separated, set apart. Yet none of the other essential attributes identified in this paper that distinguish isolation conclusively from solitude can be seen in this example.

SUMMARY

This chapter has explored the concept of isolation especially as it relates to the experience of non-English-speaking, racially diverse, rural residents. A definition of the word has been stated, and some of the relevant work in rural nursing theory, in literature, in the fields of hospital infection control, in education and sociology, as well as personal experiences have been reviewed to elucidate particular instances from which a conceptual understanding might be generated.

From this discussion, it can be seen that isolation entails many difficulties and frustrations, disadvantages and even dangers, for non-English-speaking, rural community members. Perhaps if an increased awareness of such painful experiences is stimulated by consideration of the concept, the process of concept analysis might inform clinical practice, program development, and policy-making with the sensitivity necessary to promote the well-being of *all* rural residents.

REFERENCES

Bennett, J. V., & Brachman, P. S. (Eds.). (1986). *Hospital infections* (2nd ed.). Boston: Little, Brown.

Bicknell, E. H. (1991). A rural community-based model for care delivery to chronically mentally ill elderly. In A. Bushy (Ed.), *Rural nursing* (Vol. 2, pp. 53–62). Newbury Park, CA: Sage.

Brock, T. D., Smith, D. W., & Madigan, M. T. (1984). *Biology of microorganisms* (4th ed.). Englewood Cliffs, NJ: Prentice-Hall.

Chinn, P. L., & Kramer, M. K. (1991). *Theory and nursing* (3rd ed.). St. Louis, MO: Mosby.

Coleman, D. (1987). The when and how of isolation. *RN, 50*(10), 50–55.

Dietz, M. (1991). Stressors and coping mechanisms of older rural women. In A. Bushy (Ed.), *Rural nursing* (Vol. 1, pp. 267–280). Newbury Park, CA: Sage.

Evans, B. (1968). *Dictionary of quotations.* New York: Delacorte Press.

Flexner, S.B. (Ed). (1987). *The Random House dictionary of the English language* (2nd ed., unabridged). New York: Random House.

Garner, J. S. , & Simmons, B. P. (1983). Guideline for isolation precautions in hospitals. *Infection Control, 4* (suppl), 245–325.

Klein, E. (1966). *A comprehensive etymological dictionary of the English language* (Vol. 1, A-K). New York: Elsevier.

Lee, H. J. (1991). Definitions of rural: A review of the literature. In A. Bushy (Ed.), *Rural nursing* (Vol. 1, pp. 7–20). Newbury Park, CA: Sage.

Moore, J. W. (1985). Isolation and stigmatization in the development of an underclass: The case of Chicano gangs in East Los Angeles. *Social Problems, 33*(1), 1–12.

Rodriguez, R. (1982). *Hunger of memory: The education of Richard Rodriguez.* Boston: David R. Godine.

Simpson, J. A., & Weiner, E. S. (Eds.). (1989). *The Oxford English dictionary* (2nd ed., Vol. VIII, unabridged). Oxford: Clarendon Press.

Walker, L. O., & Avant, D. C. (1988). *Strategies for theory construction in nursing* (2nd ed.). Norwalk, CT: Appleton & Lange.

Webster's new collegiate dictionary. (1979). Springfield, MA: Merriam.

22

Ethnocentrism

Julia Ann Dybbro

INTRODUCTION

This century has brought to light an ever-widening sphere of "isms." Racism and sexism are no strangers to our vocabulary. Bias, inequality, and barriers to opportunity are also experienced through ageism, ableism, and heterosexism, to name a few (Taylor, 1991). In addition, the many immigrants who come to this country, whether voluntarily or by necessity (political refugees), contribute to the ever growing diversity in which this country is immersed. The aim of this analysis is to define the concept of ethnocentrism. The analysis process used is that of Walker and Avant (1995). Dictionary definitions and uses of the concept in the literature are followed by identification of the attributes. Two cases, model and contrary, are presented.

DEFINITIONS

Ethnocentrism is the grandparent (gender neutral) of the "isms." It is defined as the basic assumption that one's own group, whether it be an ethnic, cultural, religious, or social group, is inherently superior (Simpson & Weiner, 1989). Ethnocentrism is also a way of viewing the world, that is, from the perspective of one's own world (Flexner, 1993). One's own group or world is the center, and all others are scaled and rated, and merit is assigned using one's own as an exemplar. For this chapter, a culturally distinct group consists of a collection of people sharing characteristics such as common ancestry, racial background, political or religious ideology, language, social or physical traits, geographical area, economic strata, sexual preference, education, occupation, sex, or age.

Spradley (1979) likens ethnocentrism to "naive realism," the assumption that all people, regardless of language or culture, view phenomena such as birth, death, love, marriage, and family essentially the same way. In other words, these events have the same significance and life-importance to everyone. Instead of an underlying belief of the inherent superiority of one's own culture that defines one aspect of ethnocentrism, naive realism is the equally limiting view that we are all the same.

USES OF THE CONCEPT

The word "ethnocentrism" is broken down into two parts; ethnic means pertaining to race, and centrism refers to central (Simpson & Weiner, 1989). The term, however, is broadly used and more often refers to a cultural, political, or sociological context. An example of the usage of the word comes from the *Oxford English Dictionary*: "The age at which a child normally begins to read with facility is also the age at which he turns from an autistic, egocentric individual, to a societal, ethnocentric being" (Simpson & Weiner, 1989, p. 690). Patterson (1977) uses the term ethnocentric solidarity when referring to an Afro-American's heightened cultural/ethnic consciousness. Political theorists use ethnocentrism in terms of which dominant group can exert power and establish the norms of society. Until recently, South Africa was an example of a country whose minority population, the white Afrikaners, was in a position of power to exert their ethnocentric national policies on the black majority (Dashefsky & Shapiro, 1976).

A survey of the literature available to students in the public schools during the 1960s revealed a blatant lack of non-Anglo male authors (Foster, 1987). There was scant, if any, representation from women, Native Americans, or blacks. Literature is a main source of positive role models for children, so this type of ethnocentrism by omission has far-reaching effects.

Ethnocentrism is a central theme in the academic training of field anthropologists. Ethnographers must be particularly alert to the pitfalls of ethnocentrism since the aim of good data collection is impartiality, objectivity, thoroughness, and accuracy (Fetterman, 1989). Seasoned anthropologists who have recognized the concept admit that impartiality is a huge challenge and being nonjudgemental and neutral is difficult. Humans are products of their own culture and it is impossible to separate culture from the individual. Much of our personal identity comes from a sense of belonging and being members of our culture. The danger of ethnocentrism comes from the inherent chauvinistic belief that one's own culture is superior or the only "right" one. Barrett (1984) cites that from an anthropological point of view, foreign missionaries, teachers, and aid workers are often the worst offenders for ethnocentric actions. Even after spending years in other cultures, they only solidified their own cultural biases and sense of superiority.

USES OF THE CONCEPT IN NURSING

Although rural communities and environments do not have near the heterogeneity of urban centers, there are ample examples of how cultural diversity is injected into the rural landscape: (a) many migrant agricultural workers are of Hispanic background and their work takes them to rural agricultural areas; (b) many Indian reservations are placed in remote areas; and (c) many refugee relocation sponsorship programs originate in nonurban areas. Missoula, Montana, is an example of a town where local church groups and political activist organizations (such as the Jeanette Rankin Peace Center) have sponsored Russian, Hmong, and Tibetan refugees. Missoula is also a university town that often attracts students and professors from other cultures and countries. Regardless of how culturally diverse people find themselves in a culture other than their own, they at some point may need health care and, hence, may come face-to-face with ethnocentric attitudes and assumptions about whom they are. Rural or urban, following are some examples of the concept of ethnocentrism in nursing.

Ageism is the bias inflicted on people of a certain age. It is sometimes assumed by health care workers that people over the age of 75 would not want aggressive treatment of their cancer (Yellen, Cella, & Leslie, 1994). This has not been found to be true. In studies conducted on cancer patients of all ages, there was no significant difference based on age in the desire to have aggressive cancer therapies.

Heterosexism is the assumption that everyone is heterosexual. Many studies have reported that lesbians feel barriers in using the health care delivery system because of this assumption of heterosexuality by the health care provider (HCP). Lesbians reported that often there was no comfortable way to reveal their sexuality in the history-taking or assessment process (Roberts & Sorenson, 1995; Stevens, 1995; White & Levinson, 1995). Even when strong clues were given, "I have absolutely no need for birth control," the HCP still did not recognize the opening for sexual preference disclosure (Roberts & Sorenson, 1995).

The assumption that all Native American tribes are similar and have common beliefs is incorrectly made by many health care workers (Hayes, 1995). Hayes, a prominent nurse in the Indian Health Service, states that the Chippewa Nation, for example, is very different from the Sioux Nation. Therefore, health care workers need to verify traditions and beliefs with the individual. These differences may influence the patient's care and follow-up treatment.

In this same context, not all immigrants who come to this country are here for the same reasons. A Southeast Asian woman emigrating for better economic opportunities is very different from the woman who comes here via the refugee camps. An alarming number of refugee women escaping political or ethnic persecution from their home country have been raped while escaping, and, for every one person who makes it to a safe country, another has been killed trying (Mattson, 1995). Again, these differences may greatly influence these women's health care needs and may illustrate the necessity of not assuming all immigrants have similar backgrounds, experiences, and health care needs.

Religion is a strong determinant of health care beliefs and practices. These varied beliefs and practices are sometimes misinterpreted. American health care workers often label people of other cultures as uncooperative and ignorant (Choi, 1995). This stems from a misunderstanding of fundamental cultural differences. Some Buddhists have strong beliefs in yin and yang balances, which are maintained, in part, by "hot and cold" foods and practices. An imbalance in yin and yang leads to illness. A new mother will not breast feed her baby until her milk is completely in, since doing so robs her of vital heat and fluids. This mother will bottle feed until she perceives that her milk is ready. The culturally insensitive postpartum nurse may alienate this client by pressuring her to breast feed too soon.

Some Christian Scientist followers do not believe in the power of modern medicine (Miller, 1995). Rather, they focus their energy on alternative forms of healing, such as faith healing and natural remedies. Some Hmong people, and other Buddhists as well, believe in fate and reincarnation. They may not seek out preventive health care measures, since there is much less fear of dying, and they may believe that trying to alter one's life course is useless. They also may not choose life-prolonging therapies. To ensure their health and follow their religious beliefs, Mormons and Seventh Day Adventists often focus on a strict diet, no alcohol consumption, and no smoking.

Summary of the Uses of Ethnocentrism in Nursing

Knowing all the nuances of all cultures is impossible for the health care provider. Avoiding the pitfalls of ethnocentric assumptions by remaining open to the many ways and beliefs of cross-cultural health practices is possible, though. This openness is manifested by continually evaluating the responses of the individual patient or client and by being aware when clues of a communication breakdown are occurring. It is equally important to remember that not all members of a culture or group share the same practices and beliefs (Nance, 1995). Not all Hispanics are devout Catholics, and not all devout Catholics shun divorce.

THE ESSENTIAL ATTRIBUTES OF ETHNOCENTRISM

Three attributes are common with most cases of ethnocentrism. They are (a) affiliation or membership in a culture, religion, or social group with shared traits, beliefs, or ethnic background; (b) nonrecognition of another's beliefs, cultural behaviors, ethnic background, or affiliations; and (c) placing one's culture, ethnicity, religion, or social affiliation above or superior to another's.

CASE EXAMPLES

Model Case

A woman from rural Laos comes into a health clinic in Missoula, Montana with her two-year-old child. He has a fever and has been sick for three days. The mother speaks English but not fluently. The child has a cotton scarf wrapped around his head and neck. The physician prescribes antibiotics and instructs the mother to take the child's temperature every evening and to come back for a follow-up appointment in one week. The mother keeps nodding very agreeably, "yes," to all the instructions. After the physician leaves, the nurse unwraps the scarf, tells the mother to keep the child only lightly clothed, and pats the child on the head. The mother states that she has been giving the child an herbal packing to the bottom of his feet. The nurse explains this will not help the respiratory infection, and that the antibiotics will take care of the problem. The nurse notices that the mother never made eye contact with either her or the physician. She assumes the woman is afraid and makes repeated attempts to look the mother in the eyes to reassure her and puts her arm around her shoulders. Since the mother assured the physician she understood the instructions, the nurse did not repeat them, and she handed the prescription to the mother, and they left. The mother went home, gave the antibiotics for three days but quit when her child seemed better. The infection returned, but the mother went to a different clinic this time because the nurse at the first one was rude to her.

All three attributes of ethnocentrism are present in this case. The mother and child belong to a distinct culture—rural Laotian. The nurse failed to recognize the mother's cultural behaviors. In Laos, it is considered very rude to look someone directly in the eye (Mattson, 1995). Elders and physicians have a high status of respect in Laos and to question their instructions would be considered very disrespectful. In order not to lose face, Southeast Asians may nod and agree to instructions but have no intention to carry them out. The head and shoulders are considered the seat of the soul, and one never touches the head or shoulders of another in Laos. There is also the belief that wind causes disease, not germs. That is why the child had a scarf on, to protect against wind. The nurse devalued the foot packing and stressed the superiority of the antibiotics. The mother did not understand the need to take the whole course of antibiotics, and the nurse did not use any follow-up to ensure there was mutual understanding.

Contrary Case

A non-English-speaking Mexican-American woman is five months pregnant and has come to a bilingual clinic in rural Texas for an appointment for which she is three hours late. She is found to be hypertensive. The woman's mother and grandmother have come into the examining room with her. The husband is out in the waiting room. The Spanish-speaking nurse practitioner (NP) instructs the client and the elders that the best therapy for gestational hypertension is rest. She knows that some Hispanics believe inactivity decreases amniotic fluid and leads to a sick baby, so she asks the group what they think of this recommendation (Burk, Wieser, & Keegan, 1995). The grandmother acknowledges her folk beliefs about amniotic fluid but is willing to try modern medicine. The NP also asks if they have transportation for the next visit and emphasizes the importance of being on time so the clinic can run more efficiently. They say the public bus is their transportation and they will make an afternoon appointment to make sure they can get to the appointment as close to the time as possible. The NP knows that some Mexican-Americans have a very different sense of time and acknowledges this by reassuring the client that it is the policy of the clinic to fit people in as best they can, whatever their appointment time. The NP has the client and her family watch a bilingual video on the birthing process before they go home since the elders cannot read.

This clinic actually exists and is very successful in getting pregnant Mexican-Americans in for prenatal care (Burk et al., 1995). The number one reason is because of the multicultural and bilingual staff. All the teaching materials incorporate folk beliefs with traditional medicine and are available on video and in written form.

SUMMARY

The concept of ethnocentrism has been defined and examples in different fields of study including nursing have been explored. A model case and a contrary model case were described to illustrate the concept in nursing practice. Some alternate strategies to ethnocentrism have been briefly alluded to. The literature is presently rich with nursing theories to counteract ethnocentrism in nursing. "Culture brokering" and "transcultural nursing" are middle-range theories where the nurse acts as an intermediary between the client and the health care system to resolve conflict and alleviate communication breakdowns (DeSantis, 1994; Jezewski, 1995). Culture cannot be separated out of the individual and is inherent and ever-influential when a person interfaces with the health care system. An understanding of ethnocentrism and its alternatives can only be helpful in delivering more humane health care to everyone.

REFERENCES

Barrett, S. R. (1984). *The rebirth of anthropological theory.* Toronto: University of Toronto Press.

Burk, M. E., Wieser, P. C., & Keegan, L. (1995). Cultural beliefs and health behaviors of pregnant Mexican-American women: Implications for primary care. *Advances in Nursing Science, 17* (4), 37–52.

Choi, E. C. (1995). A contrast of mothering behaviors in women from Korea and the United States. *Journal of Obstetric, Gynecological, and Neonatal Nursing, 24* (4), 363–369.

Dashefsky, A., & Shapiro, H. M. (1976). Ethnicity and identity. In A. Dashefsky (Ed.), *Ethnic identity in society* (pp. 5–9). Chicago: Rand McNally.

DeSantis, L. (1994). Making anthropology clinically relevant to nursing care. *Journal of Advanced Nursing, 20,* 707–715.

Fetterman, D. M. (1989). *Ethnography: Step by step.* (Applied social research methods series, vol. 17). Newbury Park, CA: Sage.

Flexner, S. B. (Ed.). (1993). *Random House unabridged dictionary* (2nd ed.). New York: Random House.

Foster, F. S. (1987, April). *Ethnic children's literature in the schools.* Paper presented at the Annual Conference of the Society for the Study of the Multi-Ethnic Literature of the United States, Irvine, CA.

Hayes, N. (1995, August). Interview during N 550 class, College of Nursing, Montana State University-Bozeman.

Jezewski, M. A. (1995). Evolution of a grounded theory: Conflict resolution through culture brokering. *Advances in Nursing Science, 17* (3), 14–30.

Mattson, S. (1995). Culturally sensitive perinatal care for Southeast Asians. *Journal of Obstetric, Gynecological, and Neonatal Nursing, 24* (4), 335–341.

Miller, M. A. (1995). Culture, spirituality, and women's health. *Journal of Obstetric, Gynecological, and Neonatal Nursing, 24*(3), 257–263.

Nance, T. A. (1995). Intercultural communication: Finding common ground. *Journal of Obstetric, Gynecological, and Neonatal Nursing, 24* (3), 249–255.

Patterson, O. (1977). *Ethnic chauvinism: The reactionary impulse.* New York: Stein & Day.

Roberts, S. J., & Sorenson, L. (1995). Lesbian health care: A review and recommendations for health promotion in primary care settings. *Nurse Practitioner, 20* (6), 42–47.

Simpson, J. A., & Weiner, E. S. C. (Eds.). (1989). *Oxford English dictionary: Vol. XVI* (2nd ed.). Oxford: Clarendon Press.

Spradley, J.P. (1979). *The ethnographic interview.* New York: Holt, Rinehart & Winston.

Stevens, P. E. (1995). Structural and interpersonal impact of heterosexual assumptions on lesbian health care clients. *Nursing Research, 44* (1), 25–30.

Taylor, J. (1991, January 21). Are you politically correct? *New York, 24* (3), 32–40.

Walker, L.O., & Avant, K.C. (1995). *Strategies for theory construction in nursing,* 3rd ed. Norwalk, CT: Appleton & Lange.

White, J. C. & Levinson, W. (1995). Lesbian health care: What a primary care physician needs to know. *Western Journal of Medicine, 162* (5), 463–466.

Yellen, S. B., Cella, D. F., & Leslie, W. T. (1994). Age and clinical decision making in oncology patients. *Journal of the National Cancer Institute, 86* (23), 1766–1770.

IV

SELECTED RURAL CLINICAL ISSUES

Several clinical issues related to providing care for rural clients are examined in the seven chapters comprising in this section. The first chapter (chapter 23) focuses on the needs and adequacy of resources for a specific group of rural persons. It reports the findings of a qualitative study conducted with caregivers of family members who had experienced cancer. Two themes related to adequacy and the concept of distance from those resources evolved from the data analysis and could be tested quantitatively.

Caring for persons who are different is a part of rural nursing as well as any other nursing speciality. The Native Americans, once principally a nomad population roaming the Northern Plains of which Montana is a part, are the major minority group in the state. Comparison of patterns of responses to symptoms between Caucasian and Native American women living in rural and frontier areas is the focus of the second chapter in this section (chapter 24). Contextually, the process described in this chapter captures a process that potentially is carried out in a variety of settings.

Organ procurement is the clinical issue described in chapter 25. The authors describe the second author's practice. She is a rural nurse in a specialized field who practices quite differently from her cohorts in urban settings. The distances involved, the characteristics of the rural people she serves, and her acceptance and success as an insider are eloquently described.

The author of chapter 26 describes health care providers' perceptions of issues arising while caring for Native American clients in health care facilities. These clients wish to follow their customs and traditions when they use the dominant culture's facilities for health care. Two core variables evolved from the analysis of interviews. The first variable was "containing disruption." It was evident for the informants as they provided care and as they attempted to manage the resulting problems. The second variable was "cultural awareness;" the degree of the informants' awareness influenced the process of managing disruption.

Some formerly invisible groups, the persons of gay, lesbian, and bisexual persuasion, are now becoming more visible. Gay, lesbian, and bisexual youth are the focus in chapter 27. When faced with choosing to take the responsibility of becoming an HIV educator or losing her position, the author elected to become the educator and now is recognized as an expert on HIV issues in Montana.

Chapter 28 explores the experiences of HIV infected men with rural health care. The major finding from this qualitative study was managing the barriers to the resources these men needed for care.

Homeless people, while less visible in rural areas than in urban settings, are becoming more evident in the small cities of Montana. Care for this group of people is the topic of the last chapter (chapter 29) in this section. The author saw a need, was able to use satellite grant resources, and has continued the project since funding stopped. Over the term of the project, she has provided an excellent service for the homeless and clinical experience for senior baccalaureate nursing students as well.

Taken together, these chapters provide a look at some issues and special needs of populations living in sparsely populated areas.

23

Exploration of Home Care Resources for Rural Families with Cancer*

Janice A. Buehler and Helen J. Lee

Earlier detection of cancer and advances in medical science have lengthened the trajectory of living with cancer. At the same time, changes in the health care system over the last two decades have moved caregiving from primarily a professional one within an institution to care assumed by family members in the home environment. Just how well persons with cancer and their families manage has become a concern of the health care community. Of growing concern for rural practitioners and researchers are the needs and resources available for persons in sparsely populated states, where residents live many miles from medical center resources.

The perceived needs of persons with cancer and their families have been examined in several studies. Data collected identify needs along the trajectory of illness-newly diagnosed (1–3), in treatment (4–9), and in the terminally ill (3,10–12). Needs identified include. physical care (3,5,8,11), nutrition (3,6), emotional support (3,6,9,11), social support (3,6,11), spiritual support (3,6,11), housekeeping services (8, 10,11), transportation (3,4,6,8,10), and financial assistance (3,4,6,8).

Acknowledgment: The authors wish to acknowledge the assistance of Barbara Randonis and Tammy Schuman in the development of this chapter. This study was supported by a grant from the National Institutes of Health, National Cancer Institute (IROICA46330), and an Institutional NRSA grant (5T32NRO7048–03).

Note. From "Exploration of Home Care Resources for Rural Families with Cancer," by J. A. Buehler and H. J. Lee, 1992, *Cancer Nursing, 15,* pp. 209–308.

Specific needs identified vary, depending on where the person with cancer was in his or her illness trajectory. Mor et al. (8) found that a greater degree of need was related to being older (the person with cancer and his or her caregiver), duration of disease, fewer years of education, lower income, being female, living alone, and experiencing pain. However, common to all stages of the cancer experience was the need for more information about the disease, the treatment, the prognosis, and accessing resources (1–8,12). Houts et al. specifically identified a need area called. "problems with medical staff" (3,6). Reinterviews with study participants elicited comments that physicians frequently "were not available" or "seemed to avoid us" (3).

Findings in family studies in which a member had cancer indicated that families had greater needs than their family member with cancer (1,10,13). Role changes became necessary because of the illness; in addition, the added role, that of caregiving, was assumed by a family member(s) (1,4,9,13). Particularly anguishing to caregivers was watching the person with cancer experience symptoms and deteriorate (11–14). Consequences of caregiving, particularly for older persons who have assumed that role, was the development of major health problems (15,16). In addition, the longer the illness trajectory for the person with cancer, the less likely it was that the caregiver received respite help from other family members (16).

Identification of needs occur because persons become aware that resources are unavailable to meet those needs. Based on the studies just mentioned, most of which were conducted in urban areas, it is evident that more resources for persons with cancer and their caregivers are needed. Home care and hospice are two mechanisms linking persons with cancer and their caregivers with the necessary resources to meet identified needs (17–19). Coyle et al. and Vinciguerra et al. reported on model team approach programs and concluded that home care with support is a realistic alternative to hospitalization (18,19). However, Michels found that when a caregiver is in the home, an assumption is frequently made that a home health referral is not necessary (7).

Resources are fewer in a rural environment (20,21). Frank-Stromborg and Wright conducted their study with persons in "semi rural" northern Illinois (5), and Houts et al. used randomly selected statewide samples in Pennsylvania (3,6). However, differences between urban and rural samples were not examined. The purpose of this qualitative study, was to explore the availability and perceived adequacy of formal resources to meet the needs of rural families who cared for a family member with cancer.

METHODS

Data were collected using a qualitative research procedure called focus groups. Focus groups are "carefully planned discussion(s) designed to obtain perceptions on a defined area of interest in a permissive, nonthreatening environment" (22). These group interviews were the first stage of a larger study designed to measure the longitudinal effects of caregiving in family dyads living in rural environments. The focused interviews were conducted to better understand the provision of home care to persons with cancer in such environments and to increase the validity of closed items selected and constructed for the project questionnaire. Three focus groups-two consumer groups (informal caregivers) and one provider group (formal caregivers) were interviewed. The findings reported here are from the two consumer group interviews. The authors believe that the perceptions of informal caregivers are important elements in planning and providing care for rural families.

Setting

Montana, the fourth largest state in the United States ranks 48th in population density. Forty-six of the 56 counties in the state contain less than six persons per square mile. This low population density makes the state eligible to be classified as "frontier," a designation proposed by Popper, a Rutger's University demographer (23). For the purposes of this study family caregivers residing in the more populated 10 counties (more than six but < 100 persons per square mile), were considered "rural" whereas persons from the remaining 46 counties were designated as frontier.

Resources

Medical treatment centers are located in the five populations centers of Billings, Butte, Great Falls, Kalispell. and Missoula. There are 33 home health care agencies for the state's 56 counties. Some cover more than one county; however, 14 frontier counties have no available home health care service of any, kind. The state has 20 hospice agencies, some of which also cover more than one county; however, 12 frontier counties are without any kind of hospice service. Additionally, those hospices supplying services in many frontier counties may provide no professional nursing services, only volunteers for emotional support and occasional respite.

Sample

Informal caregiver focus group participants included persons from all over the state who had experienced the giving of care for an adult with cancer in their own home. They were recruited through directors of hospices throughout the state. Ten informal caregivers (six women and four men) participated in two focus groups. Half of the sample lived in rural counties; the remaining five came from frontier counties. Two participants were in the younger age group (< 40 years), five were middle-aged (40–64 years), and three were older (≥ 65 years). Two of the caregivers experienced a short dying trajectory (< 1 year); eight experienced a trajectory lasting 1–11 years (Table 23.1).

TABLE 23.1 Length of Dying Trajectory/Adequacy of Resources

	Length of dying trajectory			
	Short		Long	
Adequacy of resources	Rural	Frontier	Rural	Frontier
Adequate	Susan (4 mo)[a]			
Somewhat adequate			William (2 yr)[a] Harold (3 yr)[a] John (5 yr)[a] Sally (7 yr)[a]	Connie (4 yr)[b]
Inadequate		Bernice (8 mo)[b]		Dick (2 yr)[c] Jeanie (11 yr)[b]
None				Nora (4 yr)

[a]Home health, hospice services available.
[b]Hospice (volunteers, no professional staff) services available.
[c]County health aide, hospice (volunteers, no professional staff) available.

Procedure

Initial contact with potential participants was by telephone. Eight individuals were recruited for each session so that, with attrition, an ideal group size of four to five was attained. If the individual accepted the invitation to participate, a letter confirming the date, time, purpose, and place of the focus group was sent. The letter also contained names of the persons who would conduct the group, and information about reimbursement for mileage. Included with each letter was a list of potential focus group questions and a map pinpointing where the session was to be held. On the day before the scheduled focus group, each participant was reminded by telephone.

The interview sessions were held in Billings and Missoula, cities located in the eastern and the western sections of the state. Two persons, one of the authors and a project research assistant who has a master's degree in counseling, facilitated the sessions. Each interview started by establishing ground rules related to the tape recording of the sessions and how confidential information was going to be handled. Focused questions developed by the project staff guided the group interview; variations in the group process occurred, dependent on content presented by the participating informants.

Audio tapes of the focus group interviews were transcribed and content validated. Data were analyzed, using the grounded theory procedures of substantive coding, constant comparative analysis, and memo writing (24). Substantive coding (open coding) involved initial coding and recoding. During initial coding, the authors independently read the transcribed data, underlined all data that captured "what was going on" (25), and placed initial codes in the right-hand margin. Frequently, these initial codes were the actual words of informants. Although the authors had not previously worked together in coding qualitative data, within a short period consistent agreement was attained.

After initial coding of the data was completed, the analysts began the constant comparative method. This involved comparing incident to incident (datum to datum), incident to initial code, and initial code to initial code. During this process, recoding occurred, with initial codes often being regrouped, collapsed, or expanded, and renamed. The codes resulting from recoding are the concepts and their properties, and relationships between concepts discussed in the findings section. These concepts are more abstract in nature than the initial codes, and account for broader phenomena and variability in the data.

Memo writing was implemented throughout the constant comparative analysis and recoding. Memo writing involved the analysts writing their ideas about the emergent concepts, properties of concepts, and relationships between the concepts. Relevant data incidents were included in memos to illustrate the concept or property from which they were derived.

FINDINGS

The analytic paradigm that emerged in the grounded theory analysis of the focus group data appears in Fig. 23.1. This paradigm sets the stage for the discussion of findings.

The home care of a family member with cancer in a rural state (Montana) was the phenomenon studied, and is the context in the paradigm. The antecedent condition was development of cancer in a family member. There were three emergent conditions: (a) the client with cancer; (b) a family caregiver, and (c) formal resources. The

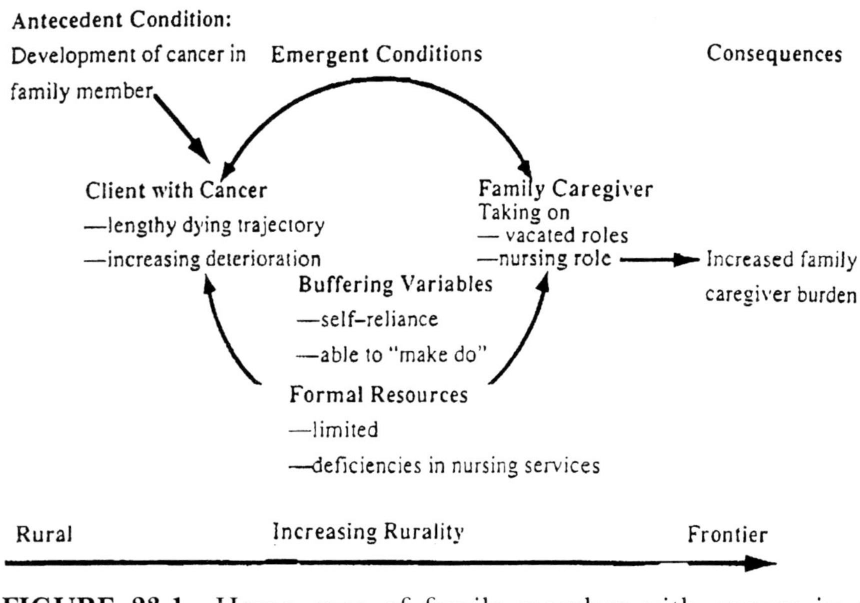

FIGURE 23.1 Home care of family member with cancer in a rural state.

"increasing rurality" continuum at the base of the figure refers to population density; it moves from rural (more than six but < 100 persons per square mile) to frontier (less than six persons per square mile). Reviewing the antecedent and emergent conditions within the variable of increasing rurality showed two major study themes. The first: the more rural the family, the more limited are the formal resources available to assist them in their care of their family member with cancer.

Limited formal resources, such as home health care, hospice services. and homemaker and respite services, became especially problematic for rural and frontier families when their loved one with cancer experienced a lengthy dying trajectory (26) and increasing deterioration. These conditions form the second major emergent theme of the study: the longer the dying trajectory of the family members with cancer and the greater their deterioration, the more resources become inadequate and the greater the family caregiver burden.

The Rural Family with Cancer

The majority of the rural persons with cancer who received care from focus group family caregivers had a lengthy dying trajectory (n = 8 of 10). Typically persons who experienced a lengthy dying trajectory also experienced considerable deterioration. The types of deterioration discussed by family caregivers were physical, social, intellectual, and/or emotional decline. There was variation in the types of deterioration suffered by any particular person with cancer. Some experienced all types of deterioration, while others experienced relatively little physical deterioration other than increasing weakness but did suffer role losses such as work and family roles. Regardless of the type of deterioration their family members suffered, caregivers consistently spoke of the psychological pain they experienced watching the decline. One focus group member, a frontier woman (Connie), described the distress she experienced during her husband's deterioration:

> *The hardest thing for me was . . . seeing someone so healthy and good-looking transformed into someone I didn't recognize, and accepting the fact that this brain tumor affected his ability to function normally. And he became very childlike and I lost my husband and had to take care of this person, and it was real hard to figure out exactly what my needs were. . . .*

This data excerpt implies that this woman's husband suffered all the types of deterioration. Later, she discussed his physical deterioration, including bladder and bowel incontinence.

For some informants, major psychological distress occurred as a consequence of social deterioration and resultant role losses for their loved one. Nora, a ranch (frontier) woman said,

> *[The hardest part] . . . was learning to take over the responsibility, because we have a ranch, and to watch my husband, where he could not control things any longer or could not handle the responsibilities, and I had to do it. . . . Really the hardest part was to watch him, that he could no longer handle these things. . . .*

Nora's comments not only indicate her distress over her husband's social deterioration, but also the necessity for role changes, which were experienced by all the family caregivers who were spouses of the persons with cancer. These role changes are categorized as taking on (a) vacated roles and (b) the nursing care role.

Taking on Vacated Roles

The assumption of roles vacated because of increasing deterioration of the persons with cancer was especially problematic for the family caregivers in this study. Their rural culture generally continues to ascribe to traditional gender roles. Men are expected to be the primary "breadwinners," and women are expected to care for family and home. Rural women may also work outside the home, but their incomes are viewed as supplemental to their primary role as homemakers.

Thus, Nora's experience of taking on the work role of her husband by operating the ranch was typical of the pre-retirement women in the sample. Another example was Susan. Her husband had worked for a large transportation company, and had owned and operated a small sports shop. When his decline prohibited his continuing to work, Susan took over running the business as well as maintaining the home and providing nursing care for her failing husband.

Likewise, pre-retirement husbands, with wives who had lengthy dying trajectories and the social deterioration of role loss, faced taking on the vacated roles of their ill and dying wives. John, a rural man, told this poignant story:

My wife passed away this spring and she'd been fighting cancer for quite a period. . . . Her last month was (at) home but. . . . it went into her spine so she was paralyzed. . . . Part of the problems were there were no registered nurses who could catheterize her and I had to do that four times a day in addition to trying to work and take care of a couple of kids; it does create quite a burden.

Although for analytic purposes the authors have separated role changes required by this sample into "taking on vacated roles" and "the nursing care role," obviously these changes are experienced and remembered as a total phenomenon. Later John reflected on how his perception of women's work changed as he took on his wife's former role tasks. He said,

. . . I took things for granted, little things like taking kids to the dentist, . . . get them registered for school, getting the clothes washed. . . . I used to come home and want to read the paper and watch the news . . . and she'd ask for a little help and I'd say I'd put in a tough day at work. Well, I didn't know what a tough day was until I'm doing both the mother and the father role!

Although retired men in the study did not have to take on the child-care role tasks discussed by John, they did become responsible for various homemaker tasks. In response to a question asking the types of tasks he had to take on during his wife's illness, William, a retired rural man said,

Well, I had to do everything. I learned to cook. I didn't even know how to hardly make coffee or boil an egg . . . and learning even how to run a wash machine and dryer . . . I never knew that . . . I just didn't do any housework [before]. . . . She worked inside and I worked out.

William reflects the traditional gender role division of labor common in a rural culture. Both men and women in the study were required to take on the roles of their spouses as well as the nursing care role.

Nursing Care Role

Parameters of the nursing care role assumed by the family caregiver were highly variable and depended on client needs and perceptions, caregiver gender, and the availability of formal and informal resources to assist the caregiver with nursing care activities. The issue of resources will be discussed in detail in a later section. However, because an inherently close relationship often exists between the family nursing care role and the needed formal resource assistance, brief reference is made to formal resources in this section.

Client needs were affected by variables, such as the type of cancer they had, the course of their illness (i.e., the amount of deterioration they experienced), side effects of treatment modalities, the length of their dying trajectory, and client and caregiver perceptions of their illness and needs.

Three examples are given to illustrate how various dimensions of client needs and other relevant parameters influenced the nursing care role of the family caregiver. Susan described her husband's illness and death as follows:

> *. . . my husband passed away eight months ago with cancer-lymphoma-and it all happened so suddenly . . . he was diagnosed in January of '88. He was an extremely strong person . . . and couldn't believe he had it and he said, "Get rid of this. I do NOT have time for it, I've got too much to do." So they really zapped him with the chemo. And the tumor disappeared miraculously, in no time really. . . . When it came back within 2 months, it came back in full force. And he said, "Let nature take its course" and he lasted . . . 5 weeks. I was very fortunate in the fact that I had him at home. He was never really incapacitated. He could always get up and use the bathroom.*

The above excerpt gives several clues about both client needs and other parameters that influence the nursing care role of the family caregiver. Susan said her husband was "never really incapacitated" and gave the example of his being able to use the bathroom. Later she indicated that his lymphoma was in his stomach and his major needs were for pain control and nutrition. The former need was apparently well met with oral medication until his last week, when a patient-controlled analgesia (PCA) pump continued effective pain control. His nutritional needs could not be met, and as Susan said, "he starved to death." At no time throughout the focus group did Susan indicate that she had any difficulty in providing the relatively minimal nursing care her husband required.

An extremely important parameter for Susan's nursing care role for her husband was his very short dying trajectory. Another significant parameter was her husband's apparent perception of his illness and ensuing death. All of Susan's comments indicate that he met his fate realistically, and with equanimity. Finally, of the 10 caregiver informants, Susan was the only one who perceived to be adequate the formal health care resources that were available to her and her husband. They received the services of a hospice nurse twice a week. The nurse monitored the husband's condition and medications, answered questions, and was in frequent communication with the physician. Susan's experience differed markedly from that of other informants. Two additional examples are given to illustrate parameters influencing the nursing role of the family caregiver.

Jeanie, an elderly woman living in a frontier area, talked about her husband's illness over an 11-year period. He had emphysema and heart disease, and then developed "cancer in the kidney area" during his last 3 years of life. Among the nursing care activities Jeanie performed for her husband were assisting with bathing, administering his medications, "fixing him nutritious meals," helping him to the bathroom during the day and night, and transporting him for occasional medical appointments. Jeanie explained that he was partially bedridden during his last years. And although she was completely devoted to his care, she found that the lack of formal resources in their sparsely populated area eventually took its toll. She said,

> *It got to the point after a few years where I felt, okay someone come along. I need help, too. Not only emotionally, but I was feeling drained physically. My youngest son said one time, 'Mother, you have to get out of here, you have to find other interests in your life. For the last two years I have watched your deterioration. I can't stand to lose you and Dad both.' If that gives you some idea of the help I did not have. I'm not saying "poor Jeanie," please understand that. I wanted to be with him, I wanted to care for him, but I also needed a little help.*

Eventually some assistance became available for Jeanie because of her husband's cancer diagnosis. Two hospice volunteers rotated, staying with her husband for short periods so she had some respite. But these volunteers did not assist with nursing care activities: she said, for example, ". . . no one came in to help with bathing him." But even more problematic for Jeanie was the feeling she had that, because her husband was old and terminally ill, his physicians were disinterested in him. She said,

> *At one time he had three doctors, permanent. Then when he was in and out of the hospital, radiologists, this type of thing, but no one said, "We'd like to have you back in 6 months." No one set up an appointment for this man. . . . I'm not pointing a finger, I don't mean to be, but it seemed to me he was just disregarded. . . . [They were] indifferent.*

Jeanie described the impact which this perceived physician indifference had upon her, ". . . I was hurt, disillusioned. . . . I would feel panicky (and) absolutely completely helpless." When asked what would have helped most during her husband's long illness, Jeanie replied, ". . . someone with a degree of medical knowledge. It was as if you had nothing but common sense."

The parameters of the nursing care role for Jeanie were more clearly influenced by her husband's many needs. His history of multiple chronic illnesses, with increasing deterioration and a lengthy dying trajectory, resulted in the nursing care role becoming Jeanie's major life role. Her other roles of wife, mother, grandmother, neighbor, and so forth became nominal. At one point, she said, "I have three children, grandchildren, all of that, but I couldn't concentrate on anything except his care."

Her story also indicates that Jeanie's life roles had followed the traditional gender roles typical of her rural background and age cohort. The probability is high that she accepted her role of nursing her husband as an extension of her other traditional roles as wife and mother, that is, family caretaker. Clearly, however, Jeanie recognized that she needed assistance with her consuming nursing care role, and found it woefully lacking. The formal resources available to assist Jeanie were indeed meager.

For the last example given to illustrate the parameters influencing a family member's nursing care role, we return to John. John's wife struggled with cancer for > 5 years. Initially, she had breast cancer, and after a mastectomy, "we thought we had it licked but it snuck back up on us." During her last months of life she became paralyzed and blind and was cared for by John and, toward the end, she also had 24-hour hospice care.

It may be recalled that John is the informant who was also responsible for the care of their two children, and who continued his work outside the home in order to support his family. Although John had hospice assistance in caring for his wife, her needs were extensive, and so he also participated in many nursing care activities. He catheterized her four times a day, a nurse coming only at noon to do this, "'cause I did have to work." He also assisted hospice staff in transferring his wife for showering and in turning her in bed. He frequently assisted her in eating, and he gave her oral medications.

During her last month of life, John's wife expressed her desire to die. "She'd kinda given up. And I can't say that I wouldn't have done the same. You can only fight so long. Finally you want to get it over. And that's what she done at the end."

In summary, the active role John assumed in providing nursing care for his wife was determined by her invasive cancer, which created severe disability and deterioration. She had a long dying trajectory, and her perception of her lingering illness culminated in a desire to die. This was a perception that John understood and accepted. Although extensive formal health care resources were available to assist John in his nursing care role, we will return to his experiences in the next section to review his evaluation of their adequacy.

Inadequate Formal Resources

The concept of inadequate formal resources derives from the perceptions of family caregivers that formal health care resources, such as hospice, home health, and physician care, and formal support services, such as respite, homemaker services, and child care, were inadequate to meet their perceived needs. All but one of the informants indicated that some formal health care resources were available and had been used to assist in the home care of their loved one. The two major dimensions of inadequate resources are limited formal services and a deficiency in existing resources.

Limited Formal Health-Care Resources

Many small rural communities and frontier areas in Montana are served by some formal health care resources. But, certainly, as rurality increases, available resources decrease. The case of Dick illustrates the property of limited health care resources. Dick lived in a small rural community and was very involved in mobilizing home care services for his father, who was dying of a brain tumor. Dick's wife provided care for her father-in-law, and "they came from the County Health Department and gave him a bath twice a week." A local volunteer hospice service also was involved. Dick described that service as ". . . more of a booster shot for our egos than anything else. It wasn't that they actually came out and did things." The time came, near the end of the father's long dying trajectory, when family and formal resources were not enough:

> *. . . We wanted my father. . . . home [to die], he wanted to be home. But it just got to the point that we were unable to do it, we couldn't physically. He was bedridden and had to be catheterized, it just got to be more than we could handle. . . .*

Had home health services been available to this family it is possible that the father would have been able to die at home. And certainly, a comprehensive hospice program with professional nurses would have been an important adjunct to the lay hospice volunteers who visited the family.

Another example of limited health care resources was the situation of Jeanie. It will be recalled that she had cared for her husband during his lengthy dying trajectory without assistance. Finally, two hospice volunteers were located who provided her with limited respite services, but no nursing care services.

Many rural and frontier areas in Montana have attempted to provide some formal services for families caring at home for ill and dying loved ones. As with many of the rural and frontier individuals discussed in this study, rural/frontier communities attempt to be self reliant and "make do" with the resources that can be mobilized. However, often the limited formal resources have serious deficiencies. Especially problematic is the lack of adequate professional nursing services.

Deficiency in Existing Resources: Nursing Services

Both rural and frontier informants discussed deficiencies they perceived in the formal home care assistance that they had received. Two closely related themes emerged from informant discussions: (a) the need for more qualified nursing staff, that is, professional nurses, rather than nursing assistants or hospice volunteers; and (b) expectations of family caregivers to provide care that did not fit their role expectations for family caregiving.

John made the following comments regarding formal nursing assistance his wife had received, which supplemented his caregiving:

> *When we were told that we could use (anonymous) Hospice, they . . . always used the term nurse, nurse, nurse, and I was assuming R.N. or L.P.N. and*

> *then it got to a point where they said, 'Well, they won't pay for registered nurses so you are going to have to do the catherization.' I said, 'Well, that's fine.' But when they said they were going to have nurses, I was expecting a lot of trained people and there were many times that I had to show a gal how to put in the suppositories, how to do this and how to do that. They were . . . good-hearted people but they were not trained. And my wife, she did go blind the last 2 months . . . and she was paralyzed, she required some care. And she heard this gal mention, 'Oh. this is my first day and what do you do?' Well, it set her off, she was frustrated. Like how can you send somebody out who doesn't know what they're doing? It bothered me, too, because I was at work and you hate to think, Jesus, this gal doesn't know what she's doing out there. . . . I think they should have explained what type of help and how much training they had prior to when we [sic] were released from the hospital.*

John clearly believed his wife required a level of professional nursing service that was unavailable to her. Other informants reiterated this theme.

Connie, a frontier woman who cared for her dying husband, said, "They [hospice] didn't have anyone that could come in and help with the medical care, which I really needed." When a focus group facilitator clarified what she meant by medical care, it became clear Connie was referring to a need for professional nursing service. She said she needed help in "getting medications [and someone] providing me with information I would need." She continued, ". . . I was kind of left with people who really cared and wanted to help, but their medical background was real limited."

Additionally, some informants discussed having to assume caregiving functions beyond their role expectations. Sally, a rural woman who provided care for her mother, summed up this theme. She said,

> *. . . I had the feeling on the medical end of hospice, the help wasn't so willing. . . . To get help I would usually be told, have you tried this, why don't you go to the drugstore and get this. You know, everything but come out and deal with the situation. . . . [I felt] she [nurse] didn't seem willing to come and that she expected me to deal with some things that I thought were more nurse related than I knew how to handle.*

Sally's comments illustrate not only the nursing service deficiency theme of unwanted family caregiver role functions, but also the dimension of wanting more professional nursing assistance.

Caregiver Burden

The whole experience of the rural caregiver in providing care for a family member was fraught with distress and burden. First, the family caregiver was faced with the deterioration of his or her loved one. This decline necessitated major role changes for the caregiver both in terms of taking on roles that the ill family member was no longer able to continue, and in the actual role of caregiver. The strain of taking on additional roles was compounded for caregivers, when they discovered that only limited formal health-care resources were available to them in their rural setting. Furthermore, when limited formal resources were available and used, caregivers found that they needed more professional nursing services.

DISCUSSION

The major conclusion of this study was that formal health care resources are woefully lacking for rural families and even more so for frontier families. A brief case study of a frontier woman illustrates this. Nora cared for her rancher husband during his illness and death. She drove her husband 100 miles round trip for his medical care, including frequent visits for chemotherapy. No home care or hospice services were available to them. Although Nora and her husband displayed a high degree of self reliance found to be typical of frontier Montana people (27), analysis of her comments showed unmet needs for home care and hospice services. For example, a home health nurse could have assisted Nora in meeting her husband's nutritional needs during chemotherapy when he experienced severe loss of appetite, vomiting, and weight loss. Likewise, a home health nurse could have assisted the couple throughout a stressful period when an error was made in the i.v. administration of a chemotherapy drug and severe damage occurred to the husband's arm. Nora indicated that for 6 weeks they did not know if he would be able to resume chemotherapy, and "they thought he might possibly lose his arm." Certainly a home health nurse could have taught the couple to care for the damaged arm, as well as provide emotional support to them. Had hospice services been available, emotional support could have been provided for the husband as he coped with role losses, and for Nora as she coped with major role changes in assuming responsibility for running the ranch and caring for her husband. And possibly, the couple would have benefited from professional support in facing and working through the husband's approaching death.

Although it is uncertain as to whether Nora and her husband would have accepted home health and/or hospice services had they been available, it is likely that they would have. The assumption is sometimes made that rural people, because of their self-reliance, do not accept or use formal health care resources. However, the authors' strong impression is that rural people do use such resources when they are available, and that, when they are unavailable, they "make do." This attribute has been noted by other authors examining rural phenomena (28,29).

In an effort to ameliorate the paucity of health care resources in rural/frontier areas, the authors suggest two models of health. care that are believed to be acceptable to rural/frontier people. These are nurse case management and mobilization of local resources, especially county extension services (30).

Although case management is a model used by independent providers, the authors believe, as do Rosenblatt and Moscovice (21), that nurse case management must be provided through existing health care agencies. Rural hospitals, home health agencies, and hospices can provide outreach opportunities for delivering case managed services to rural/frontier families. Nurse case managers are considered essential because of their knowledge base, which enables them to be client/family advocates in managing the idiosyncrasies of cancer illnesses and treatment modalities.

County extension services can provide a natural opportunity for outreach health services to rural/frontier people, if either a professional nurse is a part of the staff, or if a liaison is formed between the county health department and county extension services. Such nurses could, for example, assist community members in planning and implementing nurse-led support and information groups for persons with cancer and their families. Likewise, these nurses could organize careering classes for informal providers, similar to those developed by the University of Missouri (31,32).

The historic relationship between county extension agencies and land grant university nursing programs provide opportunities for reciprocal consultation, service, and training. Certainly, county extension agencies are respected by rural/frontier people, and could assist university faculty/students in gaining access for training and service opportunities.

REFERENCES

1. Cooper ET. A pilot study on the effects of the diagnosis of lung cancer on family relationships. *Cancer Nurs* 1984;7:301–8.

2. Derdiarian AK. Informational needs of recently diagnosed cancer patients. *Nurs Res* 1986;35:276–81.

3. Houts PS, Yasko W. Harvey HA, et al. Unmet needs of persons with cancer in Pennsylvania during the period of terminal care. *Cancer* 1988;62:627–34.

4. Blank J, Clark L, Longman A, Atwood J. Perceived home care needs of cancer patients and their caregivers. *Cancer Nurs* 1989;12:78–84.

5. Frank-Stromborg MF, Wright P. Ambulatory cancer patients' perception of the physical and psychosocial changes in their lives since the diagnosis of cancer. *Cancer Nurs* 1984;7:117–30.

6. Houts PS, Yasko JM. Kahn SB. Schelzel GW, Marconi KM. Unmet psychological, social, and economic needs of persons with cancer in Pennsylvania. *Cancer* 1986;58:2355–61.

7. Michels N. The transition from hospital to home: An exploratory study. *Home Health Care Serv Q* 1988.9:29–44.

8. Mor V, Guadagnoli E, Wool M. An examination of the concrete service needs of advanced cancer patients. *J Psychosocial Oncol* 1987.5:1–17.

9. Welch D. Planning nursing intervention for family members of adult cancer patients. *Cancer Nurs* 1981;4:365–70.

10. Grobe ME, Ahmann DI, Ilstrup DM. Needs assessment for advanced cancer patients and their families. *Oncol Nurs Forum* 1982;9:26–30.

11. Parsons J B. A descriptive study of intermediate stage terminally ill cancer patients at home. *Nurs Dimensions 1977;5:1–26.*

12. Wright K, Dyck S. Expressed concerns of adult cancer patients' family members. *Cancer Nurs* 1984;7:371–4.

13. Matson CA. Families with a terminally ill member a grounded theory of family relationships. *Am J Hospice Care 1988;5:38*–41.

14. Holing EV. The primary caregiver's perception of the dying trajectory. *Cancer Nurs* i986;9:29–37.

15. Archbold P. Impact of parent caring on middle-aged offspring. *J Gerontol Nurs* 1980;6:79–85.

16. Gavnor S. When the caregiver becomes the patient. *Geriatr Nurs 1989;10:120–3.*

17. Baird S. Nursing roles in continuing care: home care and hospice. *Semin Oncol* 1980;7:28–38.

18. Coyle N, Monzillo E, Loscalzo M, Farkas C, Massie MJ, Foley KM.

A model of continuity of care for cancer patient with pain and neuro-oncologic complications. *Cancer Nurs 1985;8:* 111–9.

19. Vinciguerra V, Degnan TJ, Sciortino A, et al. A comparative assessment of home versus hospital comprehensive treatment for advanced cancer patients. *J Clin Oncol* 1986;4:1521–8.

20. Coward R. Rural elders: Image and reality. NWGEC *Viewpoint* 1990:2:3–4.

21. Rosenblatt RA, Moscovice IS. *Rural health care.* New York: Wiley, 1982.

22. Kruger RA. *Focus groups: A practical guide for applied research.* Newbury Park, CA: Sage, 1988.

23. Elison G. Frontier areas: Problems for delivery of health services. *Rural Health Care 1986;8:1,* 3.

24. Glaser BG. *Theoretical sensitivity.* Mill Valley, CA: Sociology Press, 1978.

25. Wilson HS. *Research in nursing.* Menlo Park, CA: AddisonWesley, 1985.

26. Glaser BG, Strauss A. *Time for dying.* Chicago: Aldine, 1968.

27. Weinert C, Long KA. Understand the health care needs of rural families. *Fam Relations 1987;36:450–5.*

28. Dietz M. Stressors and coping mechanisms of older rural women. In: Busby A, ed. *Rural nursing. Vol.* 1. Newbury Park, CA: Sage, 1991:267–80.

29. Horn BM, Primomo J. Health care needs of families with children in a rural island community: Results of an ethnographic study. Proceedings of 2nd International Family Nursing Conference, Portland, OR, 1991:97.

30. Jenkins S. The future of rural communities: Mobilizing local resources. In: Bushy A, ed. *Rural nursing.* Vol. 2. Newbury Park, CA: Sage, 1991:16–28.

31. Halpen BP. Volunteer information provider program: Strategy to reach and help rural family caregivers. *Gerontologist 1988:28:* 256–9.

32. Halpert BP, Sharp TS. A model to nationally replicate a locally successful rural family caregiver program: The volunteer information provider program. *Gerontologist* 1989;29:561–3.

24

Patterns of Responses to Symptoms in Rural Residents: The Symptom-Action-Time-Line Process

Janice A. Buehler, Maureen Malone, and Janis M. Majerus

INTRODUCTION

How people identify, evaluate, and respond to symptoms is an important determinant of their health and illness behavior (Lenz, 1984). An increasing amount of literature addresses health behaviors of rural people (Lee, 1991; Long, 1993; Long & Weinert, 1989; Moon & Graybird, 1982; Weinert & Long, 1990). However, little information is available on the patterns of responses of rural people to symptom occurrence signifying actual or potential health problems. In addition, there is a paucity of information on health behaviors of certain rural groups, specifically, women and Plains Indians.

Although actual processes of health-seeking behavior are not delineated in most research of rural health behaviors, some patterns are evident. A survey of health risk prevalence in rural Montana (Moon & Graybird, 1982) revealed that participants believed in self-responsibility for health. Lee (1991) noted that the quality of hardiness may be responsible for some rural dwellers' delay in seeking assistance from the professional health care system when symptoms of illness appear. Rural people were viewed as delaying health care until they were very ill, thus often needing hospitalization at the point care was sought (Long, 1993; Long & Weinert, 1989; Rosenblatt & Moscovice, 1982; Weinert & Long, 1990).

Studies on responses to symptom occurrence, not specific to rural people, have been conducted by behavioral and social scientists. Mechanic (1960) stated that possible responses to illness include discretionary inaction, the use of medicines, seeking professional care, and using a lay network. Suchman (1966) described individual responses to symptom occurrence as proceeding in this sequential pattern: (1) the Symptom Experience Stage, (2) Assumption of Sick Role Stage, (3) Medical Care Contact Stage, and (4) Dependent Patient Role Stage.

Segall and Goldstein (1989) noted that lay persons clearly do routinely self-evaluate and self-treat many of their health problems as a part of daily living and that the nature and extent of these self-care practices are not well understood. They concluded it is not clear whether self-care behavior is equally prevalent among different social groups, whether self-care is used for both health maintenance and the treatment of illness, and whether self-care is used only in response to selected symptomatic conditions.

METHODS

The qualitative method of grounded theory was used in this study (Glaser & Strauss, 1967). Grounded theory provides a means of understanding behavioral patterns from the perspective of the participants. It enables learning about their world and the interacting influences of personal, social, and cultural characteristics without imposing the cultural biases of the interviewer (Chenitz & Swanson, 1986). Grounded theory allows for the direct examination of the world of rural residents in a naturalistic way (Schatzman & Strauss, 1973).

The convenience sample was composed of 16 rural or frontier Montana women, 8 of whom were Native American women living on a federal reservation and 8 of whom were Caucasian farm or ranch women. Elison (1986) defines rural as a population density of more than 6 but less than 100 per square mile and a driving distance to a hospital of at least 30 minutes. "Frontier" is defined as a population density of less than 6 per square mile and driving time to a hospital of either 60 minutes or severe geographic and/or seasonal climatic conditions.

The eight Caucasian farm or ranch women were married and had at least two children. Six of them were self-employed, actively farming and ranching with their husbands. Two were employed in a small city 60 miles from their homes. Four of these women lived in rural locations and four in frontier locations. Their nearest neighbors lived one-fourth mile to 8 miles away. One informant's nearest neighbor was 5 miles away but did not have a phone. For emergencies, this informant would travel 12 miles to the nearest neighbor with a telephone. The primary means of paying for health services for these women was through private pay and individual health insurance.

Of the eight Native American women, seven were classified as rural and one as frontier. Five of the informants lived on small ranches and three lived in one of two towns each with populations of less than 200 (U.S. Bureau of Census, 1987). Seven of the informants have lived on the reservation all of their lives. Three of the women were unemployed and on Aid to Families with Dependent Children, two considered themselves full-time homemakers, and the remaining three were employed in local towns. Five of the Native American women were married, two were single, and one was divorced. All informants had children, with an average number of 2.3 children per household and a range of 1–6 children per household. Five informants lived with extended family members, and three lived with only their children and husbands. All eight women used the Indian Health Service which provided free health care as entitled by treaty.

Face-to-face focused interviews were conducted in the homes of the participants. Open-ended interview questions and probes were used to stimulate free responses (Woods & Catanzaro, 1988). Topics included describing the steps used when someone in the home becomes ill, examples of when self-treatment would be used or of when someone would be consulted, signs indicating illness, examples of home remedies, length of time before seeking help, and reasons for deterrence in obtaining care from professional health resources.

The grounded theory data analysis for this study revealed a basic social process (BSP) termed the *symptom-action-time-line process* (SATL).

FINDINGS

Both Native American and Caucasian farm/ranch women used the symptom-action-time-line process to respond to symptoms of actual or potential health problems. The process consists of four stages in which symptoms are identified and actions are taken to move to a desired state of health. The stages are (a) symptom identification, (b) self-care, (c) lay resources, and (d) professional resources. Each stage has a time period (time-line) in which the participant takes actions in response to a symptom, evaluates the effectiveness of the actions in resolving the symptom, and decides whether to go on to the next stage. Time periods during stages are dependent on the intensity, duration, and amount of interference in function caused by the symptom and may be minutes, days, or years. The first stage, symptom identification, is the stimulus leading to the other stages.

Symptom Identification Stage

Symptom identification was preceded by symptom occurrence and included assessment of conditions or signs perceived as being an undesired alteration in the person's usual state of health that required actions to move the person to his or her desired state. Participants identified their desired state as being the way they were before the symptom occurred. The symptoms had three properties: physical signs and sensations, degree of interference in the ability to function, and intensity and duration. Physical signs included "fever," "vomiting," "pain," "pulling at ears," "broken bones," "hard to breathe," and "losing blood." Interference in function included "not being able to do ordinary things like housework," "I couldn't move my finger," and "unable to eat or play." Intensity and duration of symptoms were the degree and rate of change in a symptom, onset of new symptoms, and length of time they persist. Examples included "temperatures over 102 degrees for 3 days" and "a bloody nose that couldn't be stopped after 2 hours." After the symptoms were assessed, they were given meaning, and a decision was made whether to take action. This was dependent on knowledge and past experience with illness, intensity and duration of the symptoms, and degree of interference with normal functioning. A Native American woman stated, "Whenever my girl pulls at her ears and is fussy, I know from before that she probably has an ear infection and we should go in (to the clinic). . . . The first time (she was sick), I waited until she had a fever, and it went so high it really scared me." Participants in both groups stated they noticed most symptoms within minutes to a few hours after occurrence.

Variation noted between Caucasian and Native American women in symptom identification was due to meanings given to symptoms. For example, one of the Native American women, after getting no relief from headaches through use of medications prescribed by a physician, attributed her headaches to supernatural origins and sought care from a medicine man. Both groups of women described lower thresholds of tolerance for duration and intensity of symptoms in their children. This resulted in shorter symptom-action-time-line processes for children.

Self-Care Stage

The second stage of the SATL process was characterized by the initiation of self-care. Self-care involved those activities self-initiated and performed for self or family members in response to symptoms. Examples of self-care listed by respondents ranged from "getting extra rest," "slowing down," "waiting for more symptoms" to more complicated activities such as "soaking my foot three times a day." The time-line described by both groups of women for starting self-care after symptom identification was seconds for intense symptoms to a "couple of days" for minor symptoms.

The self-care stage was also characterized by using self-care tools, those items used by the respondent to resolve symptoms on their own. Both groups listed such items as nonprescription medications, leftover prescription medicine, teas, thermometers, heating pads, disinfectants, and reference books. The majority of the Native American women used traditional self-care tools to treat certain symptoms. These included sage, sweet-grass, and medicine bundles. One Native American woman used a first aid book for reference whereas half the Caucasian ranch women regularly referred to their "family health textbooks." One informant in this group stated, "I looked up symptoms my daughter had, and the book told me what I could do for her at home or if I needed to see a doctor." Another informant added, "Everyone in my family knows how to look up their illnesses in our health book." All of these informants live in the frontier area. Another self-care tool mentioned only by these frontier women was "animal" ointments to treat hand rashes resulting from feeding lambs.

Actions for this stage included initiating self-care; evaluating its effectiveness based on a decrease in the duration, intensity, or the amount of interference in the ability to function; and deciding to seek help if self-care was ineffective. A typical response, for both Native American and Caucasian informants, regarding the decision to seek help was, "I tried taking Tylenol but after two days I still had a fever, so I called my mother for advice."

Lay Resources Stage

In this, the third, stage, the participants involved their informal network of family, friends, and neighbors, that is, their lay resources, by describing the symptoms and obtaining assistance to alleviate symptoms. Properties of this stage included symptom validation, asking advice for self-care or self-care tools, receiving physical care, or seeking emotional support—particularly for deciding to go to a physician. Time-lines for consulting lay resources after symptom identification ranged from one to three days for both groups. Both groups had usually initiated a self-care activity before they consulted their lay resources.

Ranch women stated their most frequently used lay resources were their mothers, but they also consulted with neighbors. Two frontier ranch women described how they had become aware of each other having similar joint pain of the great toe. They compared their symptoms over the phone while referring to their health textbooks that guided them to diagnosing themselves as having gout. They then verified these symptoms and information with another lay resource, a neighbor who was a registered nurse. Ranch women also described an organized informal lay network of volunteer farmers and ranchers who acted as first responders to emergencies. They were called for such symptoms as "chest pain," "losing blood," and "broken bones."

Organized, volunteer networks of lay resources were not described by Native American women. The majority identified their mothers as their primary source of help. A few consulted only with their husbands, stating that they had no relatives or friends living in the area for them to contact. Participants stated they would usually consult a relative before they would consult a neighbor who was not a relative. The majority of the Native American women also consulted their lay network for advice on the use of traditional healing practices. The following described this use of a lay resource.

> *My son (nine-months-old) had been fussy for two days; he was not taking his bottle and had cold sweats. Tylenol didn't seem to be helping, so my mother suggested that I take him to my aunt because he might have colic. My aunt massaged him and blew smoke in his ear. He went to sleep and was O.K. after that.*

Actions for this stage included contacting a lay resource; evaluating whether there was a decrease in the symptom's intensity, duration, or interference with function; and deciding whether to take further action. Varying degrees of self-care continued throughout this stage.

Professional Resources Stage

Seeking help from professional resources occurred when there was failure to alleviate symptoms through the use of self-care or lay resources, or when symptoms intensified, or when new symptoms developed. Professional resources listed by both groups included physicians, registered nurses, dentists, and chiropractors. Both groups stated they consulted professional help when "nothing else helped," "there wasn't anything I could do," or "for emergencies." Nurses were sometimes consulted for advice about whether symptoms required immediate attention or could wait awhile longer. Nurses were frequently used as lay resources in this instance, since they were called at their homes when off duty. Physicians were usually not called at home unless the participant had been under physician care for a specific condition.

Time-lines, from the symptom identification stage to the professional resource stage in situations other than emergencies, were 4–7 days for rural women and 1–2 weeks for frontier women. Time-lines for Native American women ranged from 2 to 5 days in both rural and frontier areas.

Time-line variations occurred for children and in emergencies. For children, total time-line durations were much shorter, ranging from less than 1 day to 3 days. Each stage within the time-line process was shorter; lay resources were consulted sooner and often used only to help transport the child to the professional resource. Barriers to seeking professional care were minimized so that time and distance became less important for children than for adults. In emergencies, individuals tended to bypass self-care and lay resources and go directly to professionals. Barriers were minimized according to the urgency of symptom occurrence.

If symptoms were not alleviated after going to a professional resource, participants either returned to the same professional or went to a different professional. At times, symptoms were simply "tolerated." Several Native American women sought alternative care by contacting a medicine man. This occurred because they believed physicians had not helped. The medicine man was described by these participants as another type of professional. The most frequently identified barriers to professional resources were distance and transportation. Other barriers mentioned were fear of "bad news," a lack of women doctors, and the time required to see a professional, especially time spent in waiting rooms.

IMPLICATIONS

The symptom-action-time-line process clarifies response patterns rural women display when confronted with symptoms of actual or potential health problems. The process provides a framework for health care professionals that is client centered and, therefore, has powerful implications for intervention and health education; promotes culturally sensitive planning and provision of health services; and adds to the body of literature on rural use of health resources.

The SATL process provides a systematic framework for health care providers to assess patterns of response to symptoms and to develop interventions to facilitate rural residents' responses to their symptoms. For a full understanding of what actions a rural client will use to alleviate a health problem, each stage in the process must be carefully assessed on an individual basis.

CONCLUSION

Findings in this study suggest that rural residents use several indicators to identify and evaluate their symptoms. These indicators can be clarified by using the properties of the symptom identification stage as an assessment guide, which will yield information on what signs and sensations prompted symptom identification, tolerance levels for symptoms, amount of interference caused by symptoms, knowledge levels about symptoms, meanings of symptoms, and the time-line and conditions necessary for taking further actions. With these baseline data, health care providers can determine a client's capability to accurately interpret a symptom and take appropriate actions. Corresponding interventions may be aimed at increasing the client's knowledge of indicators of disease processes and the preferable time period in which to initiate an action.

Through assessment of the self-care stage of a client's symptom-action-time-line, information can be elicited regarding the client's self-care patterns. This includes the conditions under which self-care is activated and the variety of self-care tools that are available and employed by the client. Interventions can be directed at expanding a person's access to more effective self-care tools or adapting health care to the tools already available to the person. Findings in this study suggest that assessment of self-care resources leads to an evaluation of a client's lay resources, since self-care tools are often shared with a network of relatives or neighbors. Knowing whom a rural client most often relies on for symptom validation provides valuable information about functional support systems actively used by rural/frontier people. Interventions with a rural client may be more effective if key people in these networks are included.

Assessment of the professional resource stage provides information about the conditions necessary for an individual to seek professional care, appropriateness of time-lines, and barriers that prevent access to care. For example, if clients are seeking professional care for conditions that could be handled at home, interventions can be aimed at making a client's response pattern clear to both the provider and the client by using the SATL process. With this information, the client and provider can identify which response in the process is deficient and mutually determine a more appropriate response.

The multidimensionality of the SATL process increases health professionals' awareness of the dimensions and complexities involved in caring for people from diverse cultural and geographical backgrounds. A health care provider can identify cultural views of health and illness by using the SATL process. These beliefs are deeply entwined within traditional customs and culture. By gaining insight into the traditional attitudes that people have toward health and illness, health care providers can become more sensitive to the issues surrounding health care and the cultural health beliefs of the consumer, thereby providing more comprehensive health care.

Finally, the symptom-action-time-line process has important implications for research. Although research studies appear in the literature on self-care, use of lay or informal health resources, and use of formal health services, these studies tend to focus on single health resource utilization. The SATL process begins to explicate how various types of health resources are used in an integrated manner by actual rural/frontier residents. Furthermore, the preponderance of literature on consumer use of health resources focuses on urban rather than rural populations. Further research is needed to validate the use of the SATL process among rural and urban subpopulations.

REFERENCES

Chenitz, W., & Swanson, J. (1986). From practice to grounded theory. Menlo Park, CA: Addison-Wesley.

Elison, G. (1986). Frontier areas: Problems for delivery of health care services. *Rural Health Care, 8* (5), 1, 3.

Glaser, B., & Strauss, A. (1967). *Discovery of grounded theory.* Chicago: Aldine.

Lee, H. J. (1991). Relationship of hardiness and current life events to perceived health in rural adults. *Research in Nursing and Health, 14,* 351–359.

Lenz, E. (1984). Information seeking: A component of client decisions and health behavior. *Advances in Nursing Science, 6* (3), 59–72

Long, K.A. (1993). The concept of health: Rural perspectives. *Nursing Clinics of North America, 28* (1), 123–130.

Long, K. A., & Weinert, C. (1989). Rural nursing: Developing the theory base. *Scholarly Inquiry for Nursing Practice: An International Journal, 3* (2), 113–131.

Mechanic, D. (1960). Illness behavior and medical diagnosis. *Journal of Health Social Behavior, 1,* 86–94.

Moon, R., & Graybird, D. (1987). *High risk prevalence: A report card for Montana.* Helena, MT: Montana Department of Health and Environmental Sciences.

Rosenblatt, R., & Moscovice, I. (1982). *Rural health care.* New York: Wiley.

Segall, A., & Goldstein, J. (1989). Exploring the correlates of self-provided health care behaviour. *Social Science Medicine, 29* (2), 153–161.

Schatzman, L., & Strauss, A. (1973). *Field research.* New Jersey: Prentice-Hall.

Suchman, E. (1966). Health orientation and medical care. *American Journal of Public Health, 56* (1), 97–105.

United States Bureau of Census. (1987). *Statistical Abstract of the United States: 1988* (108th ed.). Washington, DC: U. S. Government Printing Office.

Weinert, C. & Long, K. A. (1990). Rural families and health care: Refining the knowledge base. *The Journal of Marriage and Family Review, 15* (1–2), 57–75.

Woods, N. F., & Catanzaro, M. (1988). *Nursing research: Theory and practice.* St Louis, MO: Mosby.

25

Organ Procurement: A Rural Nurse Generalist in a Specialized Field

Sharon R. Hovey and Debra A. Doll

The purpose of this chapter is to describe the unique rural nursing practice of the second author, a certified procurement transplant coordinator in Montana. The mission of the rural generalist in this specialized field is advocacy, support, and development of activities that will maximize the availability of organs and tissues and enhance the quality, effectiveness and integrity of the organ donation process. The information and anecdotal material contained herein reflect the lived experience of working in a rural setting.

HISTORY

A northwest regional kidney donation program, the Northwest Organ Procurement Agency (NOPA), was initiated in 1971 in Seattle, Washington. The NOPA program serves western and central Washington, Alaska, and Montana. Expansion in 1986 to include the recovery of other organs and tissue created an opportunity for a rural nursing practice made possible through a grant awarded to the Northwest Kidney Center and NOPA. These nurse coordinator positions were designed to identify, refer, and manage donors and to educate the public and professionals about organ donation.

THE RURAL MONTANA ENVIRONMENT

Expansive distances, weather extremes, and sparse population all impact this rural nursing role. Montana's 1995 population of 870,280 people live within 145,392 square miles (Montana Department of Public Health and Human Services, 1996). Montana has an overall population density of 5.5 persons per square mile. Frontier counties have a population density of less than 6 people per square mile. Forty-six of the 56 Montana counties are frontier counties. Nationwide 24% of all U.S. citizens live in rural areas. In Montana, roughly 75 percent of all people live in rural areas (Babcock, 1993).

RURAL NURSE GENERALIST IN A SPECIALIZED FIELD

The organ procurement program in Montana is divided into three geographic regions. Each region is served by a registered nurse with specialty certification as a procurement transplant coordinator (CPTC). In the urban organ procurement setting, CPTCs function in only one of four major roles: hospital education and development, procurement, community and media relations, or as a bereavement specialist. The rural CPTC is responsible for all four roles. This generalist role demands a highly self-directed and skilled practitioner. Resource mobilization responsibilities, verbal and written communication skills, and knowledge of hospital, community, and family systems are integral to the practice of this role.

Resource development within the community and hospital combined with knowledge of hospital, community, and family systems provide for smooth coordination of the organ recovery process. One mechanism to smooth coordination is the development of a donor council. In each of the three consolidated population settings in the state, key people interested in the process of organ and tissue donation have been identified to develop a donor council. Donor councils aid in maintaining continuity and accountability for in-house hospital donor programs.

The CPTC is also responsible for the education of health care professionals and the community about organ donation. The donor process consists of (a) confirming brain death documentation, (b) making sure the next-of-kin has given informed consent and the proper forms are signed, (c) blood draws for tissue typing and serology with transportation arranged to the Seattle lab, (d) donor management and organ placement instituted, (e) coordination of procurement team's arrival with hospital operating room staff, and (f) staff and family follow-up.

Through developmental efforts, NOPA featured a Great Falls, Montana, hospital and its staff in its regional newsletter (Barber & Doll, 1994). The article raised awareness and motivated the health care team to increase their efforts to offer the option of donation to families in appropriate situations. In one instance, this heightened awareness by a rural hospital member resulted in a 16–year-old involved in a fatal horseback riding incident being identified as a potential donor. The procurement nurse coordinator drove 200 miles, one way, to the hospital to work with the donor family and to coordinate the donor process.

Collaboration with nurses, physicians, social workers, pastoral care, x-ray, respiratory therapy, laboratory, pharmacy, medical records, patient accounts, and coroners provides information crucial to the nurse's care of the donor family. Support for these health team members is provided by the nurse coordinator and is essential throughout the donor process. The hospital staff had a positive donation experience related to the horseback riding fatality. Their participation resulted in giving new life to three recipients, sight to two people, and bone and skin grafts to many who needed orthopedic surgery or bone cancer treatment. This energized the staff to continue to develop the donor program. With the procurement nurse coordinator's assistance, hospital policies were updated, and a brain death policy was adopted by the medical staff.

Verbal, nonverbal, and written communication skills are all interwoven into the generalist role. Development of support systems and follow-up with donor families provides the opportunity for interaction with varied cultures and communities. The nurse must be responsive to multiple health care providers and diverse community service organizations, such as church groups, homemaker clubs, funeral homes, driver's license departments, and schools. Community awareness about donation is increased by interaction with the media. This includes newspaper features, radio public service announcements, and television talk shows.

In follow-up of the organ and tissue procurement from the horseback riding accident, members of this hospital's health care team took their positive attitudes to the community systems where they were involved. This brought about speaking engagements for the CPTC with groups such as the Lions and Kiwanas Clubs. Articles about donation were placed in the local newspaper, and programs were aired on local radio and TV. The ripples in the rural setting parallel a very similar international situation known in the media as the "Nicholas Effect." This is the well-known story of a seven-year-old American, Nicholas Green, who was killed by bandits on the autobahn while vacationing with his parents in Italy. His parents chose to donate his organs in a country (Italy) that knew little about organ and tissue donation (The Nicholas Green Foundation, 1995). Extreme sensitivity to family systems and communities in crisis is crucial to the communication role.

Bereavement care is also an integral part of the generalist's role. In assessing family grief dynamics and support systems, the rural nurse often meets unanticipated challenges. One family, experiencing the loss of a teenage daughter, had very little monetary resources. They were afraid of not being able to afford a funeral and had no money to buy a dress in which to bury their daughter. The mother asked if there was monetary compensation provided to families by procurement programs in exchange for their willingness to donate. Under strict national guidelines, organ procurement agencies are not able to reimburse families for donation. This nurse coordinator explained the guidelines to the family, but still felt a need to help. She made a call to the local ministerial council; people from a local church came to visit with the coordinator and the family. This church mobilized resources to aid the family in funeral expenses and obtained a dress for burial of this young girl. The continued bereavement needs of the family were attended to through the donor family aftercare program of "Something More." This national group collaborates with procurement programs under the direction of the CPTC and is a resource for telephone, mail, and face-to-face bereavement support. The involved donor family was followed by the nurse coordinator for several months to make sure there were support networks and to assess the family's grief work.

UNIQUENESS OF RURAL PRACTICE

Rural neighbors may be isolated geographically but not interactively. Full-sized cars or four-wheel drive vehicles are viewed as an economic necessity related to safety in long-distance travel and harsh climate conditions. During one year this nurse coordinator logged more than 17,000 miles within the state to do her job. A four-wheel drive vehicle was necessary for many of these miles. During this year, she also made seven trips to Seattle covering 35 days and made job-related flights to Alaska, Colorado, and Oregon. In that same year temperature extremes covered 147 degrees, ranging from 106 degrees Fahrenheit in the summer to 41 degrees below zero in the winter.

Mobilization of Rural Hospital and Community Resources

The mobilization of resources to remote areas is exemplified in the following story. During midwinter in below-zero weather on a moonlit snowmobiling outing, tragedy occurred when a rider was thrown and sustained a severe injury. One companion stayed with the injured while another went for emergency help 24 miles away. The local EMT response provided optimal field stabilization until transport to the area medical center was accomplished. Because of the severity of the injury, the victim became brain dead, and the family consented to multiple organ and tissue donation. Although the injured person's life ended, the quick and capable response by the EMT system preserved organ function and provided many people and their families with renewed life.

In many smaller rural hospitals, surgery and ancillary staff must be called in to facilitate the donor process. While the urban hospital may be resistant to rescheduling a busy operating room for procurement, the rural hospital quickly mobilizes resources. Rural hospitals and communities are very supportive with personnel, food, and transportation. Highway patrol, military transport, and charter airline services often assist with the transportation of donated tissues.

Because one rural family knew the connections within their community, they were able to donate. This small town family lost their son in a car accident in a remote part of the state. Because of their desire to help others, the family initiated contact with a person they knew was aware of the donor program. This ancillary health care provider then notified the organ procurement nurse coordinator who made arrangements with a small rural hospital near the accident site. The nurse coordinator (who had traveled 90 miles by car), the staff of the rural hospital, and the local general physician did the tissue recovery. There was a limited amount of time to facilitate the transport of the tissue to a commercial airport 100 miles away. The county sheriff offered police escort to hasten the travel. The commercial airline held the flight for the arrival of the nurse coordinator and the donated tissue that was to be transported to the urban out-of-state processing center.

Serology testing is vital to the donation process, especially for hepatitis and human immunodeficiency viruses. Blood for this process must be transported long distances to one of the two major cities within the state. If a potential donor is identified during the night, the process may be delayed several hours due to the lack of commercial transportation for blood specimens. The following example explicates resource mobilization related to the nurse's community connections. One rural emergency room nurse had a friend who was a pilot and volunteered to request his services for blood transport. His consent and flight during the dark hours of the night saved the donor process approximately 15 hours of crucial time.

The CPTC as "insider"

The value of the expertise and the willingness of a community to accept the CPTC is contingent upon the nurse's "fitting in" with community norms and becoming an insider. These norms include the status of the spouse's livelihood—often measured in acres farmed/ranched or numbers of livestock owned; the children's school and social activities; and elements of the nurse's personhood including personal and social interactions and dress. A presentation made by this rural procurement nurse in casual attire to a small hospital physician and nursing staff was acceptable because the coordinator was seen as a "local" whose husband was a farmer. Her appearance in a three-piece suit probably would have been met with resistance and nonacceptance. Being viewed as "too different" is often interpreted as really not understanding the needs of the rural setting. Another fear related to the potential display of wealth (the three-piece suit) is that "they're here to make money off us." These aspects of rural culture impact the willingness of rural dwellers to help their neighbors through donor decisions—and to trust the nurse they know.

Stressors

"Required request" laws compel the nurse to request anatomical gifts at the time of death. Rural donor families generally know and trust their health care providers. Separating the personal and professional roles becomes very difficult in the small, rural community setting. Friends, neighbors and their children are often the patients the local nurse must care for in the emergency room after a tragic and fatal situation. This familiarity with the potential donor and their family creates a personal agony and may complicate the stresses for the nurse. Although there is often internal anguish for the professional, this extension of care can also provide a trusting and safe environment for the grieving family.

Reverence for Preservation of Life

Birth and death are intimate parts of life in a rural setting. The violence of urban areas is often related to humans. In addition to humans, the cycle of life in rural areas often relates to animals, to the survival of species, and to the seasons in nature. An anecdote reflects rural respect for life. The eyebank was to receive donated eyes via bus transport from a distant hospital. The box containing the eyes was stolen during transport. Emergency room personnel received an anonymous call later that day, saying there was a package to be picked up on the nearby steps of the hospital. When the previously opened box was recovered by the ER staff, it was found to contain a pair of donated eyes. This box that only hours before had been stolen from the bus depot was probably thought to have contained drugs. Upon discovering the reality, the thief chose not to discard the box in a dumpster but to return the find to the hospital. The sight of another was not to be robbed.

Role Effectiveness

The rural organ recovery nurse functions in an effective and culturally sensitive way. One measure of the effectiveness of this rural nursing role may be the donor rate. The national rate of donors per million population was 19 in 1992 and 1994. According to the ongoing statistical information in the office of the Northwest Organ Procurement Agency, in western and central Washington the donor rate per million population was 13.5 in 1992, 14 in 1994, and 15 in 1996. Donor rates for the same years in Montana reached a remarkable high of 32, 25, and 25. Rural people are very generous and sharing of their resources, even human organs.

Another measure of effectiveness may be longevity in the position. This Montana nurse procurement coordinator was recently honored nationally. She was recognized for her eight-and-one-half years of service in a position that has a national average burnout rate of 18 months (UNOS Update, 1995). Perhaps the challenges and diversity of the rural generalist contributed to her longevity!

The value of the rural nurse generalist's role in rural communities may be vastly underestimated and taken for granted. Intrinsic rewards—knowing a person has sight again, a child with biliary atresia returned to her parents with a new liver, and another person is off the dialysis machine—are much greater for the rural nurse in the specialized field of organ recovery. She can connect with the family, health care team, and community through all phases of the organ recovery process. The circle is often completed as the nurse coordinator facilitates the meeting of donor and recipient families—and shares in the opportunity to transform a devastating loss into life for another human being. Organ procurement may offer a tremendous reward for the rural nurse generalist in a specialized field.

REFERENCES

Babcock, M. (1993, July 17). Urban rulemakers are out of touch. *Great Falls Tribune,* p. A5.

Barber, K. & Doll, D. (1994). New program helps hospital identify donor candidates. *Procure, 9* (Fall), p. E1.

Montana Department of Public Health and Human Services. (1996, November). *1994 and 1995 Montana Vital Statistics* (pp. 95–101). Helena, MT: Vital Statistics Bureau and Office of the State Registrar.

The Nicholas Green Foundation. (1995). PO Box 937. Bodega Bay, CA 94923. (707) 875-2263.

UNOS Update. (1995). Dedication, adrenaline, keep coordinators going: Doll, Wilson, and Hall profiled. *11*(7), 1–4. Richmond, VA: United Network of Organ Sharing (UNOS).

26

Provider Perceptions of Problems Caring for American Indians: Containing Disruption

Janice A. Buehler

This qualitative study describes health care provider perceptions of issues involved in providing care to American Indian clients in health care facilities (excluding Indian Health Service facilities) in six communities in Montana. All of these communities are within easy travel of one or more of Montana's six Indian reservations.

Most of Montana Indians are members of various Plains tribes, such as the Crow, Northern Cheyenne, Blackfeet, Gros Ventre, and Assiniboine (Snipe, 1989). Albeit, the nomadic life of following the buffalo is long gone, aspects of the traditional Plains culture have been maintained (Bryan, 1985; Buehler, 1992; Frey, 1987). Classic examples, relevant to nursing and health care, are the prime importance of extended family in daily life and the practice of traditional healing ceremonies and rituals. The importance of providing culturally sensitive nursing care continues to be a major theme of transcultural nursing literature. However, Bailey (1996) in reviewing this literature, found few empirical studies actually documenting this need.

Semistructured interviews were conducted with a convenience sample of 35 health care providers, 22 of whom were affiliated with three health care facilities in three rural cities (population less than 100,000),

Acknowledgment: funded by the Montana Consortium for Excellence in Health Care.

and 13 of whom were affiliated with three health care facilities in three small towns (population less than 2,500). Two providers were American Indian, and the remaining 33 were non-Indian. The majority of health care professionals in the sample were nurses (n = 26). Three physicians and 6 other health care providers (social worker, nutritionist, etc.) completed the sample. Informants were asked to discuss experiences in providing care to American Indian clients. Prompts included common issues and/or problems, successes, barriers, and resources.

Grounded theory data analysis (Glaser, 1992) revealed two core variables. The first is a basic social process (BSP), "*containing disruption.*" This variable is both the main problem confronted by the informants as they care for their Indian clients and the process they use to attempt to manage the problem. The second core variable is a contextual continuum, "*cultural awareness.*" This variable refers to the apparent degree of cultural awareness of individual provider-informants. Cultural awareness impacts each stage of the process of containing disruption. The next sections elaborate the substantive theory based on these emergent variables.

CONTAINING DISRUPTION

As noted in Figure 26.1, the condition giving rise to the process of containing disruption consists of the clashing of two disparate cultures. The process consists of three phases or stages. The first involves the actual disruption, the second phase entails the strategies that providers use in attempting to contain disruption, and the final stage consists of resolution of the disruption.

Condition	Stage 1	Stage 2	Stage 3
clashing cultures	disruption occurs - environment - provider comfort	containing strategies	resolution

FIGURE 26.1 Containing disruption.

ENVIRONMENT

Family
- —crowd our waiting and patient rooms
- —want information and/or expect to be included in decision making
- —"out of control" children play in our halls and elevators

PROVIDER DISCOMFORT

Demeanor Difference
Discrimination Claiming
"Noncompliance" with *our* care/treatment regimes

FIGURE 26.2 State I: Disruption.

Stage One: Disruption Occurs

The potential for disruption and the necessity for attempting to contain it can exist whenever and wherever an American Indian client/family seeks health care. The coming together of persons with cultural backgrounds as different as Indian clients and health care providers can set the stage and provide the condition for the first stage of the process, disruption.

The concept of disruption emerged as I examined the provider data discussing the problems/issues encountered in caring for Indian patients. I realized these problems related to health care providers viewing Indian clients/families as breaking implicit and explicit rules of the health care facilities and/or of the providers. Included in this rule-breaking were multitudes of examples of provider expectations being unmet by the Indian client and her or his family. As seen in Figure 26.2, two types of rule-breaking disruption were problematic: environmental and provider comfort.

Environmental disruption: The family. An Indian patient's extended family is often viewed as an environmental disruption. The culturally unaware provider, with his or her assumption of the nuclear family as the proper standard, was frequently not accepting of the larger numbers of family members accompanying an Indian patient. A culturally aware provider who plays an advocacy role for Indian patients/families in a hospital setting said:

Native American families tend to have a tremendous amount of family involvement when a patient is ill, and so they show up at the hospital, as they probably do all over Montana, in great numbers—which I think is wonderful. And the hospital doesn't appreciate that. The staff don't appreciate that; they think that's wrong.

Provider complaints of Indian families included that there were "too many of them in our small waiting rooms" and/or "too many of them staying in the patient's room." When I asked complaining providers what they thought accounted for these larger numbers of family members, rarely was there awareness of the cultural significance of the extended family to an Indian person.

An Indian provider talked about the importance of family when she told the following story:

. . . [recently there was] this one lady in particular, she had cancer, she was dying. So the family stayed with her. But that was her whole life—her family. Her life revolved around her kids and grandkids . . . they all just needed to be with her, they just needed to be together to help her and each other through that. There were a lot of them. They were coming in shifts, and some of them were staying here all the time.

An indicator of a lack of understanding of the importance of family being together during illness was displayed by the nurse who worried that Indian patients "don't receive enough rest because there's so many family in the room." Those of us who are members of the dominant society with our individualist, rather than group, orientation fail to understand or at least tend to underestimate the support and strength an ill Native American receives from the presence of her or his family.

The contrast between group and individual orientations was also seen in the observation, by a culturally aware provider, of the necessity for Native Americans to make health care decisions as a family group. The provider said:

Our Native Americans like to make group decisions by consensus, with enough time to let an answer come. And our doctors want to come in and demand a procedure be done, and that you make the decision cause I'm standing here and put your signature on that. . . . The doctors don't want to wait and talk to lots of family; they want things to click, click. And that's been a problem.

A related provider complaint was breaking the norm that information about a patient's condition is given to *only one* family member. That individual is then expected to communicate with other family members. Frequently hospital nurses complained of this norm violation. As one nurse said, "... I find it hard to know who to give information to so that you're not talking to a lot of people and repeating yourself when you have a busy day." Furthermore, the dominant society assumption that the appropriate contact person for a married patient is the spouse may not be the case with Native Americans. A nurse described this situation:

> *Say a Native American man comes in. And then you ask him, you know we usually assume that the person to contact would be the wife or husband, depending. And in this case you ask him who his wife is, he tells you who that is and you say, "Well, is that who you want contacted?" And he says, "No, you need to get hold of my mother or my [other] mother," indicating the other two women that are there with him. And when you say, "Well, is this your biological parent?" [And he says,] "Well this one is and the other is my stepmother." And then they say, "Well, but then there's my aunt and she will need to know." So in most of these cases the wife doesn't have a lot to say. She isn't necessarily the contact person; it's other adult females.*

Another frequent family disruption complaint was that of visiting Indian children "being out of control." This involved "playing in the halls" and "riding the elevators." And to compound matters, some providers said family members had become irritated when asked to control their children! Rather than being out of control, Indians tend to view their children as simply being children. Typically, Plains Indians, as well as many other tribes, tend to rear their children with minimal interference, encouraging exploration and discovery.

A comparative group used for contrast with other study facilities was an outpatient clinic staffed by providers and administrators with a special commitment to providing culturally sensitive health services to their predominately Native American clientele. I observed that the physical environment of the clinic was open, light, and airy, and the walls were filled with Native American art. The decor included an indoor garden area with a waterfall. And the waiting area contained a large glass enclosed play room with toys, books, and health education material for children of various ages. The staff I interviewed made no mention of disturbances by "out of control" Indian children. When I asked if children were ever a disturbance, I was told "no."

Disturbances by family were the norm-breaking events that created environmental disruption for health care providers in the study. The other type of disruption encountered in this first stage of the process is *provider discomfort.* Provider discomfort consists of three types: demeanor differences, discrimination claiming, and "noncompliance" with care and treatment regimes.

Provider discomfort: Demeanor differences. Among common complaints by some providers were differences in Indian patients' demeanor such as their being quiet and reserved. A young provider who worked with both inpatient and outpatient Indian patients said:

> *They tend to be very closed and don't want to talk . . . They're mostly very closed minded—I don't want to say closed minded, but they're quiet. You know, they don't want to provide a lot of information.*

Another issue of demeanor that was often misunderstood and caused provider discomfort was that of Indian patients and family members not making eye contact with providers. A nurse I interviewed talked about recently attending a cultural awareness workshop at her facility and how she had learned about the cultural meaning, to many Indians, of direct, sustained eye contact. She said, "I thought it was rude that they didn't make eye contact when talking to you. Now I know they think *that* is rude, that it is staring!"

A final demeanor creating discomfort is that of the Indian patient and/or family speaking their indigenous language in the provider's presence. A nurse described the discomfort of her peers:

> *[Another] problem that some other nurses have mentioned is that they feel real uncomfortable when they go into the room, and they say something to a patient, and then the other [family] members in the room are speaking whatever their native tongue—most of the time it's Crow. And they feel real uncomfortable because you feel like people are talking about you.*

Speaking one's native language, averting eye contact, and a quiet, reserved manner were the Indian demeanor some health care providers found discomforting. Likewise, several providers spoke of being uncomfortable with what they assumed were inaccurate, unfair claims by Indians of discriminatory behavior by providers.

Provider discomfort: Discrimination claiming. Various providers shared a perception that Indians make unfounded claims of discrimination in how an ill family member or visitors were treated. An ICU nurse spoke of Indian visitor complaints that limitation of visitors was discriminatory:

> *We've been told we've been discriminatory, you know. We limit our visitors to the intensive care unit, and because certain cultures bring mother and brother and aunt and uncle and third and fourth cousin. It's not necessary for them to hang around somebody who's recuperating . . . we do the same thing for anybody, you know, as far as whether they're white or Hispanic or black or whatever. But we've been told we're discriminating against them, and it's not true, because we do it for everybody. It's the policy.*

I found it interesting that throughout this conversation the provider never referred to the subjects of her complaint, i.e., Indians.

A provider who views a major part of his role as an advocate for Indian patients and families shared his experiences of hearing nurses complain about Indians' claims of discrimination. He said:

> *. . . the nurses, they always complain, you know, "If us white folks don't have something that we like in a hospital and we complain, you know, we go about it the proper way and try to fix it. . . . Whereas, Native Americans cry foul and prejudice no matter what's wrong and think they're gonna get better care because they scream that."*

Later in the interview with the above provider, I asked his assessment of the legitimacy of discrimination claiming by Indian patients/families. He said, "The Native American families I've worked with don't cry discrimination, don't cry prejudice, unless there is prejudice."

Provider discomfort: Noncompliance. The last discomfort discussed by providers was what they termed noncompliance. Provider complaints ranged from Indian people not seeking preventive and/or early health services to not following prescribed or recommended treatment and care regimes. Frequently the range of noncompliance complaints was made about the same patient. This was the case with a medicine man from a local tribe described by a nurse informant:

> *I think he'd been sick for quite awhile and hadn't sought health care until he was quite ill. . . . They determined he had some serious respiratory problems and required oxygen . . . we got him kind of stabilized, and he hadn't wanted to stay in the hospital for very long, he just wanted to get out right*

away. So he was discharged after about three days. . . . He came right back just a few days later that week with increasing respiratory difficulty, and he had developed some renal failure. . . . a lot of it was he didn't want to comply with what the physician was trying to get him to do.

Generally, noncompliance was an issue discussed by providers regardless of their degree of cultural understanding. The difference cultural understanding made was in defining "who has the problem." Clearly in the quote above, the nurse blamed the patient. A culturally sophisticated nurse manager of a unit recognized that compliance issues reflected her priorities, not the patient's. She said,

. . . the most difficulty is with compliance. From our perspective, there are certain issues, particularly if you're dealing with spinal cord injuries, that aren't really up for negotiation, like skin integrity, bowel retraining, being aware of things they need to do for health maintenance. And sometimes our priorities, more likely than not, are different than what the [Indian] person with the disability feels is important.

In the above quotation, the culturally aware nurse defined "who has the problem" as the staff expecting compliance.

One informant, a culturally enlightened physician, chose not to use the terms compliance and noncompliance and explained her position as follows:

I view compliance differently than I think most medical people do. I'm a person who feels that if someone makes an informed decision and decides not to do something we recommend, then I don't label them as noncompliant. I do think that the Native American population makes different choices than, say, non-Indian people would. But I still think they are informed choices, so I don't consider it noncompliance. I consider it a choice that they've made for whatever reason and deal with it that way.

Interestingly, this provider's view that an *informed decision* not to comply negates using the term noncompliance, is contrary to the taxonomic work of the North American Nursing Diagnostic Association (NANDA) (Wuest, 1993). That is, NANDA defines noncompliance as "a person's informed decision not to adhere to a therapeutic regimen" (p. 217). Regardless of these differing definitions, serious debate continues in the nursing literature over whether the term noncompliance has a place in nursing practice. In a critique of nursing research on noncompliance, Wuest finds both an ethnocentric and androcentric bias.

The discussion of provider discomfort and its properties of discrimination claiming and demeanor differences brings to an end the first phase of the process of containing disruption. To recapitulate, the first phase, "disruption occurs," involves provider perceptions of two major sources of disruption: provider discomfort and the environment. The latter refers to the issue of perceived disruption in the health care facility environment believed to be created by American Indian families.

Stage Two: Containment Strategies

The strategies discussed by providers to contain perceived disruption created by the presence of American Indian clients and families were diverse. Some were specific to particular containment issues identified in phase one; others were more general and sometimes were used for more than one containment problem. The especially relevant dimensions of the strategies were the *interactional level* of the strategy and the implied *degree of cultural awareness* implicit in the strategy. These two dimensions are cross-cut in Figure 26.3 and constitute the typology of containment strategies.

Data analysis revealed that containment strategies occur on the dyadic interactional level of *provider-client* and on the *administrative/*

Degree of Cultural Awareness	**Interaction Levels** **Provider-Client**	 **Administrative**
Aware	- clearly communicating expectations - "asking them questions" - negotiating priorities **Aware Provider**	- matching patient/provider - policies making expectations clear - attempting to change racist attitudes through mandatory training **Aware Administration**
Unaware	- avoiding client - complaining behind the scenes **Unaware Provider**	- reactive negative sanctions e.g., restrict visitors **Unaware Administration**

FIGURE 26.3 Stage II: Containment strategies.

managerial level. On each level, some strategies seem indicative of provider or administrative cultural awareness, and others do not. Examples of each are given.

Aware provider strategies. Several providers spoke of the simple strategy of "asking if you don't understand." This strategy was especially common when a provider was unclear about the cultural meaning of something to an Indian client. A nurse who had experience caring for American Indians in another region said, "If I feel I don't understand, I'm not afraid to ask." Later in the interview, this nurse gave a specific example related to the demeanor difference of eye contact that creates discomfort for some providers:

> *I've learned some things from this particular family we have right now because they don't give you eye contact. Of course that seems to be usual behavior [among many Indians] but I just needed to check it out with this family. They gave me really good information about their culture. They were listening, they just don't believe in making eye contact.*

A culturally enlightened physician, within the context of the issue of compliance, talked about the importance of asking questions about the culture of her Indian patients. She said, "I think we need to be asking questions, and we don't always ask them, about how the culture is impacting what we're seeing or the decisions that are being made."

Another example of a strategy used by culturally aware providers was *clearly communicating expectations*. An Indian nurse said, regarding the presence of large numbers of family interfering with care, "All you have to do is just ask them to step out, and they do." As will be discussed later, this strategy was also used on the culturally aware administrative level.

A final example of a strategy used by an aware provider to contain the disruption of noncompliance was *negotiating priorities*. A nurse in a rehabilitation setting discussed this strategy:

> *I have found, a lot of times, if I get [Indian people] to try to explain to me why they feel and believe certain ways for certain things. And to have them identify what they think is important and then work from that angle to get what's valuable to them versus what is valuable to us, that has saved me a lot of frustrating moments.*

Unaware provider strategies. The contrast between the strategies used by culturally aware providers compared with unaware providers is striking. Unaware providers were willing to acknowledge only two such strategies. The first was to *avoid the Indian patient.* A forthright nurse described this strategy and the environmental disruption that might prompt it. She said,

> *You know, it's very difficult because of the size of the rooms and the number of [Indian] people in the rooms. Um, to be able to get in there and to do what you need to do. And at times, it's almost easier to almost—I don't want to say ignore—but to not go in the room. Because it's so much trouble to get by everyone to get to the patient.*

The second strategy, *ignoring/complaining,* was described by a nurse in response to my asking what strategies she used or saw other providers using to contain perceived family disruption. She said,

> *Well, I think for the most part we tend to just ignore it or complain about it behind the scenes. We expect that they will comply with our rules and values. We don't do anything constructive, just be upset by it and let it go on.*

Not all complaints were behind the scenes. Both administrators and providers discussed administrative disruption containment strategies used in their facilities. I have categorized these as "aware administrative" and "unaware administrative" and will discuss the latter first.

Unaware administrative strategies. A nursing administrator discussed her facility's strategy, *reactive negative sanctions,* for attempting to manage large numbers of family members visiting an ill Indian patient. She said:

> *Often times Native American families show up with large numbers of extended family. One of their family members is hospitalized, and we've often had difficulty accommodating all of them within our facility—to the point that administration has now put a maximum on the number of people that can visit at a time. . . . I find it difficult to communicate that to them—to limit the number—they have a difficult time understanding why the whole family can't be there!*

A provider and active advocate for Indian clients shared with me his understanding of the circumstances that brought about the administrative edict. The essence of the situation was that an especially large extended family came to visit their family member in the intensive care unit [ICU]. They brought their own food to save money and overflowed the small ICU waiting room. Some of their children were found by night security riding the elevators. At some point, night security tried to get the family to leave the hospital, and they refused. According to the provider/advocate, "administration got wind of all this, took it to the board, and next thing you know there's a limit on—there can't be more than three visitors in the ICU waiting room!"

The provider/advocate in the above situation told me he spent considerable time talking with people directly involved in the imbroglio and concluded it had been managed by instituting a reactive negative sanction, i.e., restricting visitors.

Aware administrative strategies. The last category of containment strategies also occurs at the administrative interactional level and is indicative of cultural awareness of administrators and managers. Three such strategies were identified: policies making facility expectations clear, matching patient/provider, and attempting to change racist attitudes through mandatory training.

The first strategy, *making expectations clear,* was also used on the dyadic interactional level. On the administrative (managerial) level a provider described the policy on her unit for containing a source of environmental-family disruption. She said,

> *We've been working very consciously to try to intervene early on, when the patient is first admitted, to let them know that our unit has a very open visitor policy. But we expect, if children are brought in, they are either kept quietly in the room with the rest of the family or down in the waiting room. And most people, if you present it to them in that way during the initial admission, they know what to expect. We don't have a lot of problems.*

A nurse manager on a rehabilitation unit discussed her practice of regulating patient care assignments to protect Indian clients from nursing staff with racist attitudes. Her strategy is careful *matching of patient and provider* for patient care assignments. She stated:

> *Native Americans seem to have pretty good insight into the people that are not open-minded to them. And right away, you'll hear, "That person is prejudiced." And then they tend to find something to isolate that nurse from being involved with them. So my job is to make sure good matches occur with patients and*

staff. Some of my staff are very vocal that they don't want to work with Native Americans, and I feel it's better for everyone if they don't have that interaction.

Although matching patient and provider is a simple managerial strategy, it is also a culturally enlightened one.

The final strategy, *mandatory cultural awareness training,* was in place in one study site and was recommended by informants in several other sites. The two Indian health care providers and numerous non-Indian providers saw this strategy as indicative of responsible, culturally sensitive administration. One provider responded as follows to my query as to what he believed was necessary to promote culturally sensitive care for Indian clients:

To change people's attitudes and that requires institutional policies against prejudice. . . . And secondly, it requires an ongoing educational effort to create a sensitivity. I've thought a lot about what it would take to do this. Annual mandatory training . . . I think we should have an annual update—where we bring folks from the reservation, leaders and nurses and social workers, health professionals that are Native American to talk about different topics. And we need nonmandatory training, maybe a monthly brown bag lunch series. You know, one month you could talk about Native families, the next month about some other Native issue.

The facility, a hospital, that was currently presenting a series of cultural awareness seminars, did require mandatory attendance by all its managers responsible for nursing care. And as was suggested by the provider in the above quotation, Native Americans were involved in presenting the seminars.

Discussion of mandatory cultural awareness training as a strategy for containing disruption ends the second stage of the process. A word is necessary regarding whether the strategies presented are inclusive. I am certain they are not. Other health care facilities serving American Indian clients and other informants associated with facilities in this study would certainly add to the list of containment strategies. And the beauty of a substantive grounded theory is that it expands and may even be altered to account for variations in data.

Stage Three: Resolution

When resolution of disruption did occur, it was in one of three ways. First, the Indian patient left, either through discharge or death. Second, a solution to the perceived disruption was negotiated. Such negotiations were usually initiated by a person in a managerial or administrative role. For example, one patient care unit manager described family conferences she had organized to resolve issues of containing disruption such as noncompliance.

And the third type of resolution occurred when a provider increased his or her cultural awareness and consequently redefined the problem and who had it. An example of this was the nurse, who, after attending a cultural awareness workshop, realized that her discomfort over the lack of eye contact by some of her Indian patients was due to her lack of awareness of a cultural behavior specific for some Indian people.

SUMMARY

In summary, the process of containing disruption begins under the condition of two disparate cultures clashing in health care settings in which members of the dominant, non-Indian culture control rule defining and enforcing. The first stage of the containing-disruption process is the occurrence of the actual rule breaking, i.e., disruptive event(s). These may be either a perceived environmental disruption created by Indian family members or a disruption in provider comfort. Provider comfort is disrupted by demeanor differences, discrimination claiming, and noncompliance with the health care providers care/treatment regimes.

The second stage of the process consists of the use of containment strategies. These occur on the dyadic provider-client level and the administrative/managerial level and are indicative of either awareness or unawareness of Native American culture.

The third and last stage of the process occurs in one of three ways: the Indian client leaves, a solution to the disruption is negotiated, or providers and/or administrators/managers increase their cultural awareness and redefine the problem and who has it.

REFERENCES

Bailey, M. A. (1996). *Fostering cultural awareness: A workshop plan for professional nurses.* Unpublished master's professional paper, Montana State Univerity, Bozeman, Montana.

Bryan, W. (1985). *Montana's Indians: Yesterday and today.* Helena: Montana Magazine.

Buehler, J. A. (1992). Traditional Crow Indian health beliefs and practices: Toward a grounded theory. *Journal of Holistic Nursing, 10* (1), 18–33.

Frey, R. (1987). *The world of the Crow Indians: As driftwood lodges.* Norman: University of Oklahoma Press.

Glaser, B. G. (1992). *Basics of grounded theory analysis.* Mill Valley, CA: Sociology Press.

Snipp, C. M. (1989). *American Indians: The first of this land.* New York: Russell Sage Foundation.

Wuest, J. (1993). Removing the shackles: A feminist critque of noncompliance. *Nursing Outlook, 41,* 217–24.

27

Invisible Youth: Gay, Lesbian, and Bisexual Youth in Rural Montana

Sharon Kiely Howard

INTRODUCTION

Gay, lesbian, and bisexual youth are in need of attention from health care professionals. This aggregate constitutes a group underserved in the health care arena because gay, lesbian, and bisexual students living in a rural state are faced with limited resources needed to help assure their healthy achievement of developmental tasks. Movement into adolescence presents added challenges for these youth who find their sexual orientation the subject of schoolyard jokes or the focus of a national debate on military worthiness. The words of C. D. (1992, personal communication), a gay male who grew up in a small, Montana farming community, explain challenges in a rural environment:

> *The sense of isolation and confusion was overwhelming. As I realized I was different, I was desperate to find out information about myself and to understand what I was feeling. But I knew I couldn't ask questions of anyone in my community or the word would get out. I couldn't even send for information because anything that came in a brown paper wrapper to the post office would have called attention to me and my family before I even knew it had arrived.*

The purpose of this chapter is to address the rural setting and the meaning it has for gay, lesbian, and bisexual youth. Health care deficits that push gay, lesbian, and bisexual youth to look for information about their sexuality in the "brown paper wrapper" need to be addressed and alleviated. This population of youth who are underserved by nursing need recognition, understanding, advocacy, and the caring of nurses. Health care delivery to this population will be affected largely by the inclusion of knowledge and clinical experiences within nursing curriculums that is sensitive to the experience and needs of this rural population.

GAY, LESBIAN, AND BISEXUAL YOUTH

Unlike some ethnic subcultural groups, sexual orientation does not have a visible marker such as the color of skin. Because of societal stigmatization of gays and lesbians, many persons choose not to reveal their sexual orientation. Therefore, determining the number of gay, lesbian, and bisexual youth is relegated to estimations based on human sexuality studies. Earlier studies state that approximately 10% of the population could be homosexual with 2.9 million of the 29 million adolescents in the United States potential lesbian, gay, or bisexual in their sexual orientation (Kinsey, Pomeroy, & Martin, 1948; Kinsey, Pomeroy, Martin, & Gebhard, 1953). However, more recent studies have suggested the numbers may be smaller, in the 5% to 10% range (Gonsiorek & Weinrich, 1991).

Within human sexuality studies, the number of homosexuals is estimated from sexual behavior, not sexual orientation. This is problematic because sexual behavior is the participation in sexual activities/expressions. Sexual orientation is the identification of self as homosexual or heterosexual and represents a consistent, enduring self-recognition of the meanings that sexual orientation and sexual behavior have for oneself.

The distinction between sexual orientation and sexual behavior is clarified with the following example. A person may participate in vaginal-penile sex to accommodate sexual peer pressure, yet experience no physical or emotional attraction. In this scenario, participation in the behavior of sexual intercourse has nothing to do with the person's sexual attractions and feelings (orientation) but is a protective mechanism (behavior) to help a homosexual youth belong or be accepted by peers. Failure to distinguish between sexual orientation and sexual behavior further confuses discussion and study about the size of this aggregate.

Collection of data about all aspects of sexual activity and sexual orientation is difficult. Understanding the sensitivity of sexual issues is a challenge to researchers. The methods used in research designs to gather sexual information is important to the quality of data collection. Regardless of the numbers of gay, lesbian, and bisexual youth, nurses will encounter this minority group in health care and school settings.

The Rural Environment

There is a paucity of literature and research on gay, lesbian, and bisexual youth living in rural settings. "Those studies which have been conducted reveal, not surprisingly, tales of isolation, unsupportive social environments and a chronic lack of structural services and facilities" (Bell & Valentine, 1995, p.116). In a unique study on lesbians and gays, D'Augelli and Hart (1987) state,

> *In most rural areas the gay community is invisible. This invisibility is a result of justifiable fear and discomfort about others; reactions to disclosure of affectional orientation. Many rural gays fear discovery and possible rejection, worrying that any gay behavior will lead to exposure. Contacts with known gay people may be avoided due to fears of others' reactions. (p. 82)*

The impact of fear on the development of a sense of community has profound implications for health promotion activities directed toward gays (like safer sex programs) and care of homosexual people who are ill. Kathleen Rounds (1988) presents a discussion on the lack of community and its relationship to health promotion activities in rural areas. The disease of AIDS has witnessed infected individuals returning to their rural homes for care after they left for urban areas years before. Coming home presents the family and the individual with facing prejudice toward the disease and homosexuality. Poullard and D'Augelli (1989) add further support to this concept with the results of their study about health promotion activities in rural areas. They found that in rural areas that had health promotion programs, services were colored by rural attitudes among workers that suggested gay men can overcome homosexuality and/or that homosexuality is "disgusting" (p. 35).

Martin (1982) believes that the primary adaptive behavior of gay and lesbian youth is hiding with "the socialization of the gay adolescent becoming a process of deception at all levels, the ability to play a role" (p. 55). Alone, these youth face fear and often questions about their very existence, often retreating further and further into a solitary shell. In *Reflections of a Rock Lobster: A Story about Growing Up Gay,* Aaron Fricke (1981) describes his adolescence:

> *When I entered high school, I was completely isolated from the world. I had given up all hopes of ever finding love, warmth, or tenderness in the world. I did not lie to myself, but I did keep others from thinking I was homosexual . . . the only goal left to me was to hide anything that could identify me as gay . . . I withdrew from everyone and slowly formed a shell around myself. (pp. 29–30)*

The invisibility with imposed solitude referred to by these authors is enhanced by the lack of gay newspapers and books and the lack of unbiased, factual sources of information. Further, gay youth in rural settings cannot search a library or resource center for information about homosexual adolescents, an option available to youth in a large city. Urban settings have resources that can be accessed anonymously, an attractive form of gaining information for rural gay youth. S.K. (1992, personal communication) stated, "I hit the libraries when we arrived in a city. Research for a speech debate was always a good, safe excuse to search for information about myself." The coming of telecommunications may help alleviate some of the problems. However, at this time, no documentation of access by youth to online gay support groups, chat lines, and information centers has been reported in the literature.

Health Risks

Adolescence is a time of experimentation and separation from parental and family structures with establishment of identity, self-sufficiency, projection to future roles, and acceptance of body and sexual identity. The developmental tasks of adolescence are formidable, and these must be accomplished at a time when youth are undergoing physical and emotional maturation, intellectual changes, and sexual development. Inherent in the nature of youth are risk-taking behaviors that move them toward greater independence and understanding of the world around them. Within the risk-taking framework of growth and development are health consequences that can and do result in morbidity and mortality. Understanding the behaviors that youth are experiencing is critical to a community's approach to education and the structuring of community life and activities.

In Montana, information about sexual activity of gay, lesbian, and bisexual youth must be derived indirectly from existing data about sexual activity. The only existing source of data that originates with adolescents reporting their sexual activities does not include questions about same sex behaviors. This data is compiled from a survey tool developed by the Centers for Disease Control (CDC) and is used in Montana to increase knowledge about youth and the behaviors that place them at risk. This survey tool, The 1995 Montana Youth Risk Behavior Survey (YRBS), is administered by the Montana Office of Public Instruction (1995) and cosponsors. The survey is part of the surveillance and reporting system for adolescent risk behaviors developed by the Division of Adolescent and School Health, National Center for Chronic Disease Prevention and Health Promotion, United States Centers for Disease Control and Prevention (CDC). The YRBS poses eight questions related to sexual behaviors. The questions do not distinguish between same gender sexual activity or opposite gender sexual activity. Failure to ask questions about same sex activities does not preclude that sexual experimentation includes same gender sexual activity. Montana youth report sexual behaviors that are similar to the patterning of youth behaviors in the nation. From the 1995 Montana YRBS data, 47% of the Montana youth reported having sexual intercourse, and 54% of those youth reported wearing a condom during their last sexual activity. Twenty-three percent of sexually active students reported more than one sexual partner. Males were more likely to use alcohol or drugs before sex and to have multiple sex partners than female respondents. Approximately one of every three (36%) male ninth graders and one of every four (29%) female ninth graders in Montana reported having sexual intercourse. Sixty-two percent of male and female 12th graders in Montana reported having sexual intercourse at least once. Clearly, youth in rural Montana are reporting that they are sexually active; some of that sexual activity is same sex behavior.

Sexual behaviors at an early age carry the health risks of unwanted teen pregnancy and sexually transmitted disease. Social and developmental issues related to these complications arise and become more pronounced when a youth is struggling with the knowledge of being different from his or her heterosexual counterparts. According to Saddul (1996), "Without accurate information and emotional and social support, gay teens are more likely to engage in risky sexual behavior" (p. 4). Examples of risky sexual behavior are the lesbian adolescent choosing to become pregnant as a protective response to ensure her acceptance as heterosexual or the gay male seeking sexual experiences in the anonymous backdrop of the adult bookstore. If the threat of a human immunodeficiency virus (HIV) is the single factor considered when youth participate in sexual behaviors, then young males participating in same sex behaviors are at great risk for infection.

Problems including school avoidance and school dropout, family abuse, sexual promiscuity, teen pregnancy, drug abuse, and violence are more frequent among homosexuals compared with the heterosexual population. According to Cranston (1992), "Schools and other youth settings generally operate under the presumption that adolescents are heterosexual. Gay, lesbian, and bisexual adolescents in these settings may lack opportunities to practice social skills crucial to their development and to establish authentic systems of peer support for their emerging identities" (p. 253). Gay youth are in need of safe and knowledgeable resources and support that are seldom found in the community or school setting. Yet, homophobic response to the existence of these youth threatens their daily survival. To complete their developmental tasks and survive adolescence, gays and lesbians must come to know and accept who they are in a society that provides very little positive information, role models, or social support.

Another health risk is suicide, and youth are a high-risk group for suicide. Gay, lesbian, and bisexual youth belong to two high-risk groups. Gibson (1989), in a study commissioned by the United States Department of Health and Human Services, documented that gay, lesbian, and bisexual youth are two to three times more likely to attempt suicide than the general population of youth and that they comprise up to 30% of all suicides reported annually. Sutter, a registered nurse (1995), in a letter of response to the American Journal of Nursing wrote the following reflection in response to a suicide. "If we are to reach the 'souls of pain,' we must be sensitive to all aspects of a person—ethnic, cultural, sexual orientation, color—and let nothing stand in our way of acceptance of him as an individual. Only then can we help him reach optimal health" (p. 22).

Homophobia

Bias and prejudice within a population can be an insidious phenomena. Uncovering the roots of a prejudice can help move individuals beyond bias and can mark a beginning for acceptance and understanding. Hatred or fear of gay, lesbian, or bisexual individuals, termed homophobia, has its historical roots in the settling of our nation.

Homophobia in our Western culture dates from the colonization of America. Some religious communities carried intolerance toward homosexuals and bisexuals in their journey to the New World as they sought sanctuary from other forms of oppression. In the course of American history, homosexuals have been jailed as criminals, labeled as insane or neurotic by the medical community, and shunned as sinners from church pulpits. Over time, our nation has swayed back and forth in its tolerance of gays and lesbians, but the arrival of HIV/AIDS has escalated intolerance to a new high.

Hate crimes against homosexuals have increased radically in the 1990s with the name "gay bashing" given to unprovoked crimes committed against people perceived to be or recognized as gay, lesbian, or bisexual (Berrill, 1990). Adolescents are more often the victims of violence and minority violence, including that against gay youth, and these incidences have increased in relationship to HIV/AIDS. In a study of the first 500 youth seeking services at the Hetrick-Martin Institute in New York City, Hunter (1990) reported that 41% of the youths reported experiencing violent physical attacks. Of those youth who had been assaulted, 46% of the assaults were gay-related. She comments that the study was limited to study of physical attacks that occurred at home or in public and that emotional and verbal abuse was probably more predominant than physical assaults. Suicide attempts were documented frequently in this group.

Pockets of progress in the understanding and acceptance of homosexuals are noted in some realms. Within the criminal justice system, incarcerating persons because they are gay or lesbian or perceived to be gay or lesbian is no longer a common practice. In the 1960s sexual intercourse between same sex partners was a crime in all states in the union. In the 1990s, fewer than 20 states have laws remaining that mark same sex acts as criminal. In 1973, the American Psychiatric Association removed homosexuality from its listing of mental disorders and, in 1983, the American Academy of Pediatrics affirmed the responsibility of health professionals to homosexual adolescents. Within spiritual communities, some churches openly accept gay and lesbians. The Metropolitan Community Church was founded in the late 1960s and ministers directly to the gay community and sanctions relationships based on Christian commitment. Particular groups of Lutheran, Presbyterian, and United Methodists have been vocal supporters of the civil rights of gays and lesbians. Other churches have organized support for gays and lesbians to foster fellowship and counseling. Dignity and Integrity are two such groups. These examples of Christian ministering do not mean that the debate and controversy on the issue of homosexuality within the religious community have passed, but suggest an openness to gay people and the creation of opportunities for understanding and acceptance.

Personal experience verifies much of the literature previously cited. As a nurse, accepting an employment assignment that involved giving community presentations about AIDS was not without trepidation for me. Other aspects of my nursing career had exposed me to public homophobic responses and the realization that I would be addressing a social/health issue that was eliciting strong and, at times, violent, public response on a national level. Over a period of years, in the role of health educator, homophobic responses were experienced that could only be minimal when compared with a person who is attacked at the very core of his or her being for being gay. Hate mail damned me and my family, and anonymous religious groups stated they were holding prayer vigils for me. When scheduled to speak to classes of high school students in rural communities about human sexuality, groups of adults would arrive unannounced to monitor my presentations. At a public forum on AIDS, a fist fight erupted between opposing factions. On another occasion, a colleague and I were asked to present a talk to a small community in eastern Montana to clear up misinformation about AIDS and homosexuals imparted by a physician's assistant to the community that had resulted in community turmoil. Often I was accused of teaching children to be homosexual or of introducing children to intravenous drug use through discussions about the transmission routes for HIV and Hepatitis B. Personal experience has served to deepen my sensitivity to homophobia and to confirm that education holds hope for resolution.

Discrimination in Health Care Delivery

Stories abound in the popular press relating scenarios where individuals infected with HIV and perceived as gay have been refused health care or treated in a biased fashion. In a self-report study of homosexual and bisexual males conducted by Kass, Faden, Fox, and Dudley (1992), men with AIDS were significantly more likely to report refusal for treatment by a physician or dentist because of a known or suspected HIV-related condition. Study participants volunteered that they chose health care providers who were gay practitioners to avoid discrimination problems. In 1985, Douglas, Kalman, and Kalman found that almost 10% of nurses and doctors surveyed believed that those homosexuals who contracted AIDS deserved it. D'Augelli (1989) reported that fear of AIDS correlated significantly with homophobic attitudes among rural nurses. Koch, Preston, Young and Wang (1991) studied rural nurses' attitudes toward homosexuality and found the majority to express attitudes toward homosexuals as ambivalent to extremely negative. Male homosexuality was reported as obscene and vulgar by 40% of the nurses, and 51% reported being revolted by the thought of men having sex with men. Another 35% reported that homosexuality should be considered immoral. Scherer, Wu, and Haughey (1991), in a study of 581 registered nurses, found their attitude to be collectively homophobic.

Smith (1992) conducted a study of psychiatric nurses to measure attitudes toward gays and lesbians and to assess homophobia among psychiatric nurses. On the scale measuring attitudes toward gays and lesbians by heterosexual nurses, the respondents showed neutral to mildly positive scores. The results from the tool measuring homophobia showed that the majority of nurse respondents (77%) had moderate to severe homophobia. The author suggests that nurses may have "cognitive acceptance of gays and lesbians and homosexuality yet continue to have negative feelings toward gays and lesbians. This inconsistency between cognitive attitudes and feelings may negatively impact the nursing care provided to gay and lesbian patients" (p. 382).

Answering the question of whether or not people who identify as gay, lesbian, or bisexual experience prejudice in health care delivery is foggy, and determining if nurses, in particular, discriminate is vague. Eliason (1996b) states that "little empirical research has addressed the prevalence of negative attitudes toward lesbian, gay, or bisexual patients and their family members among health care workers. Virtually no research has explored whether, or how, negative attitudes might influence patient care" (p. 67). However, "consequences of negative attitudes can be compromised care, avoidance of a client, or active discrimination" (Eliason, 1996a, p. 17). Smith concludes that "homophobia in health care workers can lead to poor and mismanaged care of homosexual patients" (p. 16).

OPPORTUNITIES FOR INTERVENTION

School Nursing

Tartagni (1978) writes "one of the loneliest persons in any high school in America is the abandoned and isolated gay youth" (p. 26). Schools are faced with ever-increasing social issues on a daily basis. The cultural and ethnic diversity of the population of students, along with drug and alcohol use, teen pregnancy, violence, tobacco usage, and the changing face of the American family, places the school nurse in the position of being a health consultant, a resource person for faculty and students, and often a counselor to the student with a secret that needs sharing with a "safe" person. Students who are recognizing themselves as different in their sexual development may come to the attention of the school nurse through problematic behaviors associated with anxiety, stress, and the work of trying to stay safe in a hostile environment. Taylor and Remafedi (1993) state that the school nurse is in a unique position as a respected professional to make a difference with students, families, and faculty through action and education:

> *The school nurse who makes the effort to reach out in a sensitive and caring way to meet the needs of this unfairly treated and largely under served group of young people will better serve the needs of all youth, all school staff, and of our greater society as well (p. 37).*

Nursing Education

"In spite of nurses' awareness of social and demographic factors related to health care, there has been limited systematic education about cultural diversity in schools of nursing" (Eliason 1993, p. 14). Multicultural education has had a limited focus, generally considering racial and ethnic diversity. The complexities of human sexuality, sexual orientation, and sexual behavior need to be addressed with forthrightness and comprehensiveness across the curriculum. If the end result of educators' efforts is to be holistic, unbiased care toward all, then the interwoven concepts of homophobia, gender variations, sexual expression, sexual development, societal responses to sexuality, and the history of our moral structure need to be taught and discussed. Eliason (1993) states:

> *Negative attitudes about same-sex attractions tend to be deeply ingrained in the majority of nurses by the socialization process. . . . Failing to address prejudices and biases in adulthood is a breech of the nursing code of ethics for nurses pledge to provide non judgmental quality care to all. Education is the key . . . (p. 18)*

The attitude of students enrolled in nursing programs has been studied to a small extent. One study by Eliason and Randall (1991) found that 26% of nursing students were homophobic about lesbians and would avoid contact with lesbians at all costs. Nursing students had a lack of knowledge about homosexuality and accepted common stereotypes, such as fear that the lesbian would make sexual advances.

A curriculum that is comprehensive and integrating in approach to human sexuality has the benefit of supporting those nursing students who are gay or lesbian. Gay nursing students live with minority status, and the fears about discrimination can only add to the stress of successfully completing a curriculum. These students make the choice of staying invisible or risking identifying themselves as gay. Examination of faculty members' feelings toward gays and lesbians is critical to the role modeling process in relationship to acceptance, support, and advocacy for the rights of all. Theresa M. Stephany (1992) comments "Faculty can open the closet door and keep it open by modeling what they do best: teaching by example and empowering students to become change agents" (p. 23).

CONCLUSION

Nursing has been in the forefront of addressing many social problems and serving underserved and minority populations. The greatest of epidemiological challenge in modern times has been presented by the disease of AIDS. The growing numbers of infected individuals include increasing numbers of youth. Advocacy is accepted as an appropriate role for all nurses within the profession. The need for advocacy for gay, lesbian, and bisexual youth beckons now. The profession must view the educational formats of our schools of nursing and inspect for threads of homophobia that may permeate, ever so subtly, the core of our curriculums. The advocacy role calls for our support of the local development of safe, informed sources for human sexuality and behavioral information, health-promoting support groups for youth who identify themselves as homosexual, and support for family and friends of gay and lesbian youth.

Homosexuality as a rural issue has aspects complicated by the very characteristics of rural community life that are viewed as positive. The closeness of rural people poses a great threat to the youth who needs confidential health and supportive resources that will not single him or her out as different. Rural nurses educated about and sensitive to the full scope of human sexuality are in the unique position to help satisfy health needs of gay, lesbian, and bisexual youth.

REFERENCES

Bell, D., & Valentine, G. (1995). Queer country: Rural lesbian and gay lives. *Journal of Rural Studies, 11,* 113–122.

Berrill, K.T. (1990). Describing the problem: Anti-gay violence and victimization in the U.S.—an overview. *Journal of Interpersonal Violence, 5,* 274–294.

Cranston, K. (1992). HIV education for gay, lesbian, and bisexual youth: Personal power and the community of conscience. In K. M. Harbeck (Ed.), *Coming out of the classroom closet* (pp. 247–259). New York: Haworth Press.

D'Augelli, A. (1989). AIDS fears and homophobia among rural nursing personnel. *AIDS Education Prevention, 1,* 277–284.

D'Augelli, A. & Hart, M. (1987). Gay women, men, and families in rural settings: Toward the development of helping communities. *American Journal and Community Psychology 15,* 79–93.

Douglas, C. J., Kalman, C. M., & Kalman, T. P. (1985). Homophobia among physicians and nurses: An empirical study. *Hospital and Community Psychiatry, 36,* 1309–1311.

Eliason, M. J. (1993). Cultural diversity in nursing care: The lesbian, gay, or bisexual client. *Journal of Transcultural Nursing, 5,* 14–21.

Eliason, M. J. (1996a). Lesbian and gay family issues. *Journal of Family Nursing, 2,* 10–29.

Eliason, M. J. (1996b). Caring for the lesbian, gay, or bisexual patient: Issues for critical care nurses. *Critical Care Nursing Quarterly, 19,* 65–72.

Eliason, M. J., & Randall, C. (1991). Lesbian phobia in nursing students. *Western Journal of Nursing Research, 13,* 365–376.

Fricke, A. (1981). *Reflections of a rock lobster: A story about growing up gay.* Boston: Alyson.

Gibson, P. (1989). Gay male and lesbian youth suicide. In M. Feinleib (Ed.), *Prevention and intervention in youth suicide: Report to the Secretary's Task Force on Youth Suicide, Vol., 3,* (pp.110–142). Washington, DC: U.S. Department of Health and Human Services.

Gonsiorek, J., & Weinrich, J. (1991). *Homosexuality: Research implications for public policy.* Newbury Park, CA: Sage.

Hunter, J. (1990). Violence against lesbian and gay male youths. *Journal of Interpersonal Violence, 5,* 295–300.

Kass, N. E., Faden, R. R., Fox, R., & Dudley, J. (1992). Homosexual and bisexual men's perceptions of discrimination in health services. *American Journal of Public Health, 82,* 1277–1279.

Kinsey, A. C., Pomeroy W., Martin, C. (1948). *Sexual behavior in the human male.* Philadelphia: Saunders.

Kinsey, A. C., Pomeroy W., & Martin, C., & Gebhard, P. (1953). *Sexual behavior in the human female.* Philadelphia: Saunders.

Koch, P. B., Preston, D. B., Young, E. W., & Wang, M. (1991). Factors associated with AIDS-related attitudes among rural nurses. *Health Values, 15,* 32–40.

Martin, A. D. (1982). Learning to hide: The socialization of the gay adolescent. *Adolescent Psychiatry, 10,* 52–65.

Montana Office of Public Instruction. (1995). *Montana youth risk behavior survey.* Helena, MT: Author.

Poullard, J., & D'Augelli, A. (1989). AIDS fears and homophobia among volunteers in an AIDS prevention program. *Journal of Rural Community Psychology 10,* 29–39.

Rounds, K. (1988). AIDS in rural areas: Challenges to providing care. *Social Work,* May-June, 257–261.

Saddul, R. B. (1996). Coming out: An overlooked concept. *Clinical Nurse Specialist, 10,* 2–5.

Scherer, Y.K., Wu, Y.W., & Haughey, B.P. (1991). AIDS and homophobia among nurses. *Journal of Homosexuality, 21,* 17–27.

Smith, G.B. (1992). Nursing care challenges: Homosexual psychiatric patients. *Journal of Psychosocial Nursing, 30,* 15–21.

Smith, G.B. (1993). Homophobia and attitudes toward gay men and lesbians by psychiatric nurses. *Archives of Psychiatric Nursing, 8,* 377–384.

Stephany, T. M. (1992). Faculty support for gay and lesbian nursing students. *Nurse Educator, 17,* 22–23.

Sutter, S. (1995). Letters. *American Journal of Nursing, 95* (10), 21.

Tartagni, D. (1978). Counseling gays in a school setting. *School Counselor 26,* 26–32.

Taylor, B.A, & Remafedi, G. (1993). Youth coping with sexual orientation issues. *Journal of School Nursing, 9,* 26–37.

28

Experiences of HIV-Infected Men with Rural Health Care

Jean Ballantyne and Janice A. Buehler

HIV infection and acquired immunodeficiency syndrome (AIDS) can no longer be considered just an urban problem. Although HIV/AIDS is still more prevalent in metropolitan areas, more cases are being reported in rural states. There is an increasing presence of HIV-infected persons in many rural communities, including the most remote areas of rural states such as Montana. During the 11–year time period 1985–1996, there were 318 reported cases of persons with a diagnosis of AIDS in Montana; 62% or 198 of them have died (Montana Department of Public Health and Human Services, 1996). A phenomenon contributing to the increasing numbers of persons with AIDS in rural areas is the process of "migrating home" to be near family for care and support (Davis & Stapelton, 1991; D'Augelli & Poullard, 1989).

BACKGROUND AND SIGNIFICANCE

AIDS is not considered a priority health issue in many rural areas (White, 1994). Yet, HIV-infected persons in these settings have many of the same health care needs as their urban counterparts (Carwein,

Acknowledgment: This project was funded in part by College of Nursing, Montana State University-Bozeman.

Sabo, & Barry, 1993). Getting these needs met can be problematic in rural areas characterized by sparse populations, geographic isolation, lack of services, long distances to services, and limited access to resources (Fuszard, Sowell, Hoff, & Waters, 1991; Long & Weinert, 1989; Young, Koch, & Preston, 1989).

Despite the spread of the HIV epidemic to rural areas, few research efforts have focused on rural populations and care delivery issues in rural settings (Bushy, 1992). Professional nurses constitute the largest group of health care providers in rural areas; consequently, they need to be prepared for the complex challenges of caring for HIV infected clients.

PURPOSE

The purpose of this qualitative study was to describe the perceptions and experiences of HIV-infected men receiving rural health care. The specific aims of the study were (a) to describe informants' perceptions and experiences related to the availability, accessibility, utilization, and adequacy of health care in a rural or frontier setting; and (b) to describe health care barriers.

METHODS

No research studies were found that addressed the experiences of HIV clients with rural health care. Thus, a grounded theory design was selected for this study. The conceptual framework emerged through the data analysis in keeping with grounded theory methods.

Setting

The setting for the study was Montana, a western rural/frontier state with a large land mass and a sparse population. There are fewer than 6 persons per square mile in 45 of the 56 counties (U.S. Census, 1992). These counties with such sparse population can be classified as frontier (Elison, 1986). In keeping with this classification, communities in counties with less than 6 persons per square mile were designated as frontier, and communities with more than 6 but fewer than 100 persons per square mile were designated as rural. For this study, the communities in frontier counties were labeled "small towns," and communities in rural counties were labeled "rural cities."

Data Collection

Data were collected through focused interviews with open-ended questions. At the time of the interviews, there were fewer than 50 persons living with a diagnosis of AIDS in Montana and 360 cumulative positive HIV tests reported through the Montana Public Health Laboratory (Montana Department of Public Health and Human Services, July 1992). Given the sensitive nature of the research topic, extreme caution was taken to protect the anonymity of study participants. A convenience sample of eight men living in Montana who either were HIV positive or had a diagnosis of AIDS was contacted through a key informant. Potential participants were given information about the study and informed consent materials through the key informant. Participants then contacted the researcher, and the interviews were conducted at a location and manner (face-to-face or telephone) agreeable to the participant. Interviews were from one to two hours in length; six face-to-face interviews were tape recorded with participant permission and transcribed verbatim. The two interviews done by telephone were not tape recorded; detailed notes were taken by the researcher with the participant's permission. Before the beginning of each interview, the researcher and the participant reviewed the information about the study and informed consent. All data collection procedures were reviewed and approved by a University-level human subjects review committee before the start of data collection.

Data Analysis

Data analysis began simultaneously with data collection and followed the operations of the constant comparative method and theoretical sampling (Glaser & Strauss, 1967; Glaser, 1978; Strauss & Corbin, 1990). Coding of initial interviews provided clues for later interviews. Credibility of the findings was established through an audit trail and through peer consultation and debriefing activities that included checking for representativeness in the data and the affects of the researcher on data collection. Additionally, a process of simultaneous coding with a consultant resulted in comparable conclusions.

The major limitation of the study was the small nonrepresentative sample size. Nonetheless, data analysis produced an empirically grounded conceptual framework that can be used by other researchers in theory testing and theory development.

FINDINGS

The conceptual paradigm that emerged in the grounded theory analysis is depicted in Figure 28.1. The core variable, managing barriers in care seeking, was composed of three elements: encountering barriers, maneuvering barriers, and experiencing the consequences. Each is described in the following sections.

Core Variable: Managing Barriers in Care Seeking

The core variable emerging from the data analysis was *managing barriers in care seeking.* This theme refers to the experiences described by participants in their care seeking with rural health resources. Participants readily identified barriers encountered in accessing care, in the adequacy of care, and in negative attitudes and biases of health care providers. Participants subsequently described strategies for maneuvering around barriers to lessen their negative impact on care received. These strategies were educating oneself; dealing with the baggage; and migrating to care.

All participants believed that barriers created negative consequences for quality care. When barriers either in obtaining care or to adequacy of care were prominent, the consequence was *no care.* When attitudinal barriers were present, *stigmatized care* was the consequence. When fewer barriers of all types existed, clients received *compassionate care,* generally described as adequate or of high quality.

Encountering Barriers

Participants described three types of barriers, those related to access, adequacy, and attitudes. These barriers were often interrelated and covaried (that is, coexisted).

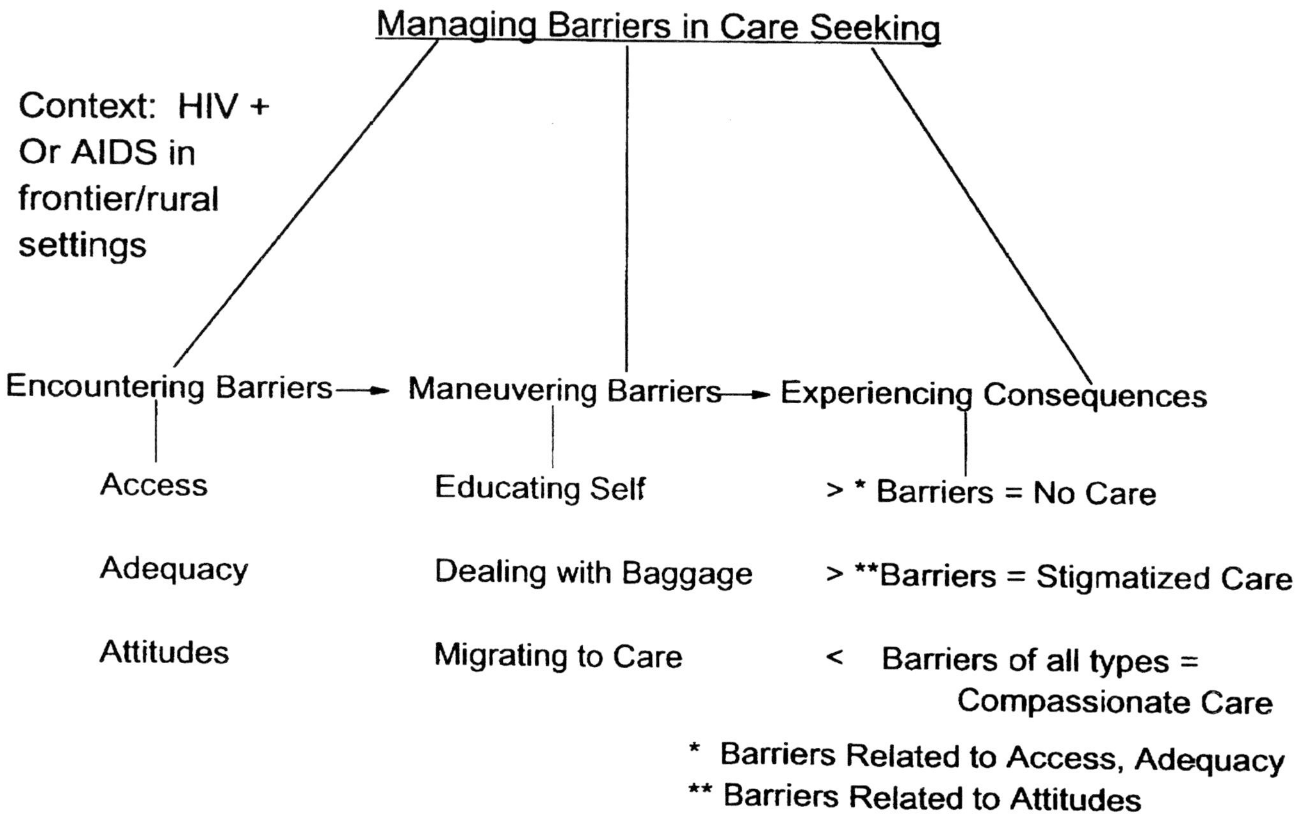

FIGURE 28.1 Conceptual model

Barriers to Accessing Care. Barriers to accessing health care included financial problems and geographic isolation. Lack of finances, both public programs and private insurance, was described as a major barrier to accessing and using health care resources in both frontier and rural areas. Responses about money problems included

> *I know the hospitals won't keep you if you have no money . . .*

> *When the place I worked changed insurance companies, I kind of hedged on the application, not knowing what else to do . . . I mean insurance, you gotta have it. I got on the insurance; I never turned in any claims.*

> *I think it was two weeks before my Mom found a doctor who could take me. I was almost dead. It had gone so far that they almost did me in. Now I'm on Medicaid, but I didn't have anything at the time.*

Geographic isolation was described as a barrier to accessing care if HIV/AIDS patients were living in frontier areas. This barrier resulted in long distances to travel to access adequate health care resources. As one participant said, "When you're really sick, you need to be in a bigger place . . . not 200 miles away."

Barriers to Adequate Health Care. The second type of barrier encountered was regarding the adequacy of care. The typical participant perceived his health care as adequate if his needs were met in a timely, knowledgeable, skilled, and compassionate manner. Indicators of barriers to adequate care included either uninformed providers or an absence of providers. Most participants, either through direct experience or through observations of the care of a friend, reported that some health care providers, particularly in small towns, lacked the knowledge and skills necessary to take care of HIV-infected patients. In some areas, there was a total lack of providers (e.g., no primary care providers and/or health care facilities). Typical responses included these statements:

> *In (small town) there were four different doctors with four different answers. They didn't know a thing about HIV. The nurses in this town don't know much, but they know as much as the doctor. They need education about the disease, how much protection they need, not to go overboard, but to do what they need to do.*

> *If you're an HIV positive person in Podunk, and there is only one Doc who doesn't know anything about HIV . . . why that's a barrier!*

Another example of small town health care providers being unprepared to care for AIDS patients was reported in a newspaper (Munzenrider & Sundby, 1992). A terminally ill patient had been cared for at home by family and a home health nurse. He described the nurse as "being afraid of AIDS." The patient subsequently repeatedly traveled 200 miles from the small town to the rural city to get adequate care.

Attitudinal Barriers to Care. The third type of barrier encountered was attitudinal. All participants expressed a keen awareness of anti-homosexual bias in both rural and frontier settings. Issues of confidentiality and anonymity were major factors described in scenarios about negative attitudes. However, the occurrence of prejudicial incidents was reported to a lesser degree in the rural city. The following were typical responses:

> *In rural areas, HIV or AIDS is still a gay disease. And, the perception here is that gays and drug users are low life anyway; they don't deserve to really live. People here know everybody else's business and are very moralistic as most rural communities are. There isn't any anonymity. Here you stand to lose your job, your house, you know, any number of things. . . . They automatically think you are gay. Being gay is a felony.*

> *The doctor was supposed to be the only one with the report about my HIV status. . . . In walked the nurse with the slip in her hand. After that it was all over town. It's a small town, about 5,000 people. So I had to leave to get health care.*

Participants also described stigmatizing experiences with health care providers who inappropriately isolated AIDS patients due to fear of contagion. Again, the participants perceived this as a greater problem in small towns than in rural cities. One participant described an experience in a small town nursing home:

> *It just seemed like being put away. They would come in with space suits on and clean the room. There was a yellow barricade across the door and a big isolation sign. Some staff didn't come in the room.*

Maneuvering the Barriers

Strategies participants used in dealing with barriers to health care included educating self, dealing with the baggage, and migrating to care.

Educating Self. All participants engaged in the "educating self" strategy from the onset of learning about being HIV positive. The strategy focused upon learning about the many complex health problems that can occur because of the infection and the current treatment modalities available. The context for this strategy was fear and uncertainty related to the diagnosis of a disease for which there is currently no known cure. There was the realization of the need to be engaged in self-advocacy and to advocate for others in a rural health care system with personnel who were often described as less knowledgeable about the disease, its treatment, and the resources available than were the participants.

Dealing with the Baggage. The second strategy for maneuvering barriers was dealing with the baggage. Besides the long-term sequelae of a physiologically devastating terminal illness, participants had to deal with the psychosocial issues that accompanied the infection. Homophobia and bias against drug users were described as baggage associated with this illness. Conservative characteristics of rural communities made finding tactics to deal with this baggage even more challenging.

One "dealing with the baggage" issue was whether or not to reveal the illness. Lack of anonymity was a concern, especially in small towns. There were benefits and risks to disclosure identified and considered individually as to social, employment, and health care consequences. Therefore, disclosure was selective and risky. There was variation among the informants in three types of disclosure tactics: concealing, distorting, and revealing. Most of the participants selectively concealed their HIV status, one distorted the illness diagnosis, and three openly and honestly revealed their illness to everyone. The tactic of distorting the diagnosis was used by one informant because of fear of the loss of his job and insurance. He told people that he had leukemia, an illness he considered socially acceptable.

The tactic of fully revealing one's HIV positive status or diagnosis of AIDs had both negative and positive consequences for informants.

Several participants said this tactic was positive in helping others, including health care professionals, gain an awareness of the humanistic aspect to this disease. As one participant said, "We are people first, human beings like everyone else . . . we have a chronic disease. . . . Why should we be treated any differently than someone with a chronic disease like cancer?" Using the tactic of revealing carried the risk of being ostracized in some way—in the home, on the job, in the community, in the health care system, or a combination of these ways.

One participant described an experience that resulted from his revealing the fact that he was HIV positive. While the experience was negative, the participant acknowledged that his perception of the health care in the rural city was currently more positive. This experience occurred in a rural city emergency room where he went to seek help for a drug overdose:

> *I told the nurse in the E.R. that I was HIV positive because I thought I should warn her. That was a big mistake. . . . They would point from the nurse's station and I could hear them talk about AIDS. . . . They isolated me. However, since that time they are getting better.*

Migrating to Care. The third strategy in maneuvering barriers was migrating to care. Most of the participants migrated back to Montana from a distant urban city to be with family and/or friends for care and support. This finding is similar to other reports that people with HIV related illnesses are returning home to families as their illness progresses and their resources decline (Davis & Stapelton, 1991; D'Augelli & Poullard, 1989). However, in this study there was the tactic of re-migrating. Several informants migrated back to small towns and then re-migrated to a rural city. In other words, informants not only came home for care but had to leave home to obtain needed health care again. This tactic was used to compensate for lack of adequate health care, lack of anonymity, and problems with confidentiality in a small town. About health care in small towns, informants said such things as "They acted scared of me;" "I was really forced to come here (to rural city);" "They didn't know a thing about HIV."

CONCLUSIONS: EXPERIENCING CONSEQUENCES IN CARE SEEKING

The three major consequences to encountering and maneuvering barriers in care seeking were "no care," "stigmatized care," or "compassionate care." These consequences also can be usefully viewed as the major outcomes of the study. The first conclusion was that no care or stigmatized care existed under specific conditions of fear, ignorance, and negative attitudes. Secondly, as rurality increased (rural to frontier), barriers to care increased. More barriers subsequently created more negative consequences in health care for HIV-infected persons in small towns. Migrating to care emerged as a key strategy in maneuvering the barriers to obtain health care. Informants reported more resources, fewer barriers, and ultimately improved, compassionate health care in *rural cities* when compared with *small towns.* An example of non-care was the refusal of health care providers to provide services. Indicators of stigmatized care included inappropriate use of protective barriers, breach of confidentiality, social isolation in health care facilities, expression of disgust, disapproval and devaluations, and superficial formalized interactions that included nurses avoiding talking about the HIV status with the patient.

The third outcome was that compassionate care existed under distinct conditions of caregivers having experience with caring for AIDS patients, a perception of caregivers having an ethic of altruism, and the presence of a patient advocate. Indicators of compassionate care included the nurse who was "a good listener," "gave accurate information about the disease and treatment," "wept with me when a friend died," and was "technically competent."

IMPLICATIONS AND RECOMMENDATIONS FOR NURSING

The empirically grounded framework that emerged through the data analysis in this study can serve as a framework for a larger study. Recommendations for further research include the integration of a quantifying instrument to test components of the theoretical framework.

In addition to the recommendations for further research, findings from this study have implications for nursing practice. First, the findings can provide insight for nurses into the perceptions of HIV-infected persons regarding health care delivery in a rural state. This insight can in turn be the impetus for interventions directed at reducing barriers to health care such as educational offerings for rural nurses and the development of case management models of health care delivery.

Tessaro and Highriter (1994) concluded that "attitudinal, normative, and professional experiences are all important in examining nurses' intentions to work with clients infected with HIV." Thus, educational offerings should include components of knowledge enhancement, clinical experience in caring for HIV-infected clients, and strategies to deal with fears and negative attitudes. Incorporating persons with AIDS into educational programs may be another helpful strategy in decreasing fear (Meisenhelder, 1994).

Case management models that include the concept of partnership with clients need to be developed to enhance continuity of care for clients with HIV infection. This may reduce access to care barriers and enhance the adequacy of care. This is especially important in the coordination of services and resources for clients who live in remote areas. Barriers could be further reduced with increasing the numbers of nurse practitioners in rural communities. There are research studies to support that nurse practitioners in consultation with physicians provide comparable quality of care to that of primary care physicians (Aiken et al., 1993). The long term management of clients with HIV infection by nurse practitioners could improve access to care and the adequacy of care.

Persons with HIV infection who live in a rural state such as Montana face the challenge of "managing barriers in care seeking." The consequences of no care or stigmatized care that HIV-infected persons experience when encountering barriers to health care is unacceptable. Nurses must work together and with other health care disciplines to eliminate these barriers. The goal of health professionals must be to provide compassionate care of the highest possible quality to each person whatever the medical diagnosis or health care setting.

REFERENCES

Aiken, L., Lake, E., Semaan, S., Lehman, H., O'Hare, P., Cole, S., Dunbar, D., & Frank, I. (1993). Nurse practitioner managed care for persons with HIV infection. *IMAGE: Journal of Nursing Scholarship, 25*(3), 172–177.

Bushy, A. (1992). Rural nursing research priorities. *Journal of Nursing Administration, 22*(1), 4–12.

Carwein, V. L., Sabo, C. E., & Berry, D. E. (1993). HIV infection in traditional rural communities. *Nursing Clinics of North America, 28*(1), 231–238.

D'Augelli, A. R., & Poullard, J. (1989). AIDS fear and homophobia among rural nursing personnel. *AIDS Education and Prevention, 1* (4), 277–284.

Davis, K., & Stapelton, J. (1991). Migration to rural areas by HIV patients: Impact on HIV-related health care use. *Infection Control and Hospital Epidemiology, 12* (9), 540–543.

Elison, G. (1986). Frontier areas: Problems for delivery of health services. *Rural Health Care, 8* (1), 1,3.

Fuszard, B., Sowell, R., Hoff, P., & Waters, M. (1991). Rural nurses join forces for AIDS care. *Nursing Connections, 4* (3), 51–61.

Glaser, B., & Strauss, A. (1967). *The discovery of grounded theory: Strategies for qualitative research.* Chicago: Aldine.

Glaser, D. (1978). *Theoretical sensitivity: Advances in the methodology of grounded theory.* Mill Valley, CA: The Sociology Press.

Long, K. A., & Weinert, C. (1989). Rural nursing: Developing the theory base. *Scholarly Inquiry for Nursing Practice: An International Journal, 3* (2), 113–127.

Meisenhelder, J. B. (1994). Contributing factors to fear of HIV contagion in registered nurses. *IMAGE: Journal of Nursing Scholarship, 26* (1), 65–69.

Montana Department of Public Health and Human Services (July 1992, October 1996). *Montana surveillance reports of resident and non-resident AIDS cases.* Helena, MT: Author.

Munzenrider, R., & Sundby, J. (1992, April 12). Coming home to die. *The Billings Gazette,* p. A1.

Strauss, A., & Corbin, J. (1990). *Basics of qualitative research: Grounded theory procedure and techniques.* Newbury Park, CA: Sage.

Tessaro, I., & Highriter, M. (1994). HIV and the work intentions of public health nurses. *Public Health Nursing, 11* (4), 273–280.

Young, E., Koch, P., & Preston, D. (1989). AIDS and homosexuality: A longitudinal study of knowledge and attitude change among rural nurses. *Public Health Nursing, 6* (4), 189–196.

U.S. 1990 Census of Population. (1992). Bureau of the Census. Washington, DC: U..S. Department of Commerce.

White, P. (1994). Providing HIV services in a rural setting. *Primary Care Perspectives, 10* (1), 1–10.

29

Levels of Prevention in a Rural Homeless Nursing Clinic

Carolyn H. Wenger

With homeless population estimates that range from six hundred thousand to three million, ignoring the homeless is no longer possible for nurses (Hunter, 1993). Regardless of practice area, nurses encounter the health problems of the homeless population. A call issued by Faye Abdellah (Abdellah, Chamberlain, & Levine, 1986), then Deputy Surgeon General and Chief Nurse of the Public Health Service, challenges nurses to deal with health care access issues by bringing nursing care directly to homeless people. With this call, universities were advised to provide opportunities for students in nontraditional practice settings. Recent literature (AACN, 1993) has also recognized the need for nursing student education to include health promotion and health maintenance in settings that target underserved populations (Kitchen, 1993). Homeless clinics have been recognized specifically as excellent sites for student learning.

In response to the 1986 call, with funding from a National Institutes of Health (NIH) Special Projects Grant, I established the Montana State University College of Nursing homeless clinic in a small city of 80,000 in south central Montana. The purpose of the clinic was threefold. The clinic was to provide direct nursing services to an underserved population, to provide a practice setting for students in an independent nurse-managed clinic, and to provide a setting for faculty practice. The goal of nursing care was to provide health maintenance and health promotion services to a vulnerable population.

The purpose of this chapter is to describe some of my experiences in developing and maintaining a nurse-managed clinic that offered nursing services to a homeless population and was a nontraditional clinical site for baccalaureate nursing students. A discussion of rural homelessness and the characteristics of the rural homeless population are included. Strategies used to gain client acceptance of the clinic are discussed. Another purpose is to discuss a record review undertaken to determine if levels of prevention were a useful framework for delivery of nursing care to a homeless population.

REVIEW OF THE LITERATURE

Homelessness and health care of the homeless have been written about extensively over the past 15 years. The general literature has evolved from basic descriptive works to relevant social policy statements and applications of theoretical models. There has been a shift from identifying prevalent pathologies to understanding and appreciating homeless people themselves. Several outstanding reviews of the homeless literature exist. One review by Snow, Anderson, and Koegel (1994) notes the tendency of homeless literature to over-pathologize. The authors specifically address (a) a tendency to regard isolated occurrences as patterns; (b) an uncritical use of psychiatric inventories; (c) decontextualized analyses, and (d) a preoccupation of researchers with documenting the existence of disabilities among homeless populations. The literature addressed here is that which relates to rural homelessness and to clinical opportunities for nursing students in homeless clinics.

The rural homeless are a subpopulation of the homeless which has not been extensively described. The lighter population densities in rural areas allow dangerous and substandard housing to seem isolated and diminish the perceived severity of rural homelessness (National Coalition for the Homeless, 1987). The National Rural Health Association (1996) discusses the members of the rural homeless as significantly underreported due to problems in defining and counting the rural homeless and due to their tendency to dwell in substandard housing and doubling up with families and friends.

Differences between rural and urban homeless include the tendency for rural homeless to be younger than their urban counterparts (Roth, Bean, Lust, & Saveanu, 1985). Patton's (1988) monograph specifically addresses rural-urban differences in homelessness. Rural homeless persons were likely to be male but had a higher proportion of women than urban homeless. They tended to be white, younger (18 to 29 years of age), and married. Disparities in gender are noted by other authors. This may be due to limited safe housing that specifically targets women.

A major theme in the rural literature is the reliance by rural homeless on families and friends. Patton (1988) notes that rural homeless were more likely to have spent the previous night with family and friends. This tendency is also discussed by First, Rife, and Toomey (1994) and by Fitchen (1992). Parvensky and Krasniewski (1988) note that 33.8% of homeless Colorado families report having stayed with friends and family prior to becoming homeless. Doubling or tripling up is one step on the road to homelessness. Gladden (1991) discusses the likelihood of this occurring on Indian reservations. The National Coalition for Homelessness (1987) suggests that this may be an imposed result of poverty rather than a cultural norm.

There are no major differences in the health care needs of rural vs. urban homeless persons. Gladden (1991) documents the major health needs of the North Dakota rural homeless population as including impaired vision requiring glasses; diagnosed mental health problems; psychological disturbances without actual diagnosed mental illness, i.e., anxiety, depression; substance abuse; dental problems; sexually transmitted diseases; hypertension; and infections. These problems do not differ significantly from those described in the urban homeless literature. Patton (1988) documents no significant differences in the health problems of rural and urban homeless.

A comparison of reported histories of mental health treatment by Nooe and Cunningham (1986) reveals no significant differences between the urban and rural groups. Rural respondents report a slightly higher rate of alcoholism than urban homeless respondents.

Homeless health care clinics have provided valuable practice sites for students and nursing faculty members. Gottesman, Lewis, Lindsey, and Brecht (1993) discuss the value of the practice site not only for clinical nursing service but also as a "social laboratory" for nurse researchers.

Anderson (1993) discusses the benefits of student work with the homeless as including conditioning to become more proactive as nurses, increased focus on holistic care, increased understanding of working with clients (as opposed to for clients), increased flexibility, increased skill in obtaining alcohol and drug histories, and decreased fear of working with hallucinating and delusional clients. Lacey and Adderly-Kelly (1993) describe work between Harvard University and the Community for Creative Nonviolence as creating learning opportunities for junior and senior nursing students in all courses. Student satisfaction from working with homeless was a major factor in facilitating the College's involvement with this project.

Turner, Bauer, McNair, McNott, and Walker's (1993) use of student journal entries capture the emotions and feelings very well of both instructor and students beginning a shelter clinic. The journals describe the culture shock and the professional growth that occur when immersing oneself in homeless populations. The journals poignantly reflect the startled thoughts of "How can I *really* help? . . . What if I were homeless?" Nurse-managed homeless clinics are not without problems, but have been reported to create excellent learning opportunities for both graduate and undergraduate nursing students.

The need for more descriptive work on the rural homeless persists. Studies of western rural homeless populations are especially needed, as the findings from studies conducted in eastern rural counties that border metropolitan areas may not be generalizable to western rural and frontier areas.

CONCEPTUAL FRAMEWORK

While most literature on homelessness focuses on acute-care needs, it was my distinct belief that the homeless could also benefit from nursing care focused on health maintenance. Because of this, the conceptual framework chosen for work at the mission was McKeown & Garrison's (1996) conceptualization of the levels of prevention (Table 29.1). The levels of prevention model bases interventions on the stages of disease, seeking to limit pathophysiological damage by early intervention. This model has helped in focusing public health nursing toward prevention and early intervention over the last three decades. Health care is divided into primary, secondary, and tertiary care.

Primary prevention is aimed at reducing susceptibility to illness and incorporating health-promoting activities. Health education was the principle mode of primary prevention in this project. For example, all patients were given blood pressure cards with blood pressure goals. Pamphlets on a variety of topics including nutrition and stress

TABLE 29.1 Levels of Prevention*

Period	Stage	Event	Preventive Measure Level	Sample Shelter Interventions
Prepathogenesis	Susceptibility	1. Interrelations host, agent, & environmental factors bring host & agent together. 2. Disease-producing stimulus is produced in host.	Primary prevention	Health promotive measures—health education, nutrition, counseling, personal hygiene Specific protection—immunization referrals
Pathogenesis	Presymptomatic disease A. Early pathogenesis	Stimulus or agent becomes established. Time and physiological changes begin.		
	B. Discernible early lesions	Clinical recognition of disease through tests that detect physiological changes is possible.	Secondary prevention	Early diagnosis & prompt treatment —screening (blood pressure, blood glucose, hematocrit), case-finding
	Clinical disease	Acute illness Disability Chronicity	Tertiary prevention	Limitation of disability—dressing changes, follow-up on chronic & acute health conditions

**Note.* Adapted from McKeon, R., & Garrison, C. (1996). Epidemological applications in community health nursing (p. 214). In M. Stanhope & J. Lancaster (Eds.), *Community Health Nursing.* St. Louis: Mosby.

reduction were used. Younger men were often interested in learning about weight training and use of nutrition supplements.

Secondary prevention through early identification of disease. The goal was to limit disease. Health screening was the principle mode of secondary prevention. Screenings included blood pressure, blood glucose, hematocrit, height/weight, and a computerized Life-Stress Analysis.

Finally, tertiary care sought to limit disability from injury or disease. Examples of tertiary care included ongoing assessment of established disease and wound care. Persons needing immediate attention were triaged to local hospitals and clinics.

LOCATION OF CLINIC

Rurality

Montana is a sparsely populated state of 800,000 (Bureau of Census, 1992) with a population density of approximately five persons per square mile. The clinic was established in Billings, the largest rural city in the state. It is a metropolitan center of 84,228 and serves as a main trade and medical center for Montana, Wyoming, and both North and South Dakota (Billings Chamber of Commerce Business Development Council, 1995).

Whether this clinic should be considered a rural facility can be questioned. Narrow definitions of rural would preclude consideration of the clinic as rural. Rural theorists Long and Weinert (1989) support the inclusion of population centers within rural states in their conceptualization of rural. Population centers such as Billings offer services to persons beyond the standard metropolitan area. Persons travel from sparsely populated areas for services that are not readily available at home. Seeing persons who have traveled 100 to 200 miles for care is usual in rural clinics and was applicable for the Billings site.

Comprehensive homeless services (i.e., shelter, food, and medical care) cannot be maintained in sparsely populated areas; therefore, rural homeless persons migrate to larger population centers. In many ways, small cities such as Billings are ideal target communities for the rural homeless. Well-established networks of supportive services provide needed resources. Agencies are large enough to protect anonymity, yet small enough to take interest in clients and not lose people in the shuffle.

Approximately one-half of the persons residing at the mission came from areas outside Billings. Some persons reported that they previously had lived with extended families or friends, but "it was no longer working out," so they traveled specifically to Billings to get help. Other persons discussed the embarrassment associated with the lack of anonymity in their small home towns; they traveled to Billings to "get their stuff together" and planned to return home later. Persons staying at the shelter included off-season farm and ranch hands and migrant workers. Off-season workers in the tourism industry were also seen.

The magnet quality of urban centers within rural states should not be overlooked when considering rural health. Small cities, such as Billings, may be considered as rural service areas due to (a) their location within large rural areas, (b) the lack of other metropolitan centers within the same proximity, and (c) their ability to attract and serve persons far beyond their urban boundaries.

Setting

A rescue mission provided a unique setting for the development of a nurse clinic for community health nursing practice. The mission had offered food, clothing, and shelter to homeless people since 1954. Located in a low socioeconomic neighborhood near railroad tracks, it was a clean facility that housed more than one hundred male and female clients.

Initially, the clinic was in the boardroom of the mission for easy access to a sink. A reticence of the homeless to enter the administrative offices and leave the residential part of the building was soon sensed by nursing faculty. The clinic was then moved to the so-called day room. The day room was the physical space where homeless men and women, primarily street people, congregated. The room was often crowded, smelly, smoky, and noisy. Street people unable to follow the structure of residential mission life (daily showers, laundered clothes, and chapel attendance) often came in to warm up and to sleep in the day room. The day room was an intimidating place for women to enter as primarily men congregated there, sharing stories and cigarettes. Despite these unfavorable conditions, faculty believed the location of the clinic to be important as it represented a willingness to practice on the turf of the homeless.

The clinic was equipped with folding tables for students and homeless clients. Portable screens provided privacy when necessary. Equipment included sphygmomanometers, stethoscopes, glucometers, educational pamphlets, an audiometer, TITMUS vision screener, portable computer, and a minicentrifuge. By placing ourselves in the center of this room, we allowed the homeless to observe us and all that we did. Some people were interested in the equipment; others observed the nursing students to be "safe" persons with whom to talk. While we were initially overwhelmed with the complexity of many health problems, we were also impressed with the interest of this group in basic health maintenance.

Clinics were held weekly. Clinics were staffed by three to five students with one supervising faculty member. Approximately 12 to 20 homeless persons were seen at each clinic.

POPULATION

The population seen at the clinic ranged in age from two days old to 94 years. Most persons seen (36%) were between the ages of 30 and 45 years. Most of the clients seen were male, with only 18.9% of the population female. This was consistent with the male-female ratio of guests at the mission. Seventy-two percent of clients seen were Caucasian, 13.6% American Indian, and 8.5% Hispanic. This reflected the predominantly Caucasian population of Montana. About 20% of the shelter residents received clinic services. This group represented a distinct group of homeless who were interested in their own health and were motivated toward improving their own health status.

Distinct subgroups within the homeless population were seen. The group often called the "new homeless" (Marion, 1991) was seen. Residents attributed their homelessness to economic trends, e.g., loss of employment. Frequently with intact families, this group was often on their way from eastern parts of Montana to the northwest, where employment opportunities were thought to be more positive. Families have been identified as the fastest growing segment of the homeless population (Marion, 1991).

The male population over age 65 was a small, but distinct, group. Some of these men received small social security payments and could pay for their beds at night. They were, however, unable to afford monthly rent, utility payments, and the required security deposits of independent living. The men had established daily routines that included going to the library, working a few hours/day in janitorial activities, walking the downtown perimeter, and drinking coffee in downtown restaurants. Maintaining their schedule was important to them. These men played a paternal role in relation to clinic nurses and newer homeless persons. For example, they told the nurses if someone coughed at night in the dorm room or if someone living on the street had a health problem. Likewise, they would tell faculty on the first clinical day of a new rotation if students looked like they were having difficulty finding the mission or its parking lot. They also made suggestions to younger homeless persons about where to find work and who to avoid on the streets.

Street people were the most readily observable subgroup. They were predominantly male, most often with mental health problems including diagnoses of posttraumatic stress disorder, alcoholism, schizophrenia, or other delusional states. While some of these men were severely crippled by their mental illness, others were quite affable. Their peculiar dress, often layered to survive the extreme temperatures, distinguished them. Unusual behaviors by some street people such as barking or yelling were tolerated by other homeless males. Homeless women with children tended to be very guarded around street people. Some homeless men attempted to protect individual street persons from ridicule or scorn by watching out for them. For example, one elderly male explained to others, "He was a prisoner of war in Viet Nam, you know," to justify the aberrant behavior of one man to observers.

RECORD REVIEW OF NURSING CARE

A three-year retrospective review of records was conducted to identify whether the levels of prevention was a useful framework for nursing care of this rural homeless population. The survey showed that primary prevention (health education independent of diagnostic need) was included in 26% of visit records. Predominant topics included safety issues for children, first aid preparedness, stress management, and making sound nutritional choices about the mission diet.

Secondary prevention was reflected in 67% of visit records. Health screening was requested by individuals interested in their health and persons with risk factors such as family history of disease. The specific values of screenings reflected a predominantly healthy population. Approximately 80% of those screened had a blood pressure less than 140/90. This was most impressive when considering the often high-fat, high-sodium diet served at the mission combined with the stresses of crowding. Sixty-five percent of persons weighed within normal weight ranges; only 4% of the population was underweight. While many envision the homeless as emaciated, donated food was in abundance at the shelter. Hematocrit testing revealed that 89% of persons were within normal limits. Blood glucose measurements were 90% within normal limits.

Health screening has been an important approach to nursing care for the rural homeless. Many persons entered the clinic requesting a simple blood pressure screen, but went on to discuss more serious health problems with student nurses. Health screening seemed to function as a testing ground of the providers by the homeless. When the provider responded seriously and with interest, the client would then begin to discuss more significant problems (many people were concerned about familial risk factors). After blood pressure screening, one woman could talk about her ongoing medical problems that resulted from many battering episodes. The woman was then referred to an appropriate service. Students and faculty were impressed with the clients' levels of knowledge about many chronic diseases, particularly heart disease and diabetes.

Tertiary care was reflected in approximately 11% of records. Usually, these clients requested assistance with trauma. Trauma most often included contusions, concussions, stab wounds, and first- to third-degree frostbite. A major nursing role with tertiary care included triage to sources of care where the client would be expected and accepted. If x-rays were needed, clients were referred to a clinic with x-ray capabilities. Avoiding possible perceptions of "being given the run-around" was important when referring clients to outside health care resources. When possible, rides to services were arranged. Case management services were conducted to verify care and to convey the message to community health care providers that there was interest in the quality of indigent care.

RURAL HOMELESS CHARACTERISTICS

Some observed characteristics of this homeless population have not appeared in the descriptive literature on homelessness. Three of these traits, however, have been discussed in the rural literature. These traits include self-reliance (Weinert & Long, 1987), self-care, and hardiness (Bigbee, 1991).

Self-reliance

Weinert and Long (1987) have discussed self-reliance in rural populations as the self-management of medical problems with assistance from families and friends, rather than reliance on formal resources. Self-reliance at the homeless clinic has been expressed and interpreted in varying ways. Many clients have discussed with student nurses the importance of caring for themselves without outside assistance. Interestingly, many of these homeless clients identified nursing students as facilitators of health and not as outside help. For some homeless, taking care of one's health was "the right thing to do," a social responsibility. One 24–year-old male stated, "I need to look out for myself. No one else is going to do that for me." Many clients sought nursing services for the reassurance that there was nothing more they should be doing for themselves. Others expressed an interest in avoiding the debt that would result from medical attention.

Not all persons who were referred to medical care sought out that care. While some practitioners have viewed this behavior as an abrogation of self-care, it can also be viewed as an avoidance of "using the system." Students were often surprised at the honesty and candor of clients who would tell them "I won't go there." Again, the nurse working within the walls of the homeless mission was not seen as outside help.

Many clients demonstrated pride in their health and their health habits. One man cut out articles on self-care that he read in the newspaper. He would often quiz me on my own knowledge of health care.

Self-reliance can also be seen in the cyclic nature of the homeless population at the shelter. The mission population declines in the warm summer months. Many persons spend summer months in nearby campgrounds. Autumn in Montana always brings an increase in mission populations. Severe cold weather renders it unsafe to stay in campgrounds and automobiles. Many persons do not seek housing until freezing temperatures make reliance on the mission absolutely necessary.

Other subtle indications of self-reliance in caring for oneself included the tendency of persons to stop at the clinic and weigh themselves. Students have been impressed with the numbers of persons who are interested in measuring their weight, but decline visiting with a nurse. Other clients were interested in learning about dietary changes they could make "once they were back on their feet."

Self-care

Some innovative attempts at self-care have initially caused clinicians to shudder but need to be viewed as "doing the best one can in a bad situation." For example, Willie R. had displaced his patella in hitching a freight train ride. His knee began to swell with increased fluid. He used his friend's insulin syringe to draw excess fluid from his knee and medicated the severe pain with wine. He immobilized his leg with a piece of the frame from his backpack. While his actions were fraught with potential problems, Willie was using the resources available to him at the time.

Hardiness

Hardiness has been associated with rural persons (Lee, 1983). Kobasa, Maddi, and Kahn (1982) define hardiness as "a constellation of personality characteristics that function as a resistance resource in the encounter with stressful life events." Many clients have visited the nursing clinic with ongoing health problems that previously warranted attention. For example, clients have reported ongoing pain of significant duration that they thought they "could tough it out." Students are often impressed with the hardiness and fortitude of homeless clients.

Hardiness was evident in mission residents' endurance of physical, social, and environmental stressors. One young Native American male reported walking 35 miles with a significant stab wound. Rural transit is seriously limited in comparison with urban transit. Long walks of one to six miles through town for medical or employment appointments are usual.

The ability of homeless persons to endure social stressors is remarkable. Homeless persons often carry money that they save; they are often victims of robberies and beatings. Homeless persons are shunned and ridiculed. One young man was forced to leave his job as a dishwasher after co-workers saw him on a television news story about holiday dinners for local homeless persons. Montana's semi-arid climate of hot summers and frigid winters results in serious thermoregulatory stresses. Montana's homeless survive a combination of severe stressors.

Many persons who stayed at the shelter worked at minimum-wage or day-labor jobs. Paying for their bed and meals was important for them. Others needed to save for several months before acquiring enough money for rental and utility deposits in the community setting. While occasionally individuals can be observed panhandling around the city, rural homeless people are more likely to be seen on their way to work. The rural homeless persons who are carrying sack lunches on their way to work may not be recognized as "homeless," a stereotype that typifies a dirty and disheveled person.

Summary

Self-reliance, interest in self-care, and hardiness have been noted characteristics at this rural shelter. Self-selection of clients attending a health maintenance clinic was probably influential in the magnitude of these observed attributes. Poverty and access issues may also be associated with self-care and self-reliance. When persons cannot afford illness care, they cope by guarding their health and utilizing adaptive strategies.

CLINIC ACCEPTANCE BY THE HOMELESS

Acceptance of the nursing clinic by the homeless was initially deemed a challenge due to a reported distrust of health care providers and the hierarchy of needs associated with homelessness and poverty (Reilly & McInnis, 1985). Pragmatism dictated that acute problems be managed immediately. For example, a 22–year-old male with pain from frostbite and a moderately elevated blood pressure would be treated for the frostbite before receiving education about blood pressure. While the purpose of the clinic was to offer health-promotion and health-maintenance services, the homeless also identified the need for acute-care services.

Nursing faculty attempted to deal with professional distrust through explicit concern with health problems as they were reported by clients. When clients were sent to other clinics or hospitals, the nurse made phone calls to the other facility to prepare them for the client. Follow-up calls were also made after the client's visit to learn what services the client had received. When clients expressed dissatisfaction with health care, students and faculty not only listened but became involved with strategies such as letter-writing or role-playing to encourage effective expression of dissatisfaction by homeless.

To foster trust, faculty practice occurred over school vacation times so there was a consistent contact between the college and the shelter population. The consistent presence of a specific faculty member over several years was believed to have been important to the establishment of trust. When faculty and students were invited to eat breakfast at the mission, they joined the homeless for breakfast. Giving something back to the students was important to residents of the mission.

In response to the interests of the homeless, health education programs were planned. Posters advertising clinics and education programs were posted around the mission. Clients immediately expressed interest in and attended clinic and educational programs that were offered. Consideration of the lifestyles of the homeless necessitated modifications in health promotive suggestions. For example, education on fitness by students did not include expensive aerobic wear but focused on stretching and walking. Audiovisual materials were screened for economic bias. This screening eliminated many resources, as most videos are geared toward an upper-middle class audience. A video on stress reduction was part of the first program offered. Shawna, a large and usually loud woman who had been released from jail to the mission, was noticed to be assiduously taking notes. When her interest was reflected upon, she stated, "You know I've been put in jail a lot, and I've lost my two sons because I get rowdy. I'll get thrown out of here if I get rowdy. This is showing me how not to get rowdy. Maybe I can get my two sons back if I pay attention to this." Shawna was able to move from the mission to independent housing later that year.

STUDENT ACCEPTANCE

To foster acceptance of this learning experience, student nurses were prepared by the faculty for this clinic. The dominant culture tends to stereotype the homeless as dangerous, lazy, and alcoholic. Students were encouraged to drive by the mission during the day so that they would not have to find it in dark early morning hours. Driving in pairs was encouraged. Students were encouraged to talk about fears, biases, or concerns about working with the homeless population. The instructor discussed with students her initial feelings of insecurity and how those feelings quickly changed to feelings of security and safety as she got to know the population.

Students were allowed to wear jeans or comfortable clothes as client foot care required working on the floor. Lab coats were worn, which promoted visibility on the street as helping professionals when student nurses walked from a nearby parking lot to the mission. Students were discouraged from wearing expensive clothing or jewelry that would amplify social and economic class differences between themselves and the homeless.

Students were offered the opportunity to practice new skills prior to entering the shelter to decrease anxiety, and they were given time immediately following their homeless experiences to debrief and discuss their experiences. Some clients participated every week, and students followed through with these same clients. When clients carried out suggested changes, students felt positive about their work. Suggestions from students about running the clinic were encouraged by the instructor; students saw the clinic as "their clinic."

While some students openly discussed their lack of enthusiasm prior to beginning this clinical experience, all students have evaluated this experience positively. Students related that the genuine gratitude expressed by homeless clients was very meaningful to them. Students also commented positively on the clinic being an independent-practice setting. An important outcome is that students became the "regular" nurses in the mission and were never overlooked until the "real" or staff nurses were available. The students believed that this experience assisted in their professional role development.

OUTCOMES

The outcome of the retrospective record survey indicated that levels of prevention was a useful framework in providing nursing care to this homeless population. While acute health needs were identified, the majority of nursing needs presented were health maintenance needs. Homeless persons were often in situational crises, but they did not want to stop taking care of their own health. Most of all, they did not want minor illnesses to develop that might require expensive physician or hospital visits.

Additionally, written evaluations of the clinic services by the clients were overwhelmingly positive. Another measure of success has included long-term relationships with clients. Many clients have continued to be seen on a regular basis. While care is not always needed, former clients will stop in with pictures of new babies, news of new jobs, or simply to say "Hi. Remember me?"

ONGOING WORK

The nursing clinic continues to provide services ten years after its inception and years after federal funding ended. One of the earliest clients continues to visit the clinic weekly. Others have been seen periodically over the last decade. In addition to the nursing clinic, a Health Care for Homeless project was recently established with federal funding to provide medical care for homeless rural Montanans at the same site. The nursing and medical clinics coordinate care to provide comprehensive health care services.

Numerous benefits have been realized over the years. Student evaluations of this experience have remained consistently high. The clinic provides an environment in which students can practice critical thinking related to the current health care environment and disenfranchised populations. The clinic, mission, and students have mutually benefitted from various service projects.

Bringing health care to the homeless has been an exceedingly meaningful experience for faculty and students at Montana State University College of Nursing. In addition to offering a service, the clinic has provided fertile ground for the profound, complex, painful, and joyous experiences associated with nursing.

REFERENCES

Abdellah, F., Chamberlain, J., & Levine, I. (1986). Role of nurses in meeting needs of the homeless: Summary of a workshop for providers, researchers, and educators. *American Journal of Public Health, 5,* 494–498.

American Association of Colleges of Nursing. (1993). *Nursing education's agenda for the 21st century.* Washington, DC: Author.

Anderson, J. (1993). The homeless populations: A clinical laboratory for students in community health and psychiatric/mental health nursing. In Hunter, J. (Ed.), *Nursing and health care for the homeless* (pp. 173–178). Albany: State University of New York Press.

Bigbee, J. (1991). The concept of hardiness as applied to rural nursing. In Bushy, A. (Ed.) *Rural Nursing, Vol. 1* (pp. 39–58). Newbury Park, CA: Sage.

Billings Chamber of Commerce Business Development Council. (1995). *Billings economic handbook.* Billings, MT: Author.

Bureau of Census, U.S. (1992). *The 1990 decennial census of the United States.* Washington, DC: Author.

First, R. J., Rife, J. C., & Toomey, B. G. (1994). Homelessness in rural areas: Causes, patterns, and trends. *Social Work, 39,* (1), 97–108.

Fitchen, J. M. (1992). On the edge of homelessness: Rural poverty and housing insecurity. *Rural Sociology, 57,* (2), 173–193.

Gladden, J. (1991). Homelessness: A rural perspective. In A. Bushy (Ed.), *Rural nursing* (Vol. 1, pp. 325–393). Newbury Park, CA: Sage.

Gottesman, M., Lewis, M., Lindsey, A., & Brecht, M. (1993). Evolution and population characteristics of a nurse-prepared health center for the homeless and high-risk, low-income families. In J. Hunter (Ed.), *Nuring and health care for the homeless* (pp. 33–50). Albany: State University of New York Press.

Hunter, J. (1993). Introduction. In J. Hunter (Ed.), *Nursing and health care for the homeless* (pp. 3–5). Albany: State University of New York Press.

Kitchen, S. (1993). The role of nurses and nursing schools in health services for the homeless. In J. Hunter (Ed.), *Nursing and health care for the homeless* (pp. 215–220). Albany: State University of New York Press.

Kobasa, S. C., Maddi, S. R., & Kahn, S. (1982). Hardiness and health: A prospective study. *Journal of Personality and Social Psychology, 42,* 168–177.

Lacey, B., & Adderly-Kelly, B. (1993). Development of a model nurse managed clinic for the homeless. In J. Hunter (Ed.), *Nursing health care for the homeless* (pp. 201–206). Albany: State University of New York Press.

Lee, H. J. (1983). Analysis of a concept: Hardiness. *Oncology Nursing Forum, 10,* 92–95.

Long, K. A., & Weinert, C. (1989). Rural nursing: Developing the theory base. *Scholarly Inquiry for Nursing Practice, 3,* 113–127.

Marion, F. (1991). Homeless families: Rebuilding connections. *Public Health Nursing, 8,* 90–96.

McKeown, R, & Garrison, C. (1996). Epidemiological application of community health nursing. In M. Stanhope & J. Lancaster (Eds). *Community Health Nursing* (4th ed.) (p. 214). St. Louis, MO: Mosby.

National Coalition for the Homeless. (1987). *Rural homelessness in America: Appalachia and the south.* New York: Author.

National Rural Health Association. (1996). *The rural homeless: America's lost population.* Kansas City, MO: Author.

Nooe, R. & Cunningham, M. (1986). Rural dimensions of homelessness: A rural-urban comparison. *Human Services in the Rural Environment, 15* (4), 5–9.

Parvensky, J. & Krasniewski, D. (1988). *In search of a place to call home: A profile of homelessness in Colorado.* Denver, CO: Colorado Coalition for the Homeless.

Patton, L. (1988). *The rural homeless.* Washington, DC: US Department of Health and Human Services.

Reilly, E., & McInnis, B. (1985). Boston, Massachusetts: The Pine Street Inn nurses' clinic and tuberculosis program. In P. Brickner, L. Scharer, B. Conanan, A. Elvy, & M. Savares (Eds.). *Health care of homeless people* (pp. 291–300). New York: Springer.

Roth, D., Bean, J., Lust, N., & Saveanu. T. (1985). *Homelessness in Ohio: A study of people in need.* OH: Department of Mental Health.

Snow, D., Anderson, L. & Koegel, P. (1994). Distorting tendencies in research on the homeless. *American Behavioral Scientist, 37*(4), 461–475.

Turner, S., Bauer, G., McNair, E., McNott, B., Walker, W. (1993). The homeless experience: Clinic building in a discovery-learning project. *Public Health Nursing, 6* (2), 97–101.

Weinert, C., & Long, K. A. (1987). Understanding the health care needs of rural families. *Family Relations, 36,* 450–455.

V

EDUCATIONAL AND PROFESSIONAL ISSUES

In the first chapter of this section (chapter 30), readers are provided with a description of how the rural research and theory development program was established at Montana State University-Bozeman College of Nursing. The author, who was a newly arrived Dean for the College when she started building the program in 1975, describes the assessment needed, the changes initiated to stimulate the growth of the College, and the structure that emerged to support the changes.

Moving to the area of continuing education, the author of chapter 31 discusses an innovative continuing-education program developed for rural nurses. Using borrowed or purchased video tapes and workbooks the participants can learn about providing nursing care for the increasing numbers of elderly in rural areas.

The construct of isolation is again addressed in chapter 31. In this chapter, the isolation pertains to professional practice. The author takes a provocative look at the concept and uses cases to illustrate the concept from her former position as a nursing administrator in a small rural hospital.

Recruitment and retention of health care professionals is the subject of chapter 32. The topic represents a cyclical problem in hospital staffing patterns; therefore, upon completion of the study, the authors found that recruitment had disappeared as a problem. Nevertheless, retention of qualified professionals is still relevant, and the findings of the study provide good information for rural hospital administrators about variables related to job satisfaction of their employees.

A frequent stumbling block in doing research in rural settings is defining "what is rural." The last chapter in this section (chapter 33) reports the construction and evaluation of an index that measures rurality by using two variables, county population and distance to emergency room.

30

Developing an Educational Structure for Rural Nursing Research and Theory

Anna M. Shannon

In 1975, the Montana State University (MSU) College of Nursing began a structural and program change that combined all its efforts in a direction focused toward issues found in a rural state. New administrative leadership and school autonomy, along with a faculty group eager for change, provided the impetus for restructuring. All aspects were examined to learn what resources were available and to decide how such resources could best be used to attain goals. Each component of the assessment will be addressed.

ASSESSMENT FOR CHANGE

The Faculty

The faculty is the heart of any program and determines program quality and the success of any change. In 1975, 65% of the school's faculty was master's prepared; the only doctorally prepared faculty were the former director (nearing retirement) and the newly-appointed administrator. Other faculty members were baccalaureate prepared and often on part-time appointments. In addition, most of the masters'-prepared faculty had been taught at MSU and therefore came from similar theoretical positions. There was no research activity on the part of the faculty, and very few had any experience at another school of nursing. The faculty had no experience in self-governance and no faculty organization or bylaws by which to form a faculty organization.

On the bright side, members of the faculty had participated in the regional organization known as The Western Commission for Higher Education in Nursing (WCHEN). Through WCHEN, some faculty members had taken part in the leadership and curricular projects of WCHEN, and a few were currently active in the Research Development Project in which the new college administrator was deeply involved. Faculty members representing each of the four campuses of the school (described in the next section) were actively involved in some aspect of the WCHEN Research Development Project.

The Campuses

The school was organized among four campuses in four of Montana's larger cities. The primary campus was in Bozeman, home of Montana State University. In addition, there were campuses with resident faculties in Billings, Butte, and Great Falls. At that time, there was no campus in Missoula because a diploma program was located there. The multiple campus structure had been adopted at the beginning of the program in 1937 and made possible the richness and diversity of a large program through use of clinical facilities in the largest of Montana's population centers.

Curricula

The curricula of the school consisted of a generic baccalaureate program into which registered nurse students could matriculate with advanced credit and a master's degree program that had been in existence since 1957. The baccalaureate program needed revision in light of changes occurring in health care delivery. Proposed changes in the masters' program were timely. Whereas MSU had been the primary provider of masters' prepared faculty for the contiguous states of North and South Dakota, Wyoming, and Idaho, each of those states had masters' program proposals in the works. Other program offerings were marginal to the central degree programs. One was a program for nursing home administrators, the other a contract-supported family nurse practitioner program in its last years.

Resources

The school was marginally funded and was one of the few programs in the country to qualify twice for federal financial distress grants. A new building, opened in 1972, had been built for the Bozeman Campus using federal construction grant monies. Space at other campuses was located in hospitals in those communities, resulting in frequent moves of the faculty as hospitals identified other uses for the space. The school's budget was inadequate, and library holdings were meager.

Clinical facilities were small but comprehensive. Clinical experiences were available in all areas of nursing except for "high tech" opportunities found typically in medical centers. The small size of clinical resources affected the school programs of the school in terms of clinical group size and faculty supervision load.

The University and the School of Nursing had an excellent reputation for the quality of its graduates. Required prerequisite courses were available and rigorous. The University had just made the school autonomous and expressed support for upgrading the qualifications of the faculty through recruitment.

Students

Academically qualified undergraduates were abundant. Students were serious, industrious, and committed. Graduate students, though fewer in number, were highly motivated, mature students.

Research

There was no faculty research extant. Research course work for the graduate program was offered through the schools of agriculture and education. Most graduate students did a professional paper or project rather than a thesis, and most theses, when done, were about nurses. There was faculty interest at the Billings campus in offering some research content in their undergraduate courses. Faculty members were aware of the need to enrich the research experience for students in the undergraduate and graduate curricula.

The State

Montana is a rural state. In 1975, the time of the proposed changes, only 14 towns in Montana had a population greater than 5,000. Two cities, Billings and Great Falls, had populations of about 70,000, with Billings growing and Great Falls losing, population. These were the urban areas where the school had campuses. The state's population of 800,000 was distributed over 147,000 square miles and 56 counties with several counties defined as frontier and the rest as rural.

Hospital facilities, as previously mentioned, were small but comprehensive in the larger towns. Hospital size in the state varied from 6 to 285 beds. Patients from outlying areas were transferred to the larger communities for care requiring more specialized medical practice. Transfers involving several hundred miles were common. For a greater degree of specialized care, patients were transferred out of state to centers such as those found in Salt Lake City, UT, Seattle, WA, or Rochester, MN.

The economy of Montana was based primarily on the extractive industries (mining, timber, and agriculture) and, to a lesser extent, on small industries, a military base, educational institutions, and a beginning tourist industry. Average incomes were low, and the large size of the state made costs for services such as highways, schools, and similar state services expensive for a low tax base.

THE INTERRELATIONSHIPS OF CHANGE

It seemed clear to the new administrator that desired changes in faculty qualifications, research productivity, and curricula would have to be made within existing resources and any available faculty upgrade monies. Additional funds would have to be solicited by the school through training grants from the Division of Nursing, the only potential source for a large project known at the time. Therefore, changes were begun using faculty enthusiasm and their desire for curricular change.

Organizational Structure

The first change was the development of a faculty organization and bylaws. This effort was aided by a parallel move occurring in the

University faculty at large. As the University faculty developed an organization and bylaws that were to replace the largely administrative structure that preceded it, the nursing faculty developed a structure congruent with it. The committee structure with representation across campuses provided the means to redo the curricula, consider research as a faculty function, and plan faculty development activities for these changed circumstances. In addition, the new organizational structure increased communication between faculty and administration and provided an avenue for consideration of faculty needs, for faculty searches, and for enlightenment about the valuable attributes more highly qualified, external faculty members could bring.

The structure and the policies that came from those faculty committees also gave guidance to the administrator during those times of faculty absence (summer and holidays). Through this mechanism, it was possible for the administrator to know faculty wishes and to make decisions that would be congruent with those wishes/policies in the absence of faculty.

The physical structure of the school was not changed until 1977 when a campus in Missoula (third largest city in the state) was opened in preparation for the closure of its nursing diploma program in 1978. Following this campus opening in the larger city, the campus in Butte was phased out over several years and finally closed in 1987.

Undergraduate Curriculum

The redesign of the undergraduate curriculum began in 1975 and was introduced at the sophomore level in 1977. Two major changes, critical to the subject of this chapter, were introduced in this design: (a) the introduction of nursing assessment as a requirement at the sophomore level; and (b) the inclusion of a research objective in every nursing course. These changes meant the faculty had to develop the knowledge and skills necessary to teach to these objectives. Recognizing their need to stay ahead of students provided a great motivation to faculty members to increase their knowledge in assessment and research.

The curriculum was ready for implementation at the upper division campuses of Billings, Butte, Great Falls, and Missoula in 1978. This meant that transition content had to be designed at the first three campuses for integrating continuing students of the prior curriculum. Since the undergraduate program at Missoula began with this curriculum, no transition courses were needed but a full complement of faculty for the campus had to be recruited.

Graduate Curriculum

In 1976, two doctorally prepared faculty members were recruited to open the Missoula campus and to play a major role in the redesign of the graduate program. Dr. Jacqueline Taylor, a nurse anthropologist and psychiatric nurse from Arizona State University, and Dr. Ruth Ludemann, a newly graduated nurse sociologist and community mental health specialist from the University of Arizona, brought the kind of experience in graduate and undergraduate nursing education and research needed both at the Missoula campus and for the school as a whole.

Even before their arrival, program needs in a state like Montana were discussed with the dean. As the only graduate program in the state, the school had the opportunity to design a program unique to the state's needs. Working with the Graduate Subcommittee of the Academic Affairs Committee, Drs. Taylor and Ludemann and the dean contemplated a program that would meet the needs of the state for graduates and would increase knowledge about rural nursing. They also discussed how those ideas could be articulated in a successful grant proposal.

This effort logically led to an examination of Montana and the nursing needs in the state. The results of this examination showed, of course, that Montana was a sparsely populated state and that health care was delivered through an interaction between the very small, rural population centers and the more urban, larger centers. In addition, it showed that the need in nursing specialties was for a broader specialist as contrasted with the "super-specialist" of metropolitan medical centers. The focus of the program needed to be preparation of "mid-level" specialists for a sparsely populated state—**rural nursing**.

An examination of nursing and related literature on rural nursing revealed a body of work in rural sociology that suggested important areas to be considered and literature describing nurse practitioners' placement in rural settings. Essentially nothing, however, was found about health care delivery in rural areas addressing the salience of the "ruralness" of the setting.

The idea then evolved that the new nursing program would be designed to derive empirical knowledge about the impact of "rural" on health and health care delivery. This major aim would be met by teaching students to apply an ethnographic approach in all of their courses in the graduate program. Data thus obtained would then feed into a larger schoolwide effort to derive rural nursing theory. A Division of Nursing advanced training grant and a National Institute of Mental Health (NIMH) complementary grant for student support in psychiatric nursing were written. These grants were approved and funded in 1978 and 1979, respectively (Division of Nursing Grant # 1 D23 NU00125 and NIMH Grant # 5 TO MH15898).

Teaching of the revised graduate curriculum began in 1977. The first research reports emanating from it were presented in a symposium at the 1982 WCHEN research conference, Communicating Nursing Research (Taylor, 1982).

Faculty Development

There were two new aspects in the revised curricula with which faculty needed assistance. To develop nursing assessment skills, the school supported faculty attendance at short courses and "in-house" sharing of knowledge and skills. Audiovisual aids were purchased. Individual faculty members assessed the skill each had and needed and established an individual development plan.

In preparation for teaching and guiding research and with the help of the Faculty Affairs Committee of the faculty, the school dedicated most faculty development and travel funds to this purpose for several years. Consultants who conveyed both an enthusiasm for research and a commitment to the notion that all educational levels of nurses can do research were brought to the school to provide intensive workshops at times when all faculty members were gathered. These workshops occurred at least twice a year for several years and eventually evolved into a research conference at which faculty members presented their research to their peers. This approach provided the more formal presentation of research knowledge. It included critiques of faculty research plans as faculty developed their skills. Not all faculty members developed a research proposal, but all faculty members developed sufficient knowledge and skill to teach beginning research.

A second approach used to help faculty members develop their research skills was theses committees. As graduate students progressed through the revised research-laden curriculum, all were urged to complete a thesis, preferably with a rural focus. Committees selected by students for thesis guidance included persons with research skills and persons expert in the relevant clinical area. In this way, less research-skilled, clinically expert faculty could learn research method application along with students.

A research methods course was introduced in the revised undergraduate program at the junior level; all students completed a small research study by the end of their senior year. Faculty preparation for this teaching task was achieved by the development efforts described above and by the active participation of the College of Nursing Research Committee, both individually and as a group. Since faculty committees all had campus representation, each unit had a member in residence. The faculty load produced by this curricular change was considerable and as faculty members developed more skill they were able to trim some of the students' research ideas and encourage group research. The faculty learning achieved by these means also resulted in an increase in faculty research, some of which is reported in this volume.

Faculty travel funds were devoted to this effort. Faculty members presenting research at nursing conferences or attending research conferences were given priority. As faculty presentations increased the school became known and faculty recruitment was aided. As faculty members attended research conferences, they developed ideas for their own research and contacts with other nurse researchers.

Rural Nursing Theory Development

Some faculty members had a greater interest in research than others and wished to participate in the development of rural theory growing out of the graduate program. Money from the Division of Nursing grant helped support early meetings of the Rural Nursing Theory Subcommittee (RNTS) group by providing travel funds to bring the group together and to bring in consultants. Working empirically from the ethnographic studies produced by graduate students, theses, and faculty studies, this group evolved a theoretical structure within which the newly generated research findings could be considered in relation to other research-derived knowledge.

The theoretical structure identified by the RNTS group was designed to organize concepts deduced from the studies so they could be retrieved by other students and faculty for further study or curricular purposes. In addition, for theory building, dimensions, constructs, and concepts thus organized would be examined for interrelationships that would lead to mid-level theory. Another obvious advantage of the structure of concept relationships was identification of neglected areas where research could help round out the view of rural nursing and rural nursing theory.

Since the graduate program rotated between the campuses and students were recruited from all areas of the state, student research studies representing the diverse populations of a large rural state were possible. Similarly, since faculty members teaching in the graduate program and participating in RNTS came from each campus, their expertise in the diversity of the state was available to the theory development effort.

SUMMARY

This is the story of a faculty's commitment to excellence in the practice and teaching of professional nursing. This effort depicts how multiple aims can be met using the same resources through planning and focus. This chapter is a tribute to the many faculty, consultants, and students who, in the tradition of Dr. Anna Pearl Sherrick, the school's founder, saw a need and met it.

REFERENCES

Taylor, J. (1982). Sparsely populated areas: Toward nursing theory: A symposium. *Communicating Nursing Research, 15,* 69–77. Boulder, CO: WICHEN.

31

Making Gerontic Continuing Education Accessible for Rural Nurses*

Shirley A. Cudney

The letter read: "I saw the advertisement for your gerontological workshop series to be presented in Great Falls in November, January, and February I will not be there, and I want to tell you why. I live in the northeast comer of Montana and, though you claim Great Falls is centrally located, it means I would have to travel over 400 miles (one way) to get there, possibly in a snowstorm given the months you have chosen. It would take me one day each way to drive, not to mention the price of gas, plus a motel bill for three nights and the registration fee (though $100 for three 2-day workshops is pretty reasonable!). Besides that, my disabled elderly mother lives with us, and I prefer not to leave my teenagers unsupervised for nearly a week. My nursing home administrator tells me I will not be paid for the days I am gone, and can't get anyone to cover for me anyway. I hope you are planning to offer the workshops again, possibly in Sidney, which is only 100 miles away."

This letter (based on actual correspondence) represents a composite of the types of problems that are faced by many nurses in Montana who would like to take advantage of gerontological continuing education programs. Conversely, for a gerontological expert to go to Sidney, as requested, would mean a similar story for the traveling instructor.

**Note.* From "Making Gerontic Continuing Education Accessible for Rural Nurses," by S. Cudney, 1991, *Journal of Gerontological Nursing, 17,* pp. 29–34. Copyright 1991 by SLACK Incorporated. Reprinted with permission.

As can be seen from this illustration, it is a real challenge to provide quality gerontological continuing education to practicing nurses who care for the elderly in rural settings. Responding to this challenge, the Nursing Approaches to Quality Care for the Elderly project developed a series of 10 self-study gerontological nursing modules, which put a wealth of current gerontic information at the fingertips of geographically isolated nurses in Montana.

PROJECT OBJECTIVES

Nursing Approaches to Quality Care for the Elderly was a continuing education project with the ultimate goal of improving the quality of nursing care received by Montana's elderly by enhancing the gerontological knowledge of nursing teams (RNs, LPNs, and nurse's aides). Funded by the Administration on Aging and jointly administered by Montana State University's College of Nursing, Office of Extended Studies, and Center of Gerontology, its objectives were to

- Define and level gerontological nursing content for each of 10 programs;
- Deliver workshops at five sites in Montana;
- Develop strategies for disseminating program content to nursing personnel unable to attend on-site workshops (self-study modules);
- Establish a financially independent program; and
- Increase the number of registered nurses who could successfully pass the American Nurses' Association (ANA) certification examination for gerontological nurses or gain continuing education credits.

BACKGROUND

Gioiella reminds us that "nurses are the principal providers of geriatric care, not just because of our numbers, but also because we offer the kind of care elderly people need."[1] Carnevali and Patrick, however, admonish us to be aware that "nursing has a long way to go in terms of achieving adequate recognition of its contribution."[2] This awareness needs to be nurtured among nurses themselves as well as in the general population of consumers of nursing's services. For this reason, one of the overall guiding principles used in developing the project programs was the emphasis on nursing approaches to maintaining the health and combating the health problems of elders.

If nursing is to deliver on its promise and potential, the ANA says that nurses who care for the elderly need to be prepared to assess the health and functional status of older adults, plan and provide appropriate nursing services, and evaluate the effectiveness of such care.[3] Implied in this statement is a strong commitment to promote health with well elders and educate those with chronic illness to live quality lives despite the limitations the illness may impose. This, then, becomes a framework within which quality nursing care for the elderly can be provided and was the structure chosen within which to present the content of each of the 10 programs.

However, many nurses who are responsible for caring for elderly clients have not been prepared in gerontology and geriatrics. Two reasons are that gerontics is a relatively new field and that its content has not been included in the curricula of nursing schools until recently. Therefore, in the opinion of Russell, the deficiencies that exist in the preparation for gerontological nursing will need to be remedied through continuing education programs long after nursing schools have learned to adequately prepare nurses in the care of the elderly.[4] The situation in Montana was no exception. A continuing education program that focused on nursing care of the elderly, including assessment, planning, treatment, health promotion, and evaluation of care, needed to be developed to provide quality nursing care to the state's aged citizens.

An even greater challenge was providing quality gerontological continuing education to practicing nurses who care for the elderly in rural settings, which characterizes most of Montana. Nurses who practice in isolated areas and very small communities are not exempt from contact with elders and are eager to deliver quality care to this segment of their case load, whether it is in hospitals, nursing homes, home care, or residential settings. Data to support these statements are found in Montana's demographics and the results of a 1986 assessment of the continuing education needs of a sample of nursing care providers who serve Montana's elderly.

Montana's Demographics and Other Statistics

The problems of preparation and availability of nurses to care for the state's elderly are compounded by the fact that Montana is a large rural state with widely varying topography, unpredictable weather, and limited transportation systems. Montana ranks 4th among the 50 states in terms of size and 44th in population; the overall population density is approximately 5.4 per square mile as compared with 64.0 for the United States, and there are only 14 towns in Montana with populations over 5,000.

The demographics of Montana's elderly are similar to the national average in terms of proportion to the population but not in distribution; i.e., 119,240 persons 60 years of age or older reside in 56 counties distributed over an area of 147,138 square miles. The distribution of the aging population throughout the vast expanse of the state means that many health-care providers work in sparsely settled areas. For most, access to continuing education is compromised by their relative isolation from major educational centers. While there are insufficient resources to send instructors to a large number of distantly scattered sites to provide the education, conversely, it is difficult for healthcare agencies to free-up employees to attend extended educational programs at distant educational centers.[5]

Transportation is time consuming and is often influenced by weather. For example, to present the 43 workshops that were associated with the project, the principal investigator traveled nearly 13,000 miles in a little more than 2 years driving within the state of Montana, not to mention the miles traveled by the participants (approximately 130,000). To illustrate the distances involved, the rural communities that participated in the needs assessment are shown in relation to their distance from the major cities of the state (Table 31.1). As can be seen, distances are great and only one of these communities is within 100 miles of a major city.

The potential influence of winter weather on access to continuing education is demonstrated through the experiences of the principal investigator, who was snowed in three times and had to reschedule two workshops during the project's activities, despite the fact that the months of December and January were deliberately avoided. Our experience in offering continuing education programs in Montana and results from the needs assessment showed that there are only five months that can be used productively for continuing education ses-

TABLE 31.1 Distances of Rural Communities from Major Cities in Montana

Distances From: Rural community	To: Billings	Butte	Great Falls	Missoula
Ekalaka	261	485	433	576
Hamilton	372	148	215	47
Lewistown	129	236	105	273
Libby	509	309	319	190
Sidney	272	495	376	545

sions. More than half the year is lost if workshops are solely depended upon for delivery of information to Montana's nurses. Although our data are limited, it is not unreasonable to suspect that continuing education delivery constraints related to weather problems do exist in other northern rural states and perhaps in the summer in desert states.

Needs Assessment

In the spring of 1986, a continuing education needs assessment was developed using the Guidelines for Conducting Training Needs Assessments developed by the Center for Public Management for the Administration on Aging in 1980. The sample included 144 nursing team care providers (53 RNs, 32 LPNs, 59 nurse's aides) involved in the care of the elderly. They lived in four widely dispersed rural communities of Montana, which represent the characteristics typical of many Montana communities: they are isolated from population centers and small in population (2,661 to 7,104 people), and one town has a population of 21,645. In addition, the health-care providers were interviewed in a town with a population of 620, representative of the size of 324 Montana communities of fewer than 1,000 people, regarding rural continuing education needs.

The results of the needs assessment were useful in planning the focus and content for the workshops and modules. For example, because 48% of the registered nurses had worked in gerontological settings for more than 10 years, many had never been exposed to the concept of "nursing process," which was introduced in the mid 1970s. This finding reinforced the decision to use the nursing process as the organizing focus for the programs and to reiterate in every workshop and module its relationship to the standards of gerontological nursing care. The nursing problems selected to be addressed in the program series were those identified in the needs assessment as areas about which information was most frequently requested.

STRATEGIES

How, then, to provide quality gerontological. continuing education to practicing nurses who care for the elderly in rural Montana? The challenge was at least two-fold: accessing the often place-bound practicing nurse while doing it cost effectively. It was postulated that one way to accomplish these ends would be a combination of presenting strategically located workshops using videotaped experts, and further using the videotaped experts by developing self-study modules based on the workshop sessions.

Consequently, the workshops and self-study modules developed by the Nursing Approaches to Quality Care for the Elderly project either allowed the nurse to come to a program closer to home, reducing travel distance and time away from the workplace, or provided an opportunity for the nurse to study at home, eliminating costly and hazardous travel and the need to leave the patient's bedside.

Each of the 10 programs was to be prepared for delivery in three modes: live sessions headlining prominent guest presenters for the initial program presentation; extended site workshops in four Montana cities featuring the videotaped experts from the live sessions and a program facilitator with expertise in gerontological nursing; and self-study modules to make the programs accessible to any group or individual unable to attend the workshops.

Nationally and regionally known experts were recruited using the assistance and resources of the Geriatric Education Centers of the Universities of Washington and Utah, University of Arizona, and Montana State University (MSU).

RESULTS

Gerontological Nursing Content Defined

Based on the needs assessment and judgment of gerontological nursing experts, the topics chosen were introduction to nursing care of

- Introduction
- Faculty
- Mind jogger (pre- and post-tests)
- Introduction to the nursing diagnosis (eg, altered nutrition in the elderly)
- Assessing the (nutritional) status of an elder
- Determining nursing diagnoses and setting objectives for treatment
- Nursing strategies for treating the elder with (nutritional) problems
- Patient/family education
- Health promotion and the elderly
- Recording, evaluating, managing, and following up nursing care of elderly clients with (nutrition) problems
- Selected references
- Certification information
- Model health promotion program

FIGURE 31.1 Representative table of contents.

the elderly with an emphasis on the ANA Standards of Gerontological Nursing Practice, the normal aging process and its implications for nursing, and in-depth nursing approaches for eight nursing diagnoses that are commonly seen in the elderly (problems with mobility, sensory/perceptual deficits, thought processes, home maintenance management, nutrition, skin, elimination, and hypoxia). Program content was organized within the framework of the ANA Standards of Gerontological Nursing Practice (nursing process) and emphasized patient education and health promotion. Figure 31.1 lists a representative table of contents.

Gerontological Nursing Content Leveled

A unique feature of the programs was the attempt to designate content for one or more levels of the nursing team, i.e., registered nurses, licensed practical (vocational) nurses, or nurse's aides. The bases for these decisions were the Montana Nurse Practice Act definitions of nursing practice for registered nurses and licensed practical nurses. Although nurse's aides are not licensed (but are currently being certified) and, therefore, are not defined in the Nurse Practice Act, they are responsible for reporting observations and carrying out delegated basic hygienic and nursing care measures. Using these descriptions as general guidelines, the programs were organized to reflect the varying responsibilities of the nursing care team members. Although none of the information in the programs was restricted to any particular member of the nursing care team, it was considered important that each member of the care team be aware of specific roles as defined by the Nurse Practice Act and that the information be used appropriately within that role.

Workshop Series

Ten workshop series were presented at five sites in Montana. Although this represented a potential of 50 workshops, 43 were actually presented; 7 were canceled because of insufficient enrollment. The initial workshop for a program was presented "live" by a nationally or regionally known topic expert in Bozeman, the location of MSU. The content from the live session was videotaped on the following day in a "Conversation with the expert" format. These videotapes became the core of the workshop, which was replicated at four other sites in Montana: Billings, Great Falls, Miles City, and Missoula. The conversational nature of the videotapes and frequent breaks with question and answer periods moderated by a "live" gerontological nurse practitioner resulted in a high level of acceptance of the videotaped segments by the workshop participants.

Program Content Disseminated Via Self-Study Modules

The strategy used for disseminating program content to nursing personnel unable to attend on-site workshops was the development of 10 self-study modules, each equivalent to one 8–contact hour session. Each program was converted to a self-study module that included the videotaped interviews and demonstrations, a 100–page booklet, and other learning materials used in the workshops. These modules are available for either purchase or rental through the MSU Office of Continuing Education for the Health Professional.

Working Toward a Financially Independent Program

To establish a financially independent program and maintain the availability of the modules after the grant funding expired required fees to be charged for workshops and for rental or purchase of the self-study modules. Income from extended site workshops did not cover the cost of presenting the workshops, even if the cost of videotape production was not included. Attendance at all the workshops totaled 634 and ranged between 4 and 28 per session with a mean attendance of 15—a figure that was not sufficient to support the cost of advertising and presenting the workshops. This information prompted the decision to limit future workshops to those requiring hands-on activities and to rely on self-study modules for the major portion ofherontic information transmission.

Limited experience has been gained in the marketing and distribution of the modules. However, it is anticipated that the self-study module will prove to be the delivery method of choice for continuing gerontological education for the nursing teams of Montana and other rural states, provided the fees can be reduced to the point where they will attract individual nurses. Group rentals are currently the most economical method for obtaining the modules, and are gaining popularity in Montana and Colorado. Larger agencies in Maine, Washington, Utah, Alaska, and Canada have purchased the modules outright.

Nurses Informed of ANA Certification Process

At this time, data are not available regarding the numbers of registered nurses who successfully' passed the ANA certification examination for gerontological nurses as a result of attending the workshops or completing the modules. Perhaps the greatest contribution made by the project was to inform nurses that certification is available to them. Sixty-four registered nurses, many of whom did not previously know about the ANA certification program, indicated an interest in eventually becoming certified as gerontological nurses.

Continuing Education Credits Earned

All programs were approved for continuing education credits by appropriate nursing groups. A total of 357.55 CEUs (equivalent to 3,575.5 contact hours) and 674.5 contact hours (without CEUs) were earned by nursing team members during the project—a total of 4,250 contact hours of continuing education for Montana's nursing caregivers in gerontological settings.

IMPLICATIONS AND SPINOFFS

This project is seen as the first phase of a broader attempt to bring continuing education opportunities in gerontological nursing to nurses in rural areas. Future plans include the production of 10 additional modules; wider distribution of the modules nationally and internationally; integration of the modules into undergraduate and graduate nursing curricula, including university credit home study options; consideration of technological strategies for transmission of the modules via television or computer networks; and other creative applications for module use.

Phase II, which has been approved and funded as a special project through the Division of Nursing, will make possible the development of 10 more modules: Issues and Trends that Impact the Giving of Nursing Care to the Elderly, Pharmacological Nursing Care of Elders, Educating Health Care Personnel to Provide Quality Care to the Aged, Supervision and Management of Health Care Personnel, Communication Skills, and Nursing the Elderly in Acute Care Settings. Four additional nursing diagnoses common in the elderly will be targeted for development in the final modules to complete the series. The original 10 modules (gerontological nursing standards, normal aging, and eight common nursing diagnoses in the elderly) will be revised and updated. Taken together, the 20 modules will address all the topics covered in the ANA certification test for gerontological nurse.

Active marketing of the modules through the MSU Office of Continuing Education for the Health Professional will be expanded to 14 other Western states initially. Based on the response to the initial marketing effort, national and international distribution may be attempted.

Use of the modules in the nursing curricula is currently being planned at MSU College of Nursing as it prepares to teach a new course, Nursing Care of Aging Adults, on three distant campuses throughout the state. A logical extension of this work would be the development of one or more home study courses for university credit that could fulfill part of the gerontology requirement in the undergraduate and graduate curricula. This opportunity would be well received by nurses in outlying areas who wish to earn a BSN or MSN.

Consideration will be given to new technological strategies. One idea is to design broadcast quality videotapes that will be compatible with television broadcast schedules, should this mode of module transmission become feasible through the auspices of the public television station housed on the university campus. Thought has been given to extracting short abstracts from the modules and converting them to half-hour to 1–hour computer assisted instruction programs that can be accessed through a computer network and to which continuing education credit could be assigned. Ways in which nurses in rural areas could problem-solve by telephone networking with gerontological nursing experts and one another or the use of interactive audio tapes within the module structure could be explored.

The modules are rich resources that lend themselves to many applications. For instance, cooperative ventures between several regional nursing homes have resulted in a consortium approach to using and sharing the modules between agencies, resulting in savings of time and money. Appropriately selected segments from the modules have already been used in 15 workshops statewide to provide continuing education programs for more than 400 in-home caregivers through the sponsorship of Montana's Area Agencies on Aging. In addition, 10 model community health promotion programs designed to be presented to community living elders (a feature of each of the workshops/modules) have been compiled and bound into a single document that focuses on health promotion.

State and regional networking, coordination, and cooperation between professional groups in the West maximized the use of gerontological resources within the project and forged cooperative relationships. It was an orchestration that contributed to the success of the project and is expected to enhance the second phase, Gerontic Continuing Education for Rural Nurses Who Serve the Aged.

And so, to our letter writer from Northeastern Montana who poignantly described the problems of accessing quality gerontic continuing education programs in rural areas, we can say the challenge has been accepted. In response to pleas, self-study modules have been developed and other strategies are being examined that allow nurses to economically access gerontological nursing content without leaving family and workplace or risking long-distance travel in questionable weather.

REFERENCES

1. Gioiella EC. The right choice for geriatric *care. Nursing and Health Care.* 1987; 8(8):439.

2. Carnevali D, Patrick M. *Nursing Management for the Elderly.* Philadelphia: JB Lippincott Co; 1979:11.

3. American Nurses' Association. *Standards and Scope of Gerontological Nursing Practice.* Kansas City, Mo: Author; 1987:23.

4. National Technical Information Service, US Department of Commerce. *Geriatric Educational Program for Nurses.* Springfield, Va: Author; 1983:9.

5. *Progress Report and Future Plans of Area Health Education Development Project at Montana State University.* Unpublished manuscript. 1986:7–8.

32

Professional Isolation: A Concept Analysis

M. Jean Shreffler

Rural health care and the unmet health care needs of rural residents have captured the attention of policy makers, researchers, and national organizations (American Hospital Association, 1992; American Nurses' Association, 1989; Wakefield, 1990; Weinert & Long, 1990). What has been described as a crisis in rural health care has resulted from two interrelated groups of problems. First, there has been an actual decline in health care services available in rural areas, e.g., rural hospital closures, loss of providers, decreased funding for community-based services. Second, the changing demographics of rural residents, e.g., increasing proportion of elderly and larger number in poverty, have resulted in a growing need for health care and, at the same time, a decreased ability to afford care (Cordes, 1989; Joint Task Force, 1989).

Recruitment and retention of professionals are major issues in maintaining access to health care for rural residents. Professional isolation is often cited in the literature as a contributor to the difficulties many rural areas have with recruiting and retaining health care providers. Despite the term's frequent use, professional isolation is rarely defined within the publications that mention it. The term is used as if readers know its meaning. A clearer definition of the term could improve our understanding of the problems faced by those providers who are experiencing professional isolation. Greater clarity in the definition might also lead to intervention strategies to prevent or reduce professional isolation and, thus, improve rural health care delivery and access.

AIM AND PURPOSE

The purpose of this chapter is to analyze the concept, "professional isolation." The ultimate aim is to clarify the meaning of the term to improve the consistency of its use in the context of rural health care. This concept analysis followed the procedures described by Walker and Avant (1988). Dictionary definitions are provided; uses of the concept related to professional isolation are summarized. Defining attributes are identified; model, borderline, and contrary cases are presented; and antecedents, consequences, and empirical referents are identified.

DEFINITIONS

According to Webster (Woolf, 1973, p. 614), isolation is defined as "the action of isolating: the condition of being isolated; syn. solitude." Isolate means

> *(verb) 1. to set apart from others, quarantine, 2. to select from among others; to separate from another substance so as to obtain pure or in a free state, 3. isolate; (adj.) being alone, solitary; (noun) the product of isolating, an individual or kind obtained by selection or separation (p. 614).*

The word isolate was originally derived from the Latin word *insula,* French *isole,* and Italian *isolato* for island. Synonyms for isolation (noun) in Roget's (Morehead, 1962, p. 196) are "separation, quarantine, loneliness, solitude, segregation, seclusion;" the antonym is "sociality."

According to Webster (Woolf, 1973), the adjective professional is defined as

> *1. a) of, relating to, or characteristic of a profession or occupation; b) engaged in one of the learned professions; c) characterized by or conforming to the technical or ethical standards of a profession; 2. a) participating for gain or livelihood in an activity or field of endeavor often engaged in by amateurs; b) engaged in by persons receiving financial return; and 3. following a line of conduct as though it were a profession (p. 919).*

As a noun, professional means "one who engages in a pursuit or activity professionally" (Woolf, 1973). Definitions for the noun profession include

> *1. the act of taking the vows of a religious community and 2. a) a calling requiring specialized knowledge and often long and intensive academic preparation; b) a principal calling, vocation, or employment; c) a whole body of persons engaged in a calling (p. 919).*

Synonyms for the noun profession in Roget's (Morehead, 1962) include vocation, occupation, and calling. Professional was originally derived from the Latin word *professus,* meaning to profess or confess, and the Middle English word *professen,* meaning having professed one's vows (Woolf, 1973, p. 918).

RELATED DEFINITIONS

Many forms of isolation exist; one that bears a close relationship with the concept of professional isolation is social isolation. Carpenito (1987) defined social isolation as a state in which an individual experiences a need or desire for contact with others but is unable to make that contact. She pointed out that it is not voluntary solitude that might be used for personal renewal or creativity but instead is a negative state of aloneness and is perceived as imposed by others. Fischer and Phillips (1982) defined social isolation as the state of "knowing relatively few people who are probable sources of rewarding exchanges" (p. 22). In an early article on social isolation in nursing literature, Black (1973) defined it as a "condition of deprivation of satisfaction-giving interpersonal and other self-actualizing activity, combined with the sensory deprivation that is a necessary concomitant" (p. 575). She used the terms isolation and deprivation interchangeably.

The subjective nature of social isolation was stressed by Black (1973) who believed that it should be assessed based upon the "patient or patient system responses" (p. 577) to being alone. Some individuals mitigate the effects of isolation with satisfying creative activities and thus do not experience deprivation. Others do not find satisfying pursuits when alone and experience social isolation. Cox, Spiro, and Sullivan (1988) differentiated between the objective and subjective properties of social isolation. Objective social isolation is the size and quality of one's social network while subjective social isolation refers to the individual's response to the social network or lack of it.

USES OF THE CONCEPT

In a study of nurse administrators of urban and rural hospitals in Texas, Hillestad (1984) found that professional isolation and loneliness and the presence of supportive professional relationships were inversely related. Nearly half (47%) of the respondents in this study reported that they were professionally isolated/lonely, and these same respondents were also more likely to indicate that their professional relationships were less supportive than they would like or felt they needed. In this study, professional isolation and loneliness were not differentiated and were defined as an affective state that results when individuals lack intimate relationships within which important aspects of their work lives can be shared.

Professional isolation has been found a challenge for nurses practicing in a variety of specialities including caring for hospice patients dying at home (Ross, 1994; Steeves, Cohen, & Wise, 1994), caring for individuals with AIDS (Pasacreta & Jacobsen, 1989), and caring for inmates in correctional facilities (Peternelj-Taylor & Johnson, 1995). Nurses practicing in an urban hospital undergoing major restructuring and the implementing of a professional nursing practice model reported feeling more isolated in their work due to changes in work and relationship structures (Wolf, 1993).

Some writers have suggested that professional isolation is inherent in certain situations, positions, and occupations. Being the only ethnic minority faculty member in an academic department (Jones, 1993), being the top academic manager or school principal (Dussault & Barnett, 1996), and being a college counselor in an American-sponsored overseas school (Rifenbary, 1996) were cited in the literature as resulting in professional isolation for those in these positions. Some authors claimed that professional isolation is an intrinsic part of being a psychotherapist (Garber, 1987; Langs, 1988), and another suggested that it is an inherent part of being a dentist (Litchfield, 1989). Aspects of a nursing administrator's role such as having power to make consequential decisions, reduced opportunities for professional intimacy, and having most of ones' available nursing colleagues as subordinates have been found to result in professional isolation (Darby, 1979; Hillestad, 1984). Another writer suggested that professional isolation and loneliness are inevitable parts of the modern work world with increasingly complex and specialized positions (Fader, 1984). In this author's view, sharing what we do in our work lives or having what we do be understood by others may no longer be possible.

Some investigators reported strategies and interventions to prevent and/or ameliorate professional isolation. Peer-coaching for students in an educational administration program was found to reduce professional isolation and enhance collegiality (Speck & Krovetz, 1996). A peer-assisted leadership program and networking study groups reduced professional isolation for other educational administrators (Dussault & Barnett, 1996; Fineman, 1996). Networking through organizational participation and electronic discussion groups were strategies reported to decrease professional isolation for nurses (Beck & Utz, 1996; Murray, 1996). The use of computer-mediated communications is often suggested as a strategy to decrease professional isolation. The effectiveness of this strategy, however, has only begun to be evaluated. A search of Internet sites using the Yahoo! Search tool revealed 3580 matches for web sites containing both the words, professional and isolation, and 165 matches were revealed for web sites containing the phrase "professional isolation." A perusal of a sample of these sites showed that while most did not define professional isolation, use of the term on these web sites was relevant to the uses discussed in this chapter. Most of the sites sampled offered services, products, or educational information for those in many occupations who were interested in preventing or reducing professional isolation.

USES OF THE CONCEPT IN A RURAL HEALTH CARE CONTEXT

In general, when isolation is used to refer to a condition, situation, or feeling in the rural context, a negative connotation is implied. Depending upon one's values, the images invoked by the term *rural* can be "a place to get away from" or "a place to get away to" (Lee, 1991, p. 7). Isolation in rural areas then could be used to refer to the privacy of the "wide-open spaces," however, usually more positive terms than isolation, such as solitude or seclusion, are used in such cases. Physical isolation from resources and supportive networks has also been cited as one factor adding stress to small rural hospitals and their professional staffs (Moscovice, 1989). To decrease isolation, prevent hospital closure, and improve quality of care, recent federal initiatives have encouraged networking and alliances between small rural hospitals and larger facilities (Campion & Dickey, 1995; Moscovice, 1989).

In rural health care literature, professional isolation is frequently cited as a contributor to difficulties in recruitment and retention of health care professionals to rural areas. In her study of rural nurse administrators, Shreffler (1992) defined professional isolation as an actual deficiency in available colleagues with whom one can relate professionally. The study findings revealed that 50% of the administrators reported feeling professionally isolated at the time of the survey and that younger, inexperienced directors in small, remote hospitals were most likely to experience isolation. Rural community health nurses interviewed by Davis and Droes (1993) described professional isolation as primarily a negative part of their practice with some positive aspects. In this study, isolation contributed to role strain, uncomfortable or potentially unsafe practice, and turnover of nurses who were not able to cope with practicing alone. At the same time, the aloneness for these nurses allowed for greater independence and autonomy not found in urban practice. In a national study of physician distribution in rural areas, it was found that most rural primary care physicians were clustered together or practicing in more populated rural areas where other physicians were located (Conner, Hillson, & Krawelski, 1995). Prevention of professional isolation was cited as the major reason for this distribution pattern. Professional isolation in rural areas was also cited for being responsible for provider shortages and role stress for professionals in other health care disciplines such as physical therapy, occupational therapy, diabetes education, and mental health (Howland, 1995; Mitchell, 1996; Shelton & Frank, 1995; Wills & Case-Smith, 1996).

Recently, communications technology is being promoted to improve some of the problems caused by rural isolation for individuals, families, communities, and facilities. Telecommunications may decrease professional isolation and provide for continuing education needs of health care professionals practicing in rural areas and thus improve recruitment, retention, and quality of care (Puskin, 1992). Technology can move the clinical training of professionals into rural areas; this practice is thought to improve recruitment potential and to provide what may be more appropriate education sites for rural practice than academic health centers (Crandell & Coggan, 1994). Some authors discussed the potential positive affects that technology can have on rural communities by reducing isolation, increasing residents' knowledge of healthful practices, improving business efficiency, and improving access to education and services (Brauer, 1992; Puskin, 1992; Rowley & Porterfield, 1993). Another author pointed out, however, that although telecommunications can overcome isolation in rural areas, bringing residents jobs, better education, and richer lives, "bootstrapping rural America into the global village involves much more than simple hard wiring. Technology is associated with change in the minds of the people there, and change has never come easy . . ." to rural America (Bleakley, 1996, p. B1).

DEFINING ATTRIBUTES

The defining attributes of professional isolation were identified from the dictionary definitions and from the uses of the concept in nonrural and rural contexts. While the attributes of *professional isolation* may be similar to other uses of the term isolation, the aspect of the attributes that differentiate its meaning from other uses is the qualifier, professional.

Five defining attributes for professional isolation are identified: (a) there exists an actual separation from or a deficiency in a resource needed to fulfill one's professional responsibilities or needs (objective component); (b) a professional need is perceived as partially or wholly unmet (subjective component); (c) the actual separation or deficiency is on a continuum; it is not a dichotomous or "all or nothing" condition but a matter of degrees; (d) the individual is not voluntarily separating her/himself from an available professional resource; and (e) while not unique to rural occupations or positions, the objective component of professional isolation is more likely to be present in rural areas.

MODEL CASE

According to Walker and Avant (1988), "the model case is one that we are absolutely sure is an instance of the concept" (p. 40). The following model case was developed from my past professional experience.

Jane Smith, RN, is the 11-7 charge nurse in a small 30-bed rural hospital. She is the only RN on duty; an LPN and Nursing Assistant are her co-workers. A physician asleep at home is on call in case of an emergency. At 2:00 a.m., she checks on Mary Jones, an 85–year-old patient, who had been stable following a postoperative bowel obstruction repair two days previously. She finds that Mrs. Jones is restless, has an elevated temperature of 100.2 F., and is slightly confused as compared with previous assessments. She is concerned about the change in Mrs. Jones' condition and wishes she had a colleague with whom to discuss her concerns and options. Uneasily, she decides that this is not an emergent situation. She gives an antipyretic according to postoperative orders and checks on Mrs. Jones every 15 to 30 minutes through the night until she can consult with a colleague or the physician in the morning.

This represents a model case of professional isolation in that the nurse has an actual deficiency of colleagues with whom to consult which she needs to fulfill her professional responsibilities, and she perceives an unmet need. She is not absolutely isolated in that she could call and wake the physician, and she has not voluntarily separated herself from available colleagues. Her nursing position is in a rural hospital where colleagues with whom to consult are less likely to be available.

ADDITIONAL CASES

Additional cases are constructed to further clarify the meaning of concepts by provided examples of "not the concept" (Walker & Avant, 1988). The following borderline, related, and contrary cases were developed based on the model case with some essential differences.

Borderline Case

Jane Smith, RN, is the 11–7 charge nurse in a small, 30–bed rural hospital. She is the only RN on duty in the hospital; an LPN and Nursing Assistant are her co-workers. There is an RN on duty in the attached 50–bed Extended Care Facility. A physician asleep at home is on call in case of an emergency. At 2:00 a.m., Jane checks on Mary Jones, an 85–year-old patient, who had been stable following a bowel obstruction repair two days earlier. She finds that Mary is restless, has an elevated temperature of 100.2 F., and is slightly confused as compared with previous assessments. Jane is concerned about the change in Mrs. Jones' condition but also does not like to consult with other nurses before making decisions. She believes this makes her appear to lack knowledge. Uneasily, she decides that this is not an emergent situation. She gives an antipyretic according to postoperative orders and checks on Mrs. Jones every 15 to 30 minutes through the night until she can report the changes to Mrs. Jones' physician in the morning.

This represents a borderline case of professional isolation in that the nurse perceives an unmet need and is in a rural setting. However, she does not have an actual deficiency of colleagues with whom to consult and voluntarily chooses to separate herself from this colleague and handle the situation alone.

Contrary Case

Jane Smith, RN, is the 11–7 charge nurse in a 30–bed Medical Surgical Unit in a large urban hospital. A physician is available in-house in case of an emergency. At 2:00 a.m., Jane checks on Mary Jones, an 85-year-old patient, who had been stable following a bowel obstruction repair two days earlier. She finds that Mrs. Jones is restless, has an elevated temperature of 100.2 F., and is slightly confused as compared with previous assessments. Jane is concerned about the change in condition of Mrs. Jones and calls her colleague Susan Hall, RN, the charge nurse on another Medical Surgical Unit to discuss her assessment and her options. Susan concurs with Mary's assessment that the situation with Mrs. Jones is not emergent at this time. Jane then gives an antipyretic according to postoperative orders and checks on Mrs. Jones every 15 to 30 minutes through the night. She reports the changes to Mrs. Jones' physician in the morning.

This represents a contrary case in that none of the defining attributes of professional isolation are present.

ANTECEDENTS AND CONSEQUENCES

Antecedents and consequences can further clarify defining attributes of the concept plus shed light on the social contexts in which the concept is used (Walker & Avant, 1988). Antecedents are events or situations that must occur before the occurrence of the concept; consequences are events or situations that occur because of the occurrence of the concept.

Antecedents

Antecedents of professional isolation include these circumstances: (a) some occupations and professional positions exist in which there is a separation from or deficiency in resources needed to fulfill professional responsibilities or needs; (b) individuals in occupations and job positions have needs for resources to fulfill their professional responsibilities; (c) individuals in occupations and job positions can make choices about the use of available resources; and (d) individuals in occupations and job positions are able to perceive whether professional needs are met.

Consequences

The consequences of professional isolation are specific to the need that is unmet and the vulnerabilities of the individual in the occupation or job position. For example, if the need that is unmet is for professional consultation and support as in the model case and if the nurse is vulnerable, the consequence may be stress, frustration, aloneness, and possible termination of employment. If the need that is unmet is educational or informational regarding current approaches to care for a health problem and if the professional providing health care is uninformed of the current approaches, the consequence may be the provision of less than optimum health care.

EMPIRICAL REFERENTS

Empirical referents are groups or categories of actual phenomena that demonstrate the occurrence of the defining attributes of the concept (Walker & Avant, 1988). Two empirical referents were identified for professional isolation: (a) the availability of the needed resource is measured and found deficient; and (b) individuals in occupations and job positions express awareness of an unmet need or exhibit signs of the consequences of the unmet need.

CONCLUSION

As is shown in this concept analysis, the concept of professional isolation, is used in many contexts. This analysis clarifies the meaning of professional isolation; potentially, it will improve the consistency of its use in the context of rural health care. A clearer definition may also improve understanding of the problems encountered by those experiencing professional isolation and suggest solutions to these problems.

REFERENCES

American Hospital Association. (1992) *Hospital closures 1980 thru 1991: A statistical profile.* Chicago: Author.

American Nurses' Association. (1989). *ANA statement on rural nursing.* Kansas City, MO: Author.

Beck, S. M., & Utz, P. K. (1996). A perioperative educators network promotes collegiality. *AORN Journal, 64* (5), 786–791.

Black, S. K. (1973). Social isolation and the nursing process. *Nursing Clinics of North America, 8* (4), 575–586.

Bleakley, F. R. (1996). Rural county balks at joining global village. *Wall Street Journal,* (Jan 4), B1.

Brauer, B. W. (1992). Telehealth: The delayed revolution in health care. *Medical Progress Through Technology, 18,* 151–163.

Campion, D. M., & Dickey, D. F. (1995). Lessons from the essential assess community hospital program for rural network development. *The Journal of Rural Health, 11* (1), 32–39.

Carpenito, L. J. (1987). *Nursing diagnosis: Application to clinical practice.* (2nd ed., pp. 563–567), Philadelphia: Lippincott.

Connor, R. A., Hillson, S. D., & Krawelski, J. E. (1995). Competition, professional synergism, and the geographic distribution of rural physicians. *Medical Care, 33*(11), 1067–1078.

Cordes, S. M. (1989). The changing rural environment and the relationship between health services and rural development. *Health Services Research, 23*(6), 757–784.

Cox, C. L., Spiro, M., & Sullivan, J. A. (1988). Social risk factors: Impact on elders' perceived health status. *Journal of Community Health Nursing, 5* (1), 59–73.

Crandall, L. A., & Coggan, J. M. (1994). Impact of new information technologies on training and education for rural health professionals. *The Journal of Rural Health, 10* (3), 208–215.

Darby, C. (1979). A lonely life at the top. *Nursing Mirror, 23,* 148–150.

Davis, D. J., & Droes, N. S. (1993). Community health nursing in rural and frontier counties. *Nursing Clinics of North America, 28* (1), 159–169.

Dussault, M., & Barnett, B. G. (1996). Peer-assisted leadership: Reducing educational managers' professional isolation. *Journal of Educational Administration, 34* (3), 5–14.

Fader, S. S. (1984). Career loneliness: If you hold a typical modern job, your friends may never understand what you do. *This World* (April 19), 12.

Fineman, M. P. (1996). Learning together. *Executive Educator, 18* (5), 34–35.

Fischer, C. S., & Phillips, S. L. (1982). Who is alone? Social characteristics of people with small networks. In L. A. Peplau & D. Perlman (Eds.), *Loneliness: A sourcebook of current theory, research and therapy* (pp. 21–39). New York: Wiley.

Garber, B. (1987). The isolation and loneliness of the child analyst. *Annual of Psychoanalysis, 15,* 193–208.

Hillestad, E. A. (1984). Is it lonely at the top? *Nursing Administration Quarterly, 8* (3), 1–13.

Howland, R. H. (1995). The treatment of persons with dual diagnoses in a rural community. *Psychiatric Quarterly, 66* (1), 33–49.

Joint Task Force of the National Association of Community Health Centers and the National Rural Health Association. (1989). Health care in rural America: The crisis unfolds. *Journal of Public Health Policy, 10* (1), 99–116.

Jones, B. B. (1993, February). *Working with the "only one" in the division.* Paper presented at the Annual International Conference for Community College Chairs, Deans, and Other Instructional Leaders, Phoenix, AZ.

Langs, R. (1988). Perspectives on psychoanalysis as a late arrival to the family of sciences. *Contemporary Psychoanalysis, 24* (3), 397–419.

Lee, H. J. (1991). Definitions of rural: A review of the literature. In A. Bushy (Ed.), *Rural nursing,* Vol. 1. (pp. 7–20). Newbury Park: Sage.

Litchfield, N. B. (1989). Stress-related problems of dentists. *International Journal of Psychosomatics, 36* (1–4), 41–44.

Mitchell, R. (1996). Perceived inhibitors to rural practice among physiotherapy students. *Australian Journal of Physiotherapy, 42* (1), 47–52.

Morehead, A. H. (Ed.). (1962). *The new American Roget's college thesaurus.* New York: New American Library.

Moscovice, I. S. (1989). Strategies for promoting a viable rural health care system. *The Journal of Rural Health, 5* (3), 216–230.

Murray, P. J. (1996). Nurses' computer-mediated communications on NURSENET: A case study. *Computers in Nursing, 14* (4), 227–234.

Pasacreta, J. V., & Jacobsen, P. B. (1989). Addressing the need for staff support among nurses caring for the AIDS population. *Oncology Nursing Forum, 16* (5), 659–663.

Peternelj-Taylor, C. A., & Johnson, R. L. (1995). Serving time: Psychiatric mental health nursing in corrections. *Journal of Psychosocial Nursing & Mental Health Services, 33* (8), 12–19.

Puskin, D. S. (1992). Telecommunications in rural America. *Annals of the New York Academy of Sciences, 670,* 67–75.

Rifenbary, D. C. (1996). College counseling in far-off lands: The American-sponsored overseas school experience. *College Board Review,* (178), 18–23, 31.

Ross, M. M. (1994). Providing palliative care to older adults: Context and challenges. *Journal of Palliative Care, 10* (4), 5–10.

Rowley, T. D., & Porterfield, S. L. (1993). Can telecommunications help rural areas overcome obstacles to development? *Rural Development Perspectives, 8* (2), 2–6.

Shelton, D. A., & Frank, R. (1995). Rural mental health coverage under health care reform. *Community Mental Health Journal. 31* (6), 539–552.

Shreffler, J. (1992). *Professional isolation and loneliness in Montana nursing administrators.* Unpublished manuscript.

Speck, M., & Krovetz, M. (1996). Developing effective peer coaching experiences for school administrators. *Spectrum, 14* (1), 37–42.

Steeves, R., Cohen, M. Z., & Wise, C. T. (1994). An analysis of critical incidents describing the essence of oncology nursing. *Oncology Nursing Forum, 21* (8), 19–25.

Wakefield, M. K. (1990). Health care in rural America: A view from the nation's capitol. *Nursing Economics, 8* (2), 83–89.

Walker, L. O., & Avant, K. C. (1988). *Strategies for theory construction in nursing* (2nd ed., pp. 35–47). Norwalk, CT: Appleton & Lange.

Weinert, C., & Long, K. A. (1990). Rural families and health care: Refining the knowledge base. *The Journal of Marriage and Family Review, 15*(1, 2), 57–75.

Wills, K., & Case-Smith, J. (1996). Perceptions and experiences of occupational therapists in rural schools. *American Journal of Occupational Therapy, 50*(5), 370–379.

Wolf, K. A. (1993). *Professionalization at work: The case of nursing at Mill City Medical Center.* Unpublished doctoral dissertation, Brandeis University.

Woolf, H. B. (Ed.). (1973). *Webster's new collegiate dictionary.* Springfield, MA: Merriam.

33

Factors Related to Retention of Health Care Professionals: Impetus for Change

Barbara A. Derwinski-robinson, Helen J. Lee, Jean Ballantyne, and Jane Ellis Scharff

The problems associated with recruitment, retention, and turnover of nurses and other health care professionals are of universal concern and have a major impact on health care facilities. Though studied in urban centers, references about the impact of these problems on rural health care are infrequent. The purpose of the study described in this chapter was to identify factors related to recruitment and retention of nurses and other health care professionals in four hospitals belonging to the Montana Consortium for Excellence in Patient Care. Specifically, the aim of the study was to identify those factors related to employees' intent to remain at their present jobs.

BACKGROUND

A review of the literature provided clear direction that certain variables influence job satisfaction and, ultimately, intent to leave and

Acknowledgment: The authors acknowledge the Montana Consortium for Excellence in Health Care, a Strengthening Hospital Nursing project (funded by the Robert Wood Johnson Foundation and Pew Charitable Trusts) for the funding of this study.

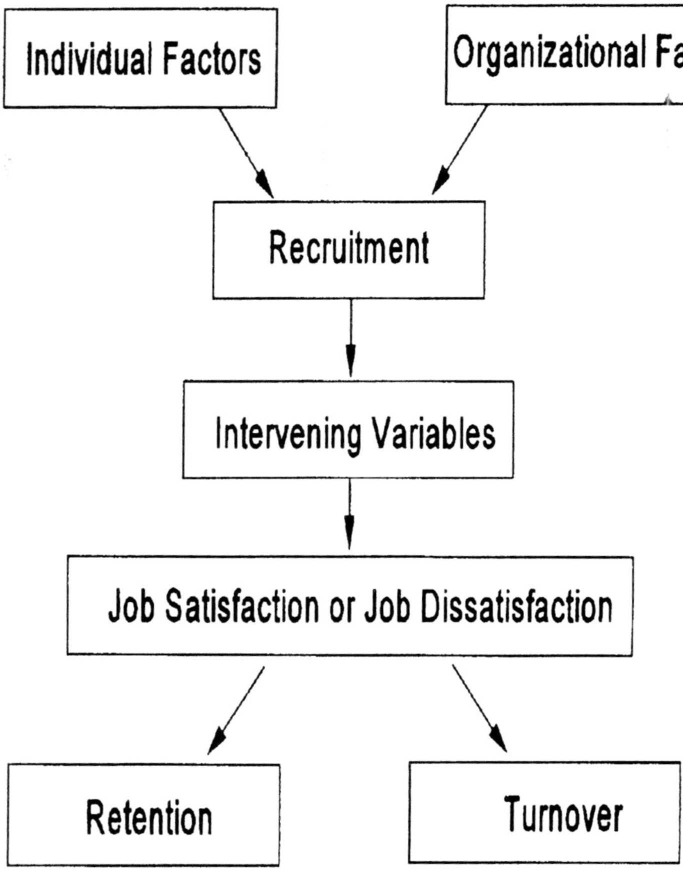

FIGURE 33.1 Conceptual framework.

actual turnover (Hinshaw, Smelzer, & Atwood, 1987; Price & Mueller, 1986). Employees who are dissatisfied with their jobs are more apt to leave. The strongest predictor of actual turnover is an indication from employees that they intend to leave the job. During employment, employees are further influenced by both individual and organizational factors (intervening variables) which lead to satisfaction or dissatisfaction with the job. Satisfaction levels (independent variable) influence intent to stay on the job (dependent variable). Figure 33.1 illustrates the conceptual framework for this study. Other researchers have used similar frameworks (Curry, Wakefield, Price, Mueller, & McCloskey, 1985; Mobley, 1977; Price & Mueller, 1986; Weisman, Alexander, & Chase, 1981). Knowledge of satisfaction levels and intent to stay empower the employer to promote organizational factors that influence retention.

SETTING

This study was a collaborative project between nursing service in hospitals in a rural state and a university-based college of nursing. Established in 1989, the Montana Consortium for Excellence in Health Care was among 19 grant holders in the nationwide Strengthening Hospital Nursing project funded by the Robert Wood Johnson Foundation and the Pew Charitable Trust. The purpose of the national project was to provide the impetus for organizational change within institutions from a departmentalized discipline-driven model to one which was unified and patient-driven.

Four of the seven hospitals in the Montana Consortium participated in this study. Hospital A was a 213-bed hospital in western Montana. Hospital B was a 146-bed hospital in eastern Montana. Hospital C was a 288-bed hospital in southcentral Montana. Hospital D was a 145-bed hospital in central Montana. The research team included one hospital consortium project director and two faculty members from the Montana State University-Bozeman College of Nursing. Consortium members from the four hospitals were actively involved in selecting individual and organizational factors for measurement.

METHODS

Design

A descriptive design using the survey method was used for this study. Following a review of the literature, more than 70 variables were identified which had some relationship to recruitment or retention of health care professionals. A modified Q-sort developed by the research team was given to consortium administrative and staff members to reduce the 70-plus originally identified variables to the 24 included in this study.

Instrument

The study questionnaire included closed-ended, open-ended, and Likert scale forced-choice response items. Content validity was established by a panel of five nurse experts. Subsequently, minor changes were made and the instrument was pilot-tested by 15 health care professionals employed at one Consortium hospital. The researchers hypothesized that the independent variable (satisfaction level) would influence the dependent variable (intent to stay or leave). Satisfaction level was measured using retention-variable items.

The questionnaire contained 24 retention variables. Nineteen of the 24 were categorized as organizational factors. The italicized acronyms in parentheses are provided for data interpretation of tables in the results section: career advancement (*cadvance*), communication (*commun*), corporate culture (*cculture*), decision making (*dmaking*), distributive justice (*djustice*), educational opportunities (*educopp*), generalist (*general*), insider-outsider (*in-out*), integration (*integrat*), job satisfaction (*jobsatis*), job stress (*jobstress*), job suitability (*jobsuit*), management style (*mgmtstyle*), role diffusion (*rolediff*), role isolation (*roleisol*), role overload (*roleover*), routinization (*routiniz*), scheduling (*schedule*), and tangible rewards (*trewards*). The remaining five variables were considered individual factors: autonomy (*autonomy*), geographic environmental desirability (*location*), personal attributes (*pattribu*), kinship responsibility (*kinship*), and professional anonymity (*privacy*).

Five of the retention variables, two organizational and three individual, were seen as particularly applicable to rural nursing. The variables of insider-outsider, professional anonymity, and generalist are concepts already identified in the seminal article on rural nursing theory by Long and Weinert (1989). Kinship responsibility was a variable identified as important to rural nurses by Ballantyne (1988). The variable geographic environmental desirability asked participants to rate the influence of geographic location on their job choice.

Data Collection

Following approval by the Montana State University College of Nursing Human Subjects Review Committee, 1,400 questionnaires were distributed to a convenience sample of health care professionals at four Consortium hospitals. Questionnaires were distributed through site visits by the research team. Questionnaires were returned directly to the research team members or the hospital consortium liaison via a locked box in the hospital cafeteria or through the mail.

Response Rate

The overall response rate was 46%, with 638 of 1,400 questionnaires returned. The individual hospital response rate ranged from 41 to 50%. At Hospital A, 400 surveys were distributed and 183 returned, a 46% response rate. Hospital B had 100 surveys distributed and 49 returned, a response rate of 49%. Hospital C had 500 surveys distributed with 206 returned, a 41% response rate. At Hospital D, 400 surveys were distributed, and 200 were returned, for a 50% response rate.

Sample

Registered nurses were 54% (n = 342) of health care professionals who participated in the study. Licensed practical nurses comprised 7.5% (n = 48). The remainder of the respondents were medical technologists (4.5%), x-ray technicians (4.4%), respiratory therapists (4.2%), pharmacists (3.1%), patient-care assistants (2.4%), physical therapists (2.4%), and occupational therapists (1.3%). Less than 1% of the sample included dietitians, emergency medical technicians, and other individuals employed in the health care setting.

Forty percent of the sample (n = 243) had their initial professional preparation at the baccalaureate level; 12% (n = 75) of these persons had a baccalaureate degree plus internship. Forty-two participants (7%) had master's degree preparation. Most of the rest of the sample had associate degree preparation.

Most of the respondents, 424 (67%), were married, 86 (14%) were divorced, 86 (14%) were never married, 19 (3%) lived with a significant other, 9 (1.4%) were separated, and 4 (0.6%) were widowed. Sixty-two percent (n = 377) identified their place of birth as rural, 25% (n = 159) listed urban as their birthplace, 11% (n = 73) listed metropolitan area as their birthplace, and 5% gave no response. Almost half (48%, n = 298) said they were "place bound." Of the 287 participants who explained their reason for being place bound, most listed multiple reasons including spouses' employment, ownership of property, and children in school.

Tenure of respondents in their current jobs had a bimodal pattern. Thirty-six percent (n = 228) had been on the job 6 to 15 years, 35% (n = 218) had been on the job 3 years or less. Smaller groups of 14% (n = 89) had been on the job for 16 or more years, and 14% (n = 87) had worked for 3 to 6 years.

RESULTS

Descriptive statistics were used to determine ranges and means for the independent organizational and individual retention variables (see Tables 33.1 and 33.2). Reliability of the retention variables containing more than one questionnaire item was established using Cronbach's

TABLE 33.1 Descriptive Statistics for Organizational Retention Variables

Variable	Range	Mean	Stay Mean	Undec Mean	Leave Mean
cadvance*	5–25	13.73	14.82[a,b,c]	11.90[a,b]	11.47[a,c]
commun*	9–45	27.89	29.80[a,b,c]	25.51[a,b,c]	22.64[a,b,c]
cculture*	5–25	14.40	15.43[a,b,c]	12.77[a,b]	11.87[a,c]
dmaking*	2–10	7.26	7.69[a,b,c]	6.60[a,b]	6.26[a,c]
djustice*	12–60	37.75	39.66[a,b,c]	35.18[a,b,c]	32.77[a,b,c]
educopp	4–10	8.10	8.24	8.18	8.05
general	10–34	23.30	23.21	23.50	23.46
in-out*	2–10	7.68	7.99[a,b,c]	7.34[a,b,c]	7.79[a,b,c]
integrat*	5–25	20.28	20.90[a,b,c]	19.58[a,b,c]	18.47[a,b,c]
jobsatis*	5–25	19.08	20.81[a,b,c]	17.08[a,b,c]	13.98[a,b,c]
jobstress*	5.24	13.38	14.18[a,b,c]	12.11[a,b]	11.49[a,b,c]
jobsuit*	8–20	16.68	17.01[a,b,c]	16.25[a,b]	15.80[a,c]
mgmtstyle*	5–25	15.80	16.99[a,b,c]	13.84[a,b]	13.21[a,c]
rolediff*	4–20	13.65	14.27[a,b,c]	12.85[a,b]	12.00[a,c]
roleisol	3–15	12.21	12.47[a,b,c]	11.75[a,b]	11.67[a,c]
roleover	2–10	5.96	6.07	5.84	5.65
routiniz*	9–25	19.36	19.84[a,b,c]	18.68[a,b]	18.17[a,c]
schedule*	4–20	18.93	19.97[a,b,c]	17.57[a,b,c]	16.18[a,b,c]
trewards*	5–25	14.41	15.27[a,b,c]	12.97[a,b]	12.60[a,c]

Denotes
*significant relationship with independent variable of intent using ANOVA
[a]significant relationship between intent variable 1 (stay), 2 (undecided), and 3 (leave)
[b]significant relationship between intent variable 1 (stay) and 2 (undecided)
[c]significant relationship between intent variable 1 (stay) and 3 (leave)

TABLE 33.2 Descriptive Statistics for Individual Retention Variables

Variable	Range	Mean	Stayer Mean	Undecided Mean	Leaver Mean
autonomy	1–5	4.25	4.27	4.16	4.31
location*	12–25	21.25	21.61[a,b,c]	20.59[a,b]	20.56[a,c]
pattribu*	21–50	40.57	41.48[a,b,c]	39.35[a,b]	38.20[a,c]
kinship	5–21	12.55	12.34	12.91	12.34
privacy	4–20	14.66	14.81	14.40	14.81

Denotes
*significant relationship with independent variable of intent using ANOVA
[a]significant relationship between intent variable 1 (stay), 2 (undecided), and 3 (leave)
[b]significant relationship between intent variable 1 (stay) and 2 (undecided)
[c]significant relationship between intent variable 1 (stay) and 3 (leave)

alpha. Alpha coefficients ranged from a high of 0.95 for management style to a low of 0.51 for role isolation.

The dependent variable was intent (to stay or leave). The intent item included five responses: (a) I definitely plan to stay in this job, (b) chances are quite good that I will stay, (c) I am undecided if I will stay or leave, (d) chances are quite good that I will leave, and (e) I have definite plans to leave. Table 33.3 shows the results for this sample.

For analysis, respondents were categorized as either "stayers," "leavers," or "undecideds" based on their response to the intent item. The five-point Likert scale for the intent item was collapsed into three categories. The responses, definitely stay and good chance of staying, became the stayer category. The responses, good chance of leaving and definitely leaving, became the leavers category. The undecideds were those who chose the item undecided. For this study, stayers comprised 64% of the participants, leavers were 16% of the participants, and 20% of respondents were undecided.

TABLE 33.3 Intent Variable (N = 612)

Item	Number	Percentage
a. Definitely stay	139	23
b. Good chance will stay	251	41
c. Undecided	123	20
d. Good chance will leave	75	12
e. Definitely leave	24	4

Mean scores for the organizational and individual retention variables were calculated for each of the three groups, stayers, undecideds, and leavers (see Tables 33.1 and 33.2) Scrutinizing the mean differences between groups revealed that, for *most* retention variables, the highest scores were obtained by the stayers, the next highest scores by the undecideds, and the lowest mean scores by the leavers. The exceptions to this trend were one organizational variable, generalist, and three individual variables, automony, kinship responsibility, and professional autonomy. For the generalist variable, the undecided group had the highest mean (23.50), the leavers obtained the next highest mean (23.46), and the stayers group had the lowest mean score (23.21). For autonomy, the highest mean was received by the leavers (4.31), the next highest mean by the stayers (4.27), and the lowest mean score was obtained by the undecideds (4.16). For kinship responsibilities, the highest mean was obtained by the undecideds (12.91); the mean score for the stayers and the leavers was identical (12.34). For professional autonomy, the highest mean score was obtained by the stayers and the leavers (14.81), and the lowest score by the undecideds (14.40).

A comparative examination of mean scores among the three groups was then performed using ANOVA; for those variables reaching significance between groups, the LSD post hoc test was used to detect significance between specific groups. Comparing the three groups, 15 of the 19 organizational retention variables and 2 of the 5 individual retention variables were statistically significant. Tables 33.1 and 33.2 show these results.

Data were then analyzed using multiple regression. In keeping with the conceptual framework for the study, a simple linear regression was performed using the independent variable of job satisfaction and the dependent variable of intent. Forty-one percent of the variance for intent was explained. Then, stepwise multiple regression was done using job satisfaction as the dependent variable, first with the organizational retention variables (Table 33.4), and second with the individual retention variables (Table 33.5).

Nine of the 19 organizational retention variables entered the regression equation for job satisfaction before the 0.05 significance criteria level for entry was reached. In order of entry, these 9 variables were job stress, insider-outsider, routinization, communication, scheduling, job suitability, career advancement, generalist, and integration. Three of the individual retention variables entered the regression

TABLE 33.4 Relation of Organizational Retention Variables with Job Satisfaction

Variable	df	beta in	R^2 Change	p
jobstress	1	.707	.294	.000
in-out	2	1.131	.404	.000
routiniz	3	.393	.463	.000
commun	4	.147	.510	.000
schedule	5	.165	.526	.000
jobsuit	6	.234	.537	.000
cadvance	7	.112	.545	.001
general	8	−.083	.550	.012
integrat	9	−.0957	.554	.018

TABLE 33.5 Relation of Individual Retention Variables with Job Satisfaction

Variable	df	beta in	R^2 Change	p
pattribu	1	.498	.344	.000
autonomy	2	−.503	.348	.000
location	3	.116	.353	.000

equation for job satisfaction. They were personal attributes, autonomy, and geographic environmental desirability.

DISCUSSION

Intent

For this study, "leavers" comprised 16% of the participants. This finding was well within the national averages which range between 10% and 30% (Curran & Miller, 1990; Hinshaw et al., 1987). This finding is supported the previous research that "leavers" were more dissatisfied with their jobs (Price & Mueller, 1986; Weisman et al., 1981).

The undecided group in this consortium study was smaller than the undecided group in a previous Montana rural hospital study (Ballantyne, 1988). In Ballantyne's study, conducted in small rural hospitals of fewer than 50 beds, the undecided group comprised 29% of the total participants (n = 116). Perhaps the larger hospital sizes in this study accounted for the smaller undecided group. For example, there is less need to be a generalist (cover all the services provided by the hospital) in a larger hospital as compared with a smaller hospital.

Organizational Retention Variables

Knowledge of intent and job dissatisfiers can give hospital administrators the data needed to start change strategies that may reduce actual turnover. The challenge for hospital managers is to identify organizational factors that contribute to job dissatisfaction. Based on the findings of this study, nine key retention factors were identified. Stayers reported a lower level of job stress than the undecided and the leavers. While most of the participants felt a sense of belonging at work and in the community (insider-outsider), stayers perceived belonging to a greater degree than did leavers or undecideds. Although scores for all groups on the routinization scale were generally high, stayers were more likely to see variety in and feel challenged by their job.

Communication scores were generally low for this entire sample (out of a possible score of 45, the overall mean score was 28). While stayers indicated they were somewhat better informed of matters at their workplace than the other two groups, a clear message was sent that something was amiss with communication. Because communication is a key element in effective organizational operations, the findings from this study suggest that management in these hospitals needs to take a closer look at communication methods.

Stayers were happier with their job schedules and were much more satisfied with their opportunities for promotion (career advancement) than the undecided or the leaver groups. Whereas integration scores were generally high for all study participants, stayers felt the strongest sense of camaraderie. There was strong agreement that reliable peer support was available. Stayers had a stronger positive feeling than leavers or undecideds that they could rely on colleagues.

Scores for the retention variable, generalist, were low, and no statistical difference was found between groups. Items for this variable include the expectation of working in and floating to more than one clinical area. Since all groups indicated unhappiness with this situation and, in particular the undecided group, those in management should assess this factor in depth and determine strategies to manage the situation.

Individual retention factors

Three individual retention factors entered the regression equation for job satisfaction. Mean scores for personal attributes for all three groups were fairly high, but stayers were significantly more likely to feel positive about their jobs, to be flexible and handle change, and to be involved in professional activities than undecideds or leavers. Autonomy, a single-item variable, measured whether respondents agreed they could practice independently within the scope of their practice. The undecideds' mean was the lowest for the sample, but the result still indicated they generally agreed that they could practice autonomously. The third individual variable entering the equation was geographic environmental desirability. Mean scores for all groups were high; however, the stayers were more happy with their environmental location than either the undecideds or the leavers. This finding indicates that where one lives does play a part in remaining satisfied with one's job.

Other organizational retention variables

While the variables of management style, tangible rewards, and role overload did not enter the organizational retention regression equation, comparison of the overall mean scores with total possible scores revealed somewhat low results for all 3 variables. For management style, the mean score for the sample was 15.80 out of a possible score of 25. Previous research has supported the proposition that middle managers play an important role in the retention of professional staff in hospitals (Taunton, Krampitz, & Woods, 1989a, 1989b). A significant finding in Taunton's (1989a,b) research was the preference of staff for participative management style. Employees appreciated being asked for their opinions on important decisions. Since responses related to corporate culture are generally negative, it is recommended that unit managers interested in participative management style do a thorough assessment of staff preferences to determine interest.

For the organizational retention variable of tangible rewards, the overall mean was 14.41 out a possible score of 25. A perception that rewards are few and far between, plus a potential for unfairness in the rewards given, leads to job dissatisfaction (Price & Mueller, 1986). Assessment and evaluation of tangible rewards available and awarded may lead to a change in management practices, thereby increasing satisfaction.

For the organizational retention variable of role overload, the mean score for the sample was 5.96 out of a possible score of 10. This result indicates that many agree that they were often asked to do extra shifts and work overtime. "Leavers" and "undecideds" were more in agreement that there was a role overload. This study was completed before the full impact of managed care was felt in Montana. Job demands should be met with appropriate staffing levels. Otherwise, burnout may result and lead to premature turnover.

Retention Variables Associated with Rural Nursing Theory Development

For the five variables that specifically addressed concepts of interest to rural nursing theory development—insider-outsider, generalist, geographic environmental desirability, kinship responsibility, and professional anonymity—some interesting trends were noted, particularly for the "undecided" group. This group received the lowest mean score for the insider-outsider variable, indicating they did not feel the sense of belonging in the organization or the community that the other two groups did. They obtained the highest mean score of the three groups for the generalist variable, showing the most unhappiness with having to work in different clinical areas from their own. Members of this group indicated less happiness with geographic location than the "stayers" did. As compared with both of the other two groups, the "undecideds" indicated a greater impact of family relationships on their ability to work. Finally, this group received the lowest mean score for professional anonymity as compared with the other two groups. Items in this variable asked participants about lack of anonymity—i.e., being recognized in public by patients and how bothered they were when neighbors or acquaintances asked for free professional advice. These findings suggest that during the recruitment process, elements of living in a rural state should be discussed to determine the prospective employees' feelings. Also, ongoing evaluation of these variables with employees may help in determining strategies aimed at retention of members of the "undecided" group.

Limitations

Two major limitations of the study are noted. One, the study used a new instrument that did not have the benefit of established reliability.

Two, the findings cannot be generalized beyond the study hospitals. In addition, the data for this study are were not analyzed separately by hospital site. While this provided protection for the study participants, hotbeds for specific problems by hospital site were not identified.

IMPETUS FOR CHANGE

When this study was conducted, the problems associated with recruitment, retention, and turnover of nurses and other health professionals were of primary concern to Consortium members. Since the completion of the study, some things have changed. Hospitals within the Consortium have felt the impact of economic influences not addressed in the study and that could not have been predicted at the outset. Some factors that have changed include:

1. The percentage of reimbursement for provision of acute care has declined dramatically;
2. A major layoff, which included nurses and other health care professionals, occurred at one study hospital;
3. Several non-Consortium hospitals in Montana have experienced layoffs as well, increasing the availability of professional nurses for other hospitals;
4. One Consortium hospital, which had a shortage of nurses at the time of study, now has a waiting list (that is, applications on file) that includes 100 new graduates from all over the country. This list also includes approximately 50 experienced nurses;
5. Two of the hospitals have experienced turnover of the top nurse executive.

While the study findings still apply, their impact has a different focus. Now, recruitment is not a priority. However, retention of committed, competent professionals still is. As many health care organizations are learning, survival depends on having high-performing, empowered staff.

Findings from this study provided a foundation for Consortium hospitals to examine the influence of their organizational factors on employee turnover patterns. Some of the factors identified by the respondents as influencing their intent to leave are within the control of the organization. Knowing which of these factors influence respondents' intent to leave can help hospital leadership in developing strategies to avert premature turnover. Key factors discovered in this study linked with intent to leave now are explored routinely as part of exit interviews.

The purpose of the Strengthening Hospital Nursing project was to provide impetus for organizational change within institutions, moving the participating hospitals toward using unified, patient-driven models. Following the knowledge of the findings of this study a process of organizational transformation at Hospital C was initiated. Key components of the restructuring, reorganizing, and organizational transformation process included

(1) use of the Interactive Planning Process (Ackoff, 1981) to plan change;
(2) use of the Five Tracks of Transformation (Kilmann, 1994) to evaluate change; and,
(3) a focus on the principles of becoming a learning organization (Senge, 1990).

The Interactive Planning Process, first described by Ackoff (1981), differs significantly from reactive, preactive, and even proactive planning usually seen in change processes. Rather than planning using predictions or projections based on the past, the process assumes stakeholders are capable of creating the future. Stakeholders are those who are affected by the planning process. The use of the Interactive Planning Process by the administrators at Hospital C is supported by this study's findings in which respondents indicated that the way information was shared was important, as were levels of staff involvement in decision making, and the way staff was informed of decisions.

The Five Tracks of Transformation proposed by Kilmann (1994) include culture, management skills, team building, strategy/structure, and reward system. Within each of these tracks, Kilmann describes a variety of concepts. Many variables in the current study have a practical relationship to one of the Kilmann tracks. For example, at Hospital C, active efforts are being made to change the organizational culture. The current study measured corporate culture and found that there was a relationship between respondents' perception of culture and their intent to leave. Again, at Hospital C, management skills are being improved through a continuing series on management and organizational development. The current study measured management style, communication of management, and management decision making and found variables that were relevant to satisfaction and intent to leave. Similar inferences can be drawn for variables that relate to each of the other tracks.

Part of the framework for change at Hospital C also includes use of principles proposed by Senge (1990), author of *The Fifth Discipline.* Principles of personal mastery and organizational learning are considered by Hospital C to be important in accomplishing organization transformation. Senge believes that individual learning is a prerequisite to organizational learning and is dependent on what he calls personal mastery. Personal mastery is described as the ability to create and sustain the creative tension necessary for change to occur. The issue is that employees need to see themselves as part of the whole organization. The findings of this study suggested that leavers do not see themselves as part of the whole, based on their report of dissatisfaction with corporate culture communication and feelings of not belonging.

CONCLUSION

While factors related to recruitment and retention are not always within the control of the organization, each must do ongoing assessments of those factors that may be within their control. Strategies to avert premature turnover can then be begun. This study provided a provocative data base for Consortium hospital administrators and appeared to lead to the initiation of a change process in one of the participating hospitals. However, it was a one-time assessment and does not replace the need for administrators to conduct continual and specific needs assessments of their staff.

One important factor in applying research findings in the practice setting was having someone from the practice setting on the research team. Such collaborative relationships should be encouraged and supported. In addition, it is strongly recommended that nurse administrators and nurse educators engage in serious dialogue about the changing job market for professional nurses in the current health care environment.

REFERENCES

Ackoff, R. (1981). *Creating the corporate future: Plan or be planned for.* New York: Wiley.

Ballantyne, J. (1988). *Determinants of intended job turnover in rural nurses.* Unpublished master's thesis, Montana State University-Bozeman.

Curran, C., & Miller, R. (1990). The impact of corporate culture on nurse retention. *Nursing Clinics of North America, 25* (3), 537–549.

Curry, J. P., Wakefield, D. S., Price, J. L., Mueller, C. W., & McCloskey, J. (1985). Determinants of turnover among nursing department employees. *Research in Nursing & Health. 8,* 397–411.

Hinshaw, A. S., Smelzer, C. H., & Atwood, J. R. (1987). Innovative retention strategies for nursing staff. *Journal of Nursing Administration, 17* (6), 8–15.

Kilmann, R. H. (1994). *Managing ego energy: the transformation of personal meaning into organizational success.* San Francisco: Jossey-Bass.

Long, K. A., & Weinert, C. (1989). Rural nursing: Developing the theory base. *Scholarly Inquiry for Nursing Practice: An International Journal, 3* (2), 113–127.

Mobley, W.H. (1977). Intermediate linkages in the relationship between job satisfaction and employee turnover. *Journal of Applied Psychology, 62* (2), 237–240.

Price, J., & Mueller, C. (1986). *Absenteeism and turnover: The case of nurses.* New York: Medical & Scientific Books.

Senge, P. (1990). *Fifth dimension: Art & practice of the learning organization.* New York: Doubleday.

Traunton, R. L., Krampitz, S. D., & Woods, C. Q. (1989a). Manager impact on retention of hospital staff: Part I. *Journal of Nursing Administration, 19* (3), 14–19.

Traunton, R. L., Krampitz, S. D., & Woods, C. Q. (1989b). Manager impact on retention of hospital staff: Part II. *Journal of Nursing Administration, 19* (4), 15–19.

Weisman, C. S., Alexander, C. S., & Chase, G. A. (1981). Determinants of hospital staff nurse turnover. *Medical Care. 21* (4), 431–443.

34

MSU Rurality Index: Development and Evaluation*

Clarann Weinert and Robert J. Boik

The word *rural* inspires a variety of images: corn fields, desert landscapes, plantation mansions, Appalachian communities, irrigation apparatus, livestock, orchards, and recreation opportunities. For some, rural means "a place to get away from," whereas for others, it means "a place to get away to" (Lee, 1991). Lee observed that there is a great diversity in present-day rural America and, thus, conceptualization and subsequent operationalization of rural also is diverse.

The definition and measurement of rurality have been stumbling blocks to researchers, theoreticians, clinicians, health care planners, and policy makers. Researchers have struggled with ways to quantify the degree of rurality and how to adequately distinguish participants based on their place of residence. There has been widespread concern regarding a health care crisis in rural areas, but little agreement as to what rural areas are (Hewitt, 1992). Coward and associates (1994) noted that the issue of a definition of rural is far from an intellectual exercise. They contended that the lack of a definition inhibits the ability to forge cohesive political coalitions, impedes a description

This work was funded by grants from the National Cancer Institute, NIH (ROICA46330), the National Fraternal Order of Eagles, the National Institute for Nursing Research, NIH (RO1 NR01 852), and the Office for Research on Women's Health (RO1-NR 01 852).

**Note.* From "MSU Rurality Index: Development and Evaluation," by C. Weinert and R. J. Boik, 1995, *Research in Nursing and Health, 18,* pp. 453–464.

of the distinctive health care needs of rural populations, and obstructs the search for solutions to the problems of rural dwellers.

Like the general rural literature, the definition and measurement of rurality also varies across rural nursing research. In a review of the literature on rural health and health-seeking behaviors, Weinert and Burman (1994) found little consistency of measurement across studies, and in some studies no definition of rural was provided. Definitions for rural appear to be chosen in a somewhat arbitrary manner to meet the needs of the particular study. For example, in one nursing study in the southwest United States rural was defined as communities of less than 100,000 (Hinshaw, Atwood, Gerber, & Erickson, 1986), whereas in a study in Montana it was defined as counties having a mean density per square mile of 5.9 or fewer persons (Weinert & Long, 1991).

Two of the most widely used typologies are those of the Census Bureau and the Office of Management and Budget (OMB). The Census Bureau defines urban as places of at least 2,500 inhabitants and rural as those not categorized as urban (U.S. Bureau of Census, 1987). The OMB designates areas as metropolitan or nonmetropolitan. Metropolitan areas (MSA) have a city of at least 50,000 or an urbanized area of 50,000 in a county of at least 100,000 (OMB, 1983).

The OMB and Census Bureau typologies share problems common to all dichotomous topologies: they oversimplify the urban/rural continuum. In particular, they fail to capture in any detail the range of variation that exists within rural areas (Office of Technology Assessment, 1990). In geographically large counties with concentrated metropolitan areas, large sparsely populated areas may be included in a MSA. Likewise, a county may be excluded from a MSA even though it contains a suburban area adjacent to the MSA (Hewitt, 1992). Interpretations of survey or census data can be highly dependent on which of the two typologies is employed. Hewitt (1992) cited an example in which the elderly make up a larger proportion of the total population in nonmetropolitan than in metropolitan areas. Nevertheless, if the Bureau of Census urban/rural categories are used then the converse is true; there is a greater proportion of elderly residents in urban rather than rural areas.

Increasing the number of categories in a typology is one way to better capture the variation inherent in the urban/rural continuum. Some urban/rural topologies, however, do not have mutually exclusive categories. For example, the National Rural Health Association's typology describes frontier counties as less than six persons per square mile and urbanized rural counties as populations of 25,000 or more not adjacent to an MSA. A county can meet both criteria resulting in a dual classification (Hewitt, 1992). Hewitt (1989) reviewed nine county-based typologies and concluded that although it is desirable to have a standardized typology to portray the diversity of rural areas. the uses of typologies vary and require the inclusion of different measures.

THE MSU RURALITY INDEX

The Montana Family Cancer Project research team at Montana State University recognized three general problems that arise when rural research is based on the commonly used definitions and typologies.

First, the definitions and typologies fail to adequately capture the variability inherent in the urban/rural continuum. An entire state like Montana could be considered as rural based on the large land mass, sparse population (less than 800,000), low population density (average of fewer than 5 persons per square mile), only two metropolitan areas (Billings with population 81,151 and Great Falls with population 55,097), and primary economies of farming/ranching, mining, logging, and recreation. By the OMB designation, all but two of Montana's 56 counties are classified as nonmetropolitan, yet on many dimensions the 54 nonmetropolitan counties are very different from each other. For example, a nonmetropolitan county in eastern Montana may have a population density of less than I person per square mile. County residents may have to travel great distances to a town large enough to have even marginally adequate retail, health, and other necessary services, whereas a nonmetropolitan county in western Montana may be much smaller in square miles and have a more dense population. Residents of these counties may have easy access to a small city, a university, retail services, health care, and all other needed services. Clearly, to examine relationships between rurality and health care variables (e.g., resource utilization, support networks, cost of managing illness) in states such as Montana, an index that has finer delineations than the conventional metropolitan/nonmetropolitan or urban/rural classifications is necessary. The conventional classifications also are minimally effective in studies of densely populated states where most counties are classified as metropolitan.

Second, most of the commonly used definitions are county-based. All residents within a county are assumed to be equal with respect to the urban/rural continuum. This is particularly problematic in counties that cover a large geographic area. For example, many families in the Montana Family Cancer Project lived in rural areas. Some families lived in remote rural areas of large counties that contain a major population center and would be classified as urban by the commonly employed indicators. Other families lived in counties that do not contain a major population center, yet their degree of social, economic, and cultural isolation varied widely. These families would be classified as rural by the commonly employed absolute indicators, without regard to their degree of isolation.

Third, urban/rural definitions and typologies are usually intended for application to the national population. Nationally normed measures, such as those used by the Census Bureau, assign the degree or category of rurality based on how the participant compares to the national population on selected characteristics. When a nationally normed measure is used in a study of a subpopulation, the degree of rurality is assigned without regard for the composition of the group under study. As a result, the measure may fail to indicate how rural or how urban a participant is, compared to the others in the study. The opportunity to detect relationships between health related variables and degree of rurality then is lost.

The MSU Rurality Index represents an attempt to surmount the preceding three problems. First, the MSU Rurality Index is a quantitative index that assigns a value (degree of rurality) to each family on the urban/rural continuum and avoids artificial categorization. Second, the MSU Rurality Index is a family-based rather than a county based measure, and thus residents within a county are not assumed to be equal on the urban/rural continuum. Third, this new index is locally normed. That is, the index is normed with respect to the subset of the population under study. Thus, as a research instrument, the index can discriminate among study participants even if they are relatively homogeneous with respect to the urban/ rural dimension, e.g., all the study participants live in sparsely populated western states.

The purpose of this article is to describe the development of the MSU Rurality Index and to report the psychometric properties (reliability and construct validity) of the new measure.

RATIONALE UNDERLYING THE MSU RURALITY INDEX

Various strategies for developing a locally normed index of rurality are feasible. Carney, Bums, and Slinkmen (1991) developed an economic index by performing a principal components analysis on eleven county-based variables measured on each county in Texas, This strategy required substantial effort in county-based data collection followed by somewhat standard data analytic techniques. The development of the MSU Rurality Index used an alternative strategy. Two key variables, one at the county level and one at the resident level, were carefully selected. Data collection efforts at the county and resident levels are minimal because in each case only a single, easily obtained, measure is required. By using resident level data, the resulting index is able to differentiate among residents within a county. To ensure that the MSU Rurality Index possesses desirable statistical properties, a slightly more complex data analytic technique than that used by Carney et al. is employed.

The two key variables of the MSU Rurality Index are population of the county of residence (as reported in the census) and distance to emergency care as indicated by self-report of study participants. The first of these variables is a proxy for diversity, which was one of the dimensions emphasized by Lee (1991) as important when defining rurality. In particular, county population reflects the availability of various types of health care services. For example, tertiary care or radiation treatment centers require large population bases to make them economically feasible. Population also is associated strongly with population density, which has been identified as a critical dimension for measuring rurality (Cordes, 1985; Hewitt, 1992; Weinert & Long, 1990). For Montana counties, the correlation between log(population) and log(population density) is $r = 0.90$. Cordes (1985) notes that population density is an important dimension because of its influence on communication and transportation patterns, one's sense of community, and the availability of specialized services.

Accessibility to various types of care and treatment will vary for people living within the same county. Thus, there is a need to differentiate among residents within the same county as well as across counties. The MSU Rurality Index employs the second key variable, distance to emergency care, to achieve this differentiation. Emergency assistance in a rural state is provided in a variety of ways ranging from an Emergency Room in a small hospital to the office of a sole provider such as a nurse practitioner or family practice physician. Distance to emergency care is a simple measure of the proximity to urban areas. Proximity to (and relationship with) urban areas was one of the dimensions noted by Hewitt (1992) to be useful for developing urban/rural typologies.

Distance to emergency care was selected over distance to other health care services because in an emergency (e.g., a serious laceration), a person tends to seek the nearest source of assistance. For nonemergency conditions, rural residents are known to by-pass the local hospital or health care provider and to seek help in a larger or more specialized facility, even though it may be a further distance to travel.

The procedures underlying the MSU Rurality Index were designed to yield a quantitative index that is reliable, valid, and approximately normal in distribution regardless of the group under study. Reliability and construct validity of the index are addressed empirically in a later section. Approximate normality is a property that will be built into the index. A measure of departure from normality is automatically obtained while constructing the index.

Before describing how normality is built into the index, it seems prudent to answer the question—why build in normality? It is intended that the MSU Rurality Index be used as a research tool; that is, it is to be used in subsequent analyses as a dependent or as an independent variable. When used as an independent (i.e., predictor) variable, normality is not ordinarily required. Nonetheless, approximate normality ensures good separation of the cases, especially in the tails of the distribution. For some analyses, however, normality of the predictor variables is required. For example, a researcher might attempt to discriminate between clinically depressed and nondepressed individuals on the basis of a set of socioeconomic variables that includes rurality. To employ ordinary linear discriminate analysis, the assumption of multivariate normality of the socioeconomic variables must be tenable. When used as a dependent variable, approximate normality is ordinarily required for valid statistical inferences (e.g., confidence intervals and hypothesis tests). For example, a researcher might have interest in the question—is tobacco use related to rurality of the user? A standard *t* test for comparing users and nonusers on rurality assumes that the rurality index is normally distributed.

MATHEMATICAL OPERATIONS ON DISTANCE AND POPULATION

In essence, the MSU Rurality Index is a set of procedures for constructing an index of rurality using county population and distance to emergency care. A researcher in possession of a data set containing them measures can, by following the procedures outlined below, construct an index of rurality tailored to the particular study group. To construct the MSU Rurality Index, four mathematical operations are performed on distance and population.

1. Distance and population measures are transformed to make the distribution of the resulting index as normal as possible.
2. The transformed distance and population measures are standardized so that each has a standard deviation of one.
3. The standardized transformed distance and population measures are weighted to produce an initial index of rurality that assigns high scores to rural families and low scores to urban families.
4. The initial index constructed in operation #3 is restandardized to have a mean of zero and a standard deviation of one.

The four operations are outlined below. Additional technical details can be obtained from the authors.

Operation #1: Transforming Distance and Population

For the ith family, denote the distance measure by D_i and denote the population measure by P_i. These measures are special cases of variables known as amounts and counts. Tukey (1977) noted that transforming amounts and counts to a log scale often helps to "normalize" the measures. A convenient way of denoting the log transformation is the following:

$$P_i \text{—>} \log(P_i) \text{ and } D_i \text{—>} \log(D_i),$$

where the arrow, —>, is read as "is transformed to." The log transformation was employed by Carney et al. (1991) to construct their county based index of rurality for Texas counties. In practice, however, there is little reason to expect that the log transformation will be optimal.

One way to expand the menu of possible transformations is to employ the Box-Cox power family (Box & Cox, 1964). Stoto and Emerson (1983) provided a tutorial on the use of power transformations in the social sciences. In the present application, the Box-Cox transformation requires that one choose two numbers. The first number, λ_1, is the power to which each distance measure is raised. The second number, λ_2, is the power to which each county population measure is raised. Specifically, the power transformations are as follows:

$$D_i \longrightarrow \text{sign}(\lambda_1) D_i^{\lambda_1} \text{ and } P_i \longrightarrow \text{sign}(\chi_2) P_i^{\lambda_2},$$

where

$$\text{sign}(\lambda_j) = \begin{cases} 1 & \text{if } \lambda_j \geqslant 0 \\ -1 & \text{otherwise,} \end{cases}$$

for $j = 1$ and $j = 2$.

For example, the square root transformation for distance is obtained by setting λ_1 to ½ and the reciprocal transformation for distance is obtained by setting λ_1 to −1. It can be shown that, after standardization in operation #2, a power of zero corresponds to taking the natural log. Note that when λ_1 is negative, as in a reciprocal transformation, $D_i^{\lambda_1}$ decreases as distance increases. The multiplier, sign(λ_1), corrects this change in direction. That is, sign$(\lambda_1) D_i^{\lambda_1}$ increases as distance regardless of the value of λ_1. Comparable remarks can be made concerning λ_2 and population.

Operation #2: Standardizing the Transformed Distance and Population Measures

Operation #2 consists of scaling the transformed measures to have a standard deviation of one. The reason for performing operation #2 is that the scales of transformed distance and transformed population (from operation #1) depend on the values for λ_1 and λ_2, respectively. For example, for $\lambda_2 = 10$, the variability of P_i^{10} gets very large whereas for $\lambda_2 = 0.001$, the variability of $P_i^{0.001}$ gets very small. Standardizing the transformed measures keeps them on the same scale regardless of the values of λ_1 and λ_2. The first two mathematical operations combined can be written as

$$D_i \longrightarrow \text{sign}(\lambda_1)\ \frac{D_i^{\lambda_1}}{\text{Std}(D^{\lambda_1})}$$

and

$$P_i \longrightarrow \text{sign}(\lambda_2)\ \frac{P_i^{\lambda_1}}{\text{Std}(P^{\lambda_1})},$$

where $\text{Std}(D^{\lambda_1})$ is the sample standard deviation of $D_1^{\lambda_1}, D_2^{\lambda_1}, \ldots, D_n^{\lambda_1}$. Identical notation is used for the county population measure.

Operation #3: Weighting the Standardized Transformed Measures

Together, operations #1 and #2 produce n pairs of standardized transformed distance and population measures. In operation #3, the two measures in each pair are weighted and summed to give an initial index of rurality. In principle, there are no restrictions on how the two transformed measures are weighted. In practice, however, it is most sensible to assign a positive weight to the distance measure and a negative weight to the population measure. This ensures that the rurality index will increase with increasing distance from emergency care and will decrease with increasing county population. The present authors recommend assigning greater weight to county population because population is a good overall indicator of available services (Hewitt, 1992, pp. 41). Distance to emergency care is a proxy for access to services and plays a secondary role by differentiating among families within a county. In this article, population is weighted twice as much as distance (i.e., distance is weighted ½ and population is weighted –1). Other researchers might want to weight distance and population differently and the MSU Rurality Index allows for such flexibility. Using the suggested weights, the initial rurality index for the ith family is denoted by I_i and is given by

$$I_i = (1/2)\left[\text{sign}(\lambda_1)\ \frac{D_i^{\lambda_1}}{\text{Std}(D^{\lambda_1})}\right] - \left[\text{sign}(\lambda_2)\ \frac{P_i^{\lambda_1}}{\text{Std}(P^{\lambda_1})}\right]. \tag{1}$$

Operation #4: Standardizing the Initial Rurality Index

The MSU Rurality Index is obtained by standardizing the initial rurality index to have a mean of zero and a standard deviation of one. The result is

$$\text{MSU Rurality Index for } i^{\text{th}} \text{ family} = \frac{I_i - \text{Mean}(I)}{\text{Std}(I)} \tag{2}$$

where I_i is defined in Equation 1.

OPTIMAL CHOICES FOR λ_1 AND λ_2

The numbers λ_1 and λ_2 are selected so that the MSU Rurality Index follows a normal distribution as closely as possible. This selection ought to be performed separately in each health study for which the index is to be employed. A selection of λ_1 and λ_2 that is optimal for one study group cannot be expected to be optimal for all studies because the distributions of distance to emergency care and county population vary from study to study. In particular, the distribution of these variables in a densely populated eastern state will differ substantially from the distributions of these same variables in a sparsely populated western state. Accordingly, the MSU Rurality Index is actually a family of rurality indices, each member of the family having a unique pair of numbers (λ_1, λ_2). To employ the MSU Rurality Index, one selects the member of the rurality index family whose distribution is closest to a normal distribution.

There are several criteria for selecting optimal transformation powers. Box and Cox (1964) selected the optimal power for a single variable by maximizing the likelihood function. In the present case, the maximum likelihood method would choose λ_1 and λ_2 so that the joint distribution of the transformed distance and population measures would follow a bivariate normal distribution as closely as possible. The maximum likelihood approach is well known and related software is available to compute optimal values for λ_1 and λ_2 (e.g., Bozdogan & Ramirez, 1988). Nonetheless, maximum likelihood estimation does not quite solve the problem at hand. It is the index in Equation 2 that is to be approximately normal, not necessarily the transformed distance and population measures themselves. Approximate bivariate normality of the transformed distance and county population scores is a sufficient but not a necessary condition for approximate normality of the rurality index. Therefore, an alternative approach is recommended.

Anderson and Darling (1952, 1954) proposed a useful test of the hypothesis that a random sample of data has been sampled from a normal distribution. Their test statistic is usually denoted by A_n^2 and is a measure of the squared distance between the distribution function of the sample of n data points and a normal distribution function. Details on the computation of A_n^2 can be found in Snedecor and Cochran (1989). Large values of A_n^2 correspond to large departures of the data from normality whereas small values of A_n^2 (i.e., values near zero) correspond to minimal departures from normality. In a typical application, the hypothesis of normality is rejected at the α level of significance if $A_n^2 \geqslant A_{n,\alpha}^2$ where $A_{n,\alpha}^2$ is the α level critical value. For moderate to large sample sizes, the critical values for 0.05 and 0.01 level tests can be approximated by $A_{n,0.05}^2 \approx 0.7514(1 - 0.79/n - 0.89/n^2)$ and $A_{n,0.01}^2 \approx 1.0348(1 - 1.013/n - 0.93/n^2)$.

The optimal values for λ_1 and λ_2 are those that minimize the Anderson-Darling statistic, A_n^2, computed on the MSU Rurality Index. To use the MSU Rurality Index, a researcher must be able to compute the optimal values for a given data set. A SAS IML (SAS Institute, 1990) program for computing optimal transformation values is available from the authors.

INTERPRETATION OF THE MSU RURALITY INDEX

The numerical value of the MSU Rurality Index increases with the degree of rurality. For residents within a single county, the index value increases (greater rurality) as distance from emergency care increases. Also, for individuals from different counties who live equidistant from emergency care, the index value increases as county population decreases. A score of zero reflects average rurality for the group under study. Positive scores reflect a rural residence and negative scores reflect an urban residence, relative to the group of residences under study. The MSU Rurality Index can be rescaled to have a mean other than zero and/or a standard deviation other than 1, but the suggested standardization puts the index on the familiar Z scale.

Thus, a family having an index score equal to +1 is one standard deviation above the mean and a family having an index score equal to –1 is one standard deviation below the mean.

Tables of the standard normal distribution can be used to find percentiles and probabilities for the MSU Rurality Index. For example, approximately 68% of the index scores of the group under study are in the interval –1 to +1 and the 50th and 95th percentiles are approximately 0 to 1.645, respectively.

RELIABILITY AND VALIDITY OF THE MSU RURALITY INDEX

To examine the reliability and construct validity of the MSU Index, data from two health-related surveys were used. The distributions of distance to emergency care and county population differ substantially between the two studies, thus lending generality to the results.

Study Descriptions

Mid-Life Women's Survey (MLWS). The first sample is a group of 295 women who participated in the study "Mid-life Women: Chronic Illness and Health Seeking" funded by the Office of Research on Women's Health. The Mid-life Women's Survey was designed to examine the transition to menopause for women ages 35 to 50 who had multiple sclerosis or whose spouse had the disease. The women were primarily Caucasian (98%), married (97%), with a mean annual family income of $45,000 to $50,000, a mean age of 43.5 years, and with a mean of 14.2 years of education. The 228 women with multiple sclerosis and the 67 women whose partners had the disease lived in 40 states across the country. Because the participants in the MLWS are essentially a national sample, conventional measures of rurality might be applicable. Nonetheless, this study is included here to demonstrate that the MSU Rurality Index can be constructed on any study group.

The Mid-life Women's Survey is a supplement to the parent project "Families Living with a Long-term Illness: A National Study" which is a 5-year study (1989–1993) funded by NIH/National Institute for Nursing Research. Data specific to the MLWS were collected in 1992. Distance to emergency care and residence data were collected on many of the MLWS participants during the remaining years of the parent study.

Montana Family Cancer Project (MFCP). The second sample is a group of 828 households from the four arms of the study "Home Care of Rural Cancer Patients in Montana" funded by NIH/National Cancer Institute. The study is commonly referred to as the Montana Family Cancer Project. The major goals of this longitudinal study were to describe the current health care of Montana's cancer patients; to explore the contributions of the family, the informal, and the formal health care system to care giving; and to examine the effects of the illness on the well-being of families who are managing cancer.

Usable data from the primary arm of the MFCP consisted of 390 families managing cancer who met the study criteria and lived in Montana. Data from the second arm of the MFCP consisted of 73 individuals with cancer who were living alone. Caregivers who had recently lost a loved one comprised the third arm of the MFCP, with data from 69 participants. The fourth arm of the MFCP was a group of 296 individuals who participated in a methodological study to establish baselines for some of the measures used in the MFCP. The participants in the combined sample of 828 observations lived in Montana, were primarily white (99%), with a median annual family income of $20,000 to $39,000.

Distance and Population Statistics

Descriptive statistics for distance to emergency care and county population for the two study samples are presented in Table 34.1. Skewness and kurtosis coefficients (Madansky, 1988, pp. 3640) for normally distributed

TABLE 34.1 Summary Statistics for Distance and Population in Two Studies

	Distance (Miles) to Emergency Care		County Population	
Statistic	MLWS[a]	MFCP[b]	MLWS	MFCP
Mean	7.66	9.82	423,726	45,362
Std. deviation	8.76	15.92	869,494	38,254
Skewness	3.06	4.27	5.23	0.63
Kurtosis	14.44	31.03	37.27	−0.88
Median	5	4	119,659	47,495
Interquartile range	8	9	423,895	67,413

[a] $n = 295$. [b] $n = 828$.

random variables are both zero. As one might expect, participants in the MFCP study, on average, live in counties having smaller populations than do participants in the MLWS. The mean distance to emergency care is larger for MFCP participants than for MLWS participants. The median distance to emergency care, however, is smaller for MFCP participants than for MLWS participants. This reversal in direction is explained by the larger skewness coefficient for the MFCP study group. The mean distance for the MFCP group is pulled upward by the large distances in the right tail of the distribution.

Rurality Indices for MLWS and MFCP

For the Mid-life Women's Survey, the optimal transformation powers for distance to emergency care and county population were computed to be $\lambda_1 = -0.20$ and $\lambda_2 = -0.05$, respectively. For the Montana Family Cancer Project, the corresponding optimal transformation powers were computed as $\lambda_1 = 0.15$ and $\lambda_2 = 0.55$. Using Equations 1 and 2. the final form of the indices are

MSU Rurality Index for *i*th family =

$$-\frac{D_i^{-0.20}}{0.343} + \frac{P_i^{-0.05}}{0.052} - 0.8534$$

for the MLWS, and

$$\frac{D_i^{0.15}}{0.588} - \frac{P_i^{0.55}}{209.509} - 0.595 \tag{3}$$

for the MFCP. Measures of the degree to which these transformations help to "normalize" the index are reported in Table 34.2. For a comparative evaluation of the effectiveness of the transformations to normality, measures of departure from normality for two competing rurality indices also are reported for each study group. The first competing index, the Raw Rurality Index, is computed like the MSU Rurality index except that the first mathematical operation (transformation of distance and population measures) is omitted and nontransformed distance and population measures are employed in operations #2 to #4. The second competing index, the Log Rurality Index, is computed like the MSU Rurality Index except that log trans-

TABLE 34.2 Measures of Departure From Normality for Various Rurality Indices

Study	Measure of Departure From Normality	MSU Index[a]	Competing Indices Raw[b]	Competing Indices Log[c]
Mid-life Women's Survey				
Skewness		0.11	−3.27	0.04
Kurtosis		0.26	22.74	0.22
χ^2 Departure from normality		1.40	7,213.95	0.59
A_n^2 Departure from normality		0.09	21.84	0.14
Montana Family Cancer Project				
Skewness		0.13	0.21	0.66
Kurtosis		−0.65	1.06	−0.05
χ^2 Departure from normality		17.58	45.23	61.38
A_n^2 Departure from normality		2.39	10.58	8.42

[a]Opimal transformation. [b]No transformation: $\lambda_1 = 1$ and $\lambda_2 = 1$. [c]Log transformation: $\lambda_1 = 0$ and $\lambda_2 = 0$.

formations on distance and population are substituted for optimal transformations in operation #1.

For each index, coefficients of skewness and kurtosis are reported. The two degree-of-freedom χ^2 statistic reported in Table 34.2 is a crude measure of departure from normality. It reflects nonnormality with respect to skewness and/or kurtosis. The Anderson-Darling statistic is a more comprehensive index of departure from normality and also is reported in Table 34.2. Critical values for the Anderson-Darling statistic for the MLWS are $A^2_{295.0.05} \approx 0.7494$, and $A^2_{295.0.01} \approx 1.0312$. For the MFCP, the critical values are $A^2_{828.0.05} \approx 0.7507$, and $A^2_{828.0.05} \approx 1.0334$. According to the Anderson-Darling test, the rurality index computed on nontransformed distance and population measures departs substantially from normality in both studies. Log transformations normalize the index nearly as well as optimal transformations in the Mid-life Women's Survey, but not in the Montana Family Cancer Project. The MSU Rurality Index in the MFCP departs from normality even though optimal transformations are employed. Nonetheless, the transformations did substantially decrease the departure from normality in the MFCP; the Anderson-Darling statistic decreased by nearly 80%. The degree of non-normality remaining in the MFCP index is sufficient that caution is needed if normal-theory based statistical in-

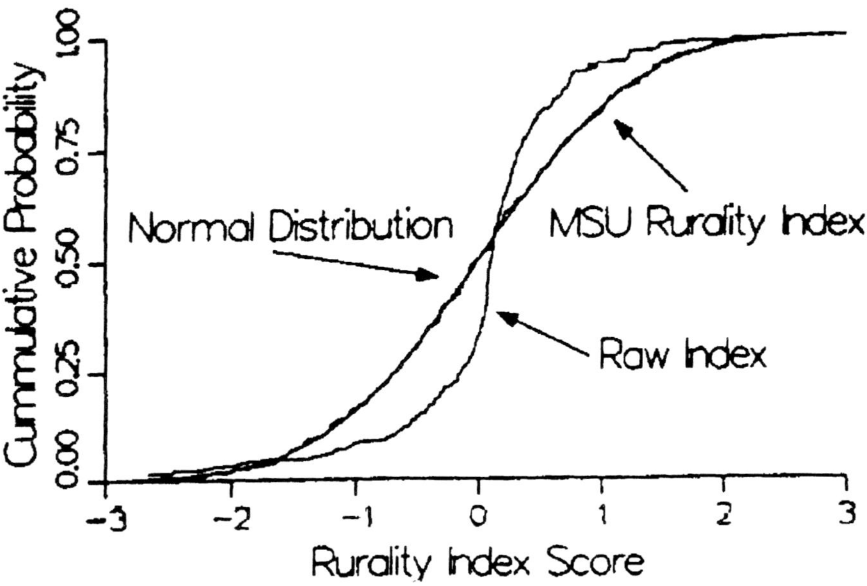

FIGURE 34.1 Distribution functions of the raw and MSU rurality indices in the Mid-life Women's Survey compared to the standard normal distribution function.

ference procedures are to be employed. The mild skewness and absence of large outliers, however, indicates that the usual descriptive statistics (e.g., means, standard deviations, correlations) are still appropriate.

The effect of the transformations in "normalizing" the rurality index for the Mid-life Women's Survey is graphically illustrated in Figure 34.1. The three curves in Figure 34.1 are probability distribution functions for the raw rurality index, and, for comparison, a standard normal random variable. The distribution function for the MSU Rurality Index population follows the normal distribution function so closely that they are hard to distinguish. The primary difference is that the normal distribution function is smooth whereas the MSU Rurality Index function consists of small steps. The raw rurality index distribution function, however, does not follow the normal distribution closely at all. The corresponding distribution curves for the MFCP are not displayed. They are similar to those in Figure 34.1 except that the raw rurality index for the MFCP deviates substantially less from normality than the raw rurality index for the MLWS and the MSU

Rurality Index for the MFCP deviates slightly more from normality than the MSU Rurality Index for the MLWS.

A scatterplot of county population (on the $\log_{10}$ scale) against the MSU Rurality Index for the Montana Family Cancer Project is displayed in Figure 34.2. The role that distance to emergency care plays in differentiating among families within a county is illustrated by the scatter plot. For example, the column of data points in the lower right-hand comer of Figure 34.2 corresponds to 140 families from Yellowstone County. Yellowstone County (population 113,419) includes the city of Billings and is the most highly populated county in Montana. For these 140 families, the index in Equation 3 simplifies to $D_i^{0.15}/0.588 - 3.472$. The value of the index ranges from –1.77 to –0.57 and the mean value is –1.42. By using the approximate normality of the index, these scores can be converted to percentiles. The rurality percentile for the average Yellowstone County resident is 8 and the percentile varies from 4 to 28. The corresponding scatterplot for the MLWS is not displayed. It is similar to Figure 34.2 except that the data points are not organized into distinct columns (corresponding to counties) as strongly as in Figure 34.2.

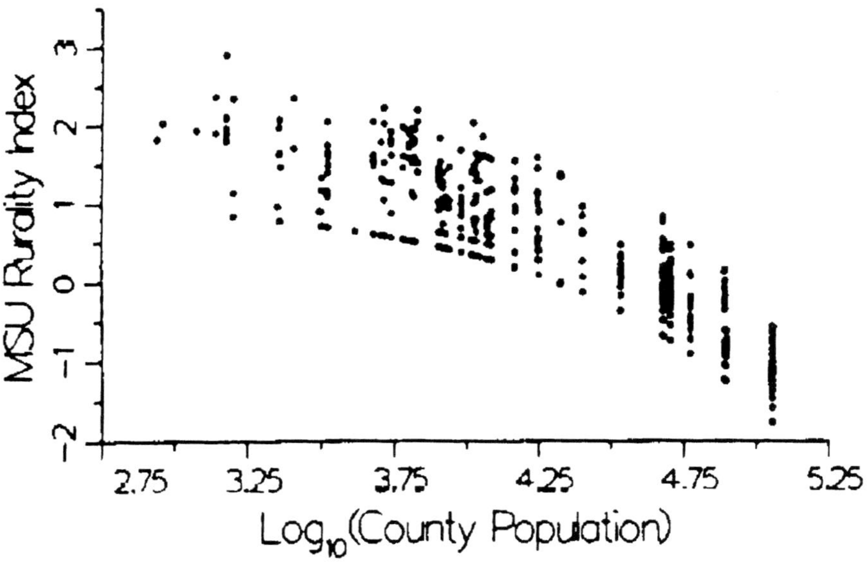

FIGURE 34.2 Scatterplot of the MSU rurality index scores against county population (Log_{10} scale) in the Montana Family Cancer Project.

Reliability Analyses

Measures of distance to emergency care for the MFCP participants were collected at a single point in time, eliminating the possibility of computing test-retest reliability coefficients. For the MLWS participants, test-retest reliability coefficients were computed for each pair of years from 1989 to 1993. Each reliability coefficient was based on women who had not changed residence over the time period in question and who had participated in the parent study both years. The MSU indices for 1989 and 1990 were computed using 1980 census data (the most recent census data available at that time). The indices for 1991 to 1993 were computed using 1990 census data. Overall, the MSU index was very reliable. All 10 of the test-retest coefficients were 0.94 or larger.

Validity Analyses

Identical validity analysis could not be conducted for the two studies because, other than distance to emergency care and county population, comparable measures were not obtained. Specifically, families in the MLWS classified their residence locations into one of eight categories, but these data were not obtained on MFCP families. Conversely, county-based measures of health-care and economic variables were available for all counties in Montana, but not for all counties represented in the MLWS. The following sections report separate, but equally useful, construct validity analyses for the MLWS and the MFCP studies.

Validation: Mid-life Women's Survey. Each respondent in the MLWS was asked to classify her place of residence into one of eight categories ranging from farm/ranch to major metropolitan area. The results are presented in Table 34.3. For each category, the mean MSU Rurality Index score is given. To evaluate the effects of weighting distance and population, mean rurality index scores based on two competing indices also are reported. The competing indices were computed in the same manner as the MSU Rurality Index except that either county population or distance to emergency care was given a weight of zero in operation #2. For example, the index that is labeled "Distance" in Table 34.3 was obtained by following the four mathematical operations, but assigning a weight of zero for county population.

TABLE 34.3 Mean Rurality Indices in the Mid-life Women's Survey According to Location of Residence

Location of Residence	n	MSU Index	Competing Indices: Distance	Competing Indices: Population
1. Farm/ranch	22	1.12	0.85	0.89
2. Rural area	55	0.58	0.66	0.36
3. Small rural town	36	0.49	0.15	0.51
4. Small town	46	0.18	−0.43	0.44
5. Medium size city	47	−0.30	−0.48	−0.10
6. Large city	17	−0.40	−0.32	−0.31
7. Suburban area	59	−0.78	−0.17	−0.85
8. Major metropolitan area	12	−1.29	−0.19	−1.47
Multiple R^2		0.41	0.22	0.39

A sensible index of rurality on average ought to have a monotonic relationship with the ordered categories in Table 34.3. Neither the Distance Rurality Index nor the Population Rurality Index has such a relationship. The Distance Rurality Index scales a "medium sized city" as more urban than any other location, including a "major metropolitan area." The Population Rurality Index scales a "rural area" as more urban than either a small rural town" or a "small town." The MSU Rurality Index, however, does have a monotonic relationship with the ordered categories. The reported R^2 values are the squared multiple correlations obtained by regressing the rurality indices on the eight categories. The eight categories explain 41% of the variability in the MSU Rurality Index and about the same percentage of the variability in the population index. A smaller percentage of the variability of the distance index is explained by the categories.

Overall. the findings in Table 34.3 support the validity of the MSU Rurality Index because the mean MSU Rurality Index increases from Major Metropolitan Area to Farm/Ranch, and because the MSU Rurality Index is as strongly or more strongly associated with the eight categories as are indices computed from distance or population alone.

Validation: Montana Family Cancer Project. Correlations between the MSU Rurality Index and county population and between the MSU Rurality Index and various health care variables for the Montana Family Cancer Project families are reported in Table 34.4. For comparison,

TABLE 34.4 Correlations Between Rurality Indices and Health Care Variables In the Montana Family Cancer Project

	Rurality Index	
Variable	MSU	Economic
$(\text{County pop.})^{.25}$	−0.91	−0.95
$-1/(\text{Dist to emergency care})^{.2}$	0.49	0.09
$-1/(\text{Dist to routine care})^{.2}$	0.42	0.16
$(\text{No. nurses in county})^{.2}$	−0.91	−0.93
$(\text{No. beds in county})^{.2}$	−0.87	−0.82

correlations between these same variables and an index constructed according to Carney et al. (1991) also are reported. Their index was computed as the first principal component based on the matrix of correlations among the following eleven economic variables observed on each county in Texas: total employment, population density, number of secondary farm operators, population, agricultural employment, median income, number of principal farm operators, population growth, concentration, average adjacent population, and percent below poverty level. The Economic Index in Table 34.4 was computed in the same fashion except that the eleven economic variables were observed on each county in Montana. Following Carney et al. (1991), each of the 11 variables was transformed to the log scale prior to analysis. The Economic Index was scaled to have a mean of zero, a variance of one, and such that rural counties are assigned positive scores. Prior to computing the correlations in Table 34.4, county population and the health care variables were transformed to approximate normality using the maximum likelihood estimate of the optimal power.

Although not reported in Table 34.4, the MSU Rurality Index for the MFCP is correlated strongly with the county-based Economic Index ($r = 0.85$). Both indices are related strongly to county population. The MSU Rurality Index is more strongly correlated with distance to emergency care and with distance to routine care than is the Economic Index. This is no surprise because the MSU Rurality Index is based, in part, on a distance measure. Both indices have strong negative correlations with the number of nurses and with the number of hospital beds in the county.

TABLE 34.5 Mean Rurality Indices in the Montana Family Cancer Project According to the Number of Hospitals in the County of Residence

Number of Hospitals	*n*	Rurality Index MSU	Rurality Index Economic
Zero	41	1.46	1.71
One	453	0.43	0.30
Two	158	−0.31	−0.17
Three	176	−1.17	−1.01
Multiple R^2		0.52	0.41

The 56 counties in Montana were classified according to the number of hospitals in the county. For each classification level, the mean scores of the MSU Rurality Index and the Economic Index were computed. The results are reported in Table 34.5. Both indices show the type of relationships that one would expect. The multiple R^2 values reveal that the MSU Rurality Index is more strongly related to the number of hospitals than is the Economic Index. The difference between R^2 values is significant, $Z = 4.09$, $p < .01$, according to Pitman's (1939) test (applied to the residual variances).

From the findings presented in Tables 34.4 and 34.5, it appears that the MSU Rurality Index is associated with various health-care variables as strongly or more strongly than the Economic Index. Thus, the validity of the MSU Rurality Index does not appear to be compromised by its parsimony.

DISCUSSION

The MSU Rurality Index was motivated by the need for a careful characterization of the degree of rurality of the participants in the Montana Family Cancer Project. The conventional classifications were not adequate for an analysis of the relationships between rurality and various health care variables because of the geographically large, sparsely populated nature of Montana.

The MSU Rurality Index is a research tool that gives a locally normed resident-based measure of the degree of rurality. The advantage of a locally versus a nationally normed index of rurality is that a locally normed index differentiates among study participants regardless of how they might compare to an outside normative group. The advantage of a resident-versus a county-based index is that a resident-based index differentiates among study participants within as well as between counties. If all participants in a study live in the same county, however, then the MSU Rurality Index will reflect distance to emergency care only, unless the index is modified. One suitable modification is to partition the county into smaller units (e.g., county subdivisions). Population of these smaller units is then substituted for county population in the MSU Rurality Index.

A noteworthy feature of the index is that it is based on only 2 variables, yet appears to be as valid as a competing index based on 11 variables. The statistical analysis that is required to construct the index is somewhat more intensive than usual, but this tradeoff between data collection and data analysis seems sensible. Data collection is generally more expensive than data analysis.

The Index can be used either as a predictor variable or as a dependent variable in investigations of the relationships between rurality and health-care variables or between rurality and family variables. Initial analyses indicated that the MSU Rurality Index is reliable and is suitably related to various health-care variables, various rural/urban variables, and to an existing county-based index of rurality. The MSU Rurality Index appears to provide a more sensitive research measure than conventionally used nationally normed indicators such as rural versus urban or metropolitan versus nonmetropolitan.

REFERENCES

Anderson, T. W., & Darling, D. A. (1952). Asymptotic theory of certain "goodness of fit" criteria based on stochastic processes. *Annals of Mathematical Statistics, 23,* 193–212.

Anderson, T. W., & Darling, D. A. (1954). A test of goodness of fit. *Journal of the American Statistical Association, 49,* 765–769.

Box, G. E. P., & Cox, D. R. (1964). An analysis of transformations. *Journal of the Royal Statistical Society,* Series B, *26,* 211–252.

Bozdogan, H., & Ramirez, D. E. (1988). UTRANS and MTRANS: Marginal and joint Box-Cox transformations of multivariate data to "near" normality. *Multivariate Behavioral Research, 23,* 131–132.

Camey, K., Bums, N., & Slinkmen, C. (1991). Index of demand: An economic index of rurality. *Texas Journal of Rural health,* 3rd quarter, 1-14.

Cordes, S. (1985). Biopsychosocial imperatives from the rural perspective. *Social Science and Medicine,* 21, 1373–1379.

Coward, R., Bull, C., Kukulka, G., & Galliher, J. (1994). *Health services for rural elders.* New York: Springer.

Hewitt, M. (1989). *Defining rural areas: Impact on health care policy and research.* (Staff paper, Office of Technology Assessment, Y3 T22/2: 2R88). Washington, DC: U.S. Government Printing Office.

Hewitt, M. (1992). Defining rural areas. In W. Gesler & T. Ricketts (Eds.), *Health in rural North America* (pp. 25–54). New Brunswick, NJ: Rutgers University.

Hinshaw, A., Atwood, I., Gerber, R., & Erickson, J. (1986). Contrasting models of job satisfaction and anticipated turnover among urban and rural nursing staff. [Abstract]. In *New frontiers in nursing research* (p. 177). (Proceedings of the International Nursing Research Conference, Edmonton, Alberta, Canada).

Lee, H. (1991). Definitions of rural: A review of the literature. In A. Bushy (Ed.), *Rural nursing: Vol. I* (pp. 7–20). Newbury Park. CA: Sage.

Madansky, A. (1988). *Prescriptions for working statisticians.* New York: Springer-Verlag.

Office of Management and Budget (1983). *Metropolitan statistical areas* (NTIS No. PB83–218891). Washington. DC: Executive Office of the President. Office of Technology Assessment (1990). *Health care in rural America,* (OTA-H-434). Washington, DC: U.S. Government Printing office.

Pitman, E. J. G. (1939). A note on normal correlation. *Biometrika. 31,* 9–12.

SAS Institute. (1990). *SAS/IML software: Usage and reference* (Version 6 1st ed.). Cary, NC: Author.

Snedecor, G. W., & Cochran, W. G. (1989). *Statistical methods* (8th ed.). Ames, IA: Iowa State University Press.

Stoto, M. A., & Emerson, J. D. (1983). Power transformations for data analysis. In S. Leinhardt (Ed.), *Sociological methodology: 1983–1984* (pp. 126168). San Francisco: Jossey-Bass.

Takey, J. W. (1977). *Exploratory data analysis.* Reading MA: Addison-Wesley.

U.S. Bureau of the Census (1987). *Statistical abstract of the United States: 1988,* (108th ed.). Washington, DC: Government Printing Office.

Weinert, C., & Bunnan, M. (1994). Rural health and health-seeking behaviors. *Annual Review of Nursing Research, 12,* 65–92.

Weinert, C., & Long, K. (1990). Rural families and health care: Refining the knowledge base. *Journal of Marriage and Family Review, 15,* 57–75.

Weinert, C., & Long, K. (1991). The theory and research base for rural nursing practice. In A. Bushy (Ed.), *Rural nursing: Vol. I* (pp. 21–38). Newbury Park, CA: Sage.

VI

LOOKING AHEAD

More than 20 years has passed since Anna Shannon had the vision to develop the rural nursing clinical and theoretical base at Montana State University-Bozeman. Because of her foresight and commitment, doing a literature search on rural nursing today yields a plethora of possible references. Nevertheless, the inquiry cannot stop here. This book is only one more step in the continuing work on rural nursing theory development.

Silva, Sorrell, and Sorrell (1995) challenge nursing faculty, nursing students, and practicing nurses to "understand how to learn rather than how to hoard knowledge, how to critique rather than how to accept, [and] how to expand rather than how to contract." (p. 12). The editor of this book and the members of the editorial board invite all involved in rural nursing and in rural theory development to continue to learn and to share their valuable knowledge. The last chapter (chapter 35), written by the author of one of the early significant articles on rural nursing theory, suggests direction for future work.

This book represents the work of dozens of people. It is a stopping point but not an ending point. Much more work in theory and research needs to be done. The many authors of the chapters in this book and the editorial board invite objective, experiential, and insightful critique. We challenge you to expand your horizons.

REFERENCES

Silva, M. C., Sorrell, J. M., & Sorrell, C. D. (1995). From Carper's patterns of knowing to ways of being: An ontological philosophical shift in nursing. *Advances in Nursing Science, 18* (1).

35

Future Directions for Rural Nursing Theory

Kathleen Ann Long

BACKGROUND

It is an interesting perspective indeed to look back on 20 years of rural nursing theory development in an effort to examine the processes, to evaluate the outcomes, and to project the future possibilities. An array of individuals and circumstances have been involved in shaping this theory of nursing as understood and practiced in sparsely populated areas. The chapter by Shannon (chapter 30) provides a context for understanding both the supportive structure and the impetus for rural nursing theory by detailing its tie to a faculty and a nursing education program.

The chapter by Long and Weinert (chapter 1), "Rural Nursing: Developing the Theory Base," has been widely quoted and referenced. It describes a ten-year process of generating ideas and frames of reference and the emergence of the beginning rudiments of a theory. What this chapter cannot capture, of course, is the lived experience of those ten years, which included a struggle to find *any* theory to guide faculty members and students in rural nursing education and practice. Review of the limited relevant literature produced through the late 1970s led to the conclusion that, in fact, there was no theoretical base for rural nursing. The creative process that followed was energizing and challenging. While centered at Montana State University, it was enriched by participants, consultants, and authors from many rural locations including Arizona, Colorado, the eastern shore of Maryland, Oregon, Mississippi, and Georgia. The fact that so many early participants had been, and often continued to be, rural residents and rural nurses, that is "old-timers" or "insiders," added an important component of realism to the academic endeavor of theory development. The early work groups, however, resisted the temptation to focus only on descriptions and anecdotes and instead developed concepts and basic premises, supported by data, and amenable to both conceptual and empirical analyses. This resulted in a beginning conceptual framework for rural nursing theory.

RURAL NURSING THEORY NOW

As this text so amply demonstrates, there is now a rich descriptive theory of rural nursing. Qualitative data from diverse rural populations have been collected and analyzed. The initially identified *key* concepts, such as isolation (chapter 5) and insider-outsider (chapters 10 and 11) have been thoroughly examined and analyzed. Significant progress has been made in clarifying and defining these concepts so that variables related to them can be identified and measured. Additional important concepts, such as familiarity (chapter 7) and hardiness, (chapter 20), have been described and their relevance in rural nursing theory examined. Populations and sub-populations of rural dwellers and rural nurses have been interviewed, described, and differentiated, and considerable work has been done in examining an important question underpinning the theory, namely, "What is rural?"

Rural nursing theory has developed from a series of personal descriptions and anecdotes to a coherent framework that is increasingly used in writing about, discussing, and researching rural health, rural health care, and the practice of rural nursing. Major questions remain regarding the viability of the theory. Are the topic broad and dense enough for the theory to be fully developed? What does a *rural* nursing theory add to, or how does it compliment, other broader nursing theories? How generalizable is the theory to the variety of rural populations? The idiosyncratic nature of much of what has been collected from and described about rural populations may not translate well across age, ethnic, or health status categories. Finally, the issue of the applicability of the theory to improving nursing practice must be addressed. Ultimately a nursing theory should be evaluated on its usefulness, not only as a framework for thinking, writing and studying problems but also as a mechanism for improving patient care.

THE NEXT STEPS IN THEORY DEVELOPMENT

Rural nursing theory can be advanced by a number of logical next steps. First, there needs to be a careful examination of and closure on a definition or definitions of "rural" as used in the theory. A theory of *rural* nursing will be limited to the extent that its most central concept remains vague, misunderstood, or variously defined. Considerable previous work (Elison, 1986; Hewitt, 1992) has addressed this definitional issue from both conceptual and practical perspectives. Weinert and Boik's "rurality index" (chapter 34) provides one example of an operational approach to the definition.

Population-based approaches will continue to be useful in helping researchers and clinicians understand types of rural settings, such as frontier verses rural/suburban. Individual studies will always require specific and relatively narrow definitions of rural. However the *theory* of rural nursing must capture the concept of rurality from a broad, inclusive, and yet consistent perspective. Rural nursing theory will be strengthened by greater attention to describing, specifying, and defining the sociocultural features that are both necessary and sufficient for the definition of a population as rural. While gradations and subcategories will inevitably be necessary in describing both population-based and socioculturally determined types of rural, specific parameters for these subcategories are necessary for testing rural theory and applying it across national and possibly international settings. In fact, the most important concept analysis in rural nursing theory may still remain to be done, that is, the analysis of rural itself.

With definitional clarity, the process of synthesizing rural nursing knowledge across rural settings that are geographically, economically, and culturally diverse can begin. Comparisons across rural settings are important, not only for enriching rural nursing theory but also for setting its boundaries and parameters. Differences of geography, climate, work patterns, traditions, beliefs, and social mores must be carefully examined to determine those characteristics that are an essential part of the term rural as used in the theory. Ultimately, a theory of rural nursing that fits well only within the mountain west of the United States is a theory destined to be of marginal significance.

Additional next steps to be taken include key concept comparisons, clarification of the unique aspects of rural nursing theory and their relationship to more global nursing theories, and the initiation of theory testing based on hypotheses that can be generated from existing data and premises. Each of these steps can be considered in light of the work already completed and summarized in this text, particularly in Parts II and III.

Several key theoretical concepts are described, analyzed, or compared in Part II of the text. A unique feature that emerges in the concept descriptions is the significance of the *perceptions* of rural people in ultimately defining the concept. This result speaks to the manner in which rural nursing theory was initially developed and is continuing to grow. A retroductive approach has been used, combining deductive and inductive reasoning. Rural respondents themselves have had a major role in informing the theoretical process. Thus Henson, Sadler, and Walton's (chapter 4) analysis of the concept of distance includes thoughtful consideration of data indicating how rural dwellers themselves view distance, and the ways in which life in rural areas colors and influences the meaning of distance. Similarly, Chafey, Sullivan, and Shannon (chapter 13) describe and analyze self-reliance primarily from the perspective of rural women. The incorporation of data not simply *about* but actually *from* rural residents is significant in the development of rich and realistic concept descriptions. The notion, for example, that spaces of several hundred miles are not considered distance by many rural dwellers captures an important frame of reference and typifies the unique concept definitions that are a part of rural nursing theory.

The concept definitions of outsider/insider and newcomer/old-timer by Caniparoli, Sutermaster, Myers, and Bailey (chapters 8 through 11) followed by concept comparison by the working group of the Rural Nursing Theory Special Committee (chapter 12) focus on describing how individuals fit within a rural community. The identified differences and similarities in these concept pairs are important in understanding individuals and groups in rural settings. Long time residents can, for example, still be community outsiders, and clarifications such as this have real significance for theory development, research definitions, and practice in rural areas. Comparisons are useful in moving the concepts of rural nursing theory from isolated pieces to more coherent and meaningful parts of an emerging puzzle. More concept comparisons are needed, and the analysis of relationships among selected concept groups such as isolation/distance/self-reliance, and familiarity/lack of anonymity/generalist could prove to be particularly meaningful.

Further development of rural nursing theory will also require that the unique features of this theoretical approach to nursing be more clearly identified and the interrelationships of this theory with broader nursing theories be articulated. The uniqueness of rural theory has begun to be addressed in this text. Certain concepts are clearly more important in rural nursing theory than in global nursing theories, and some concepts have significantly unique definitions. There is now evidence that nursing care for rural persons can be improved by the application of both theoretical constructs and research findings derived from rural nursing theory. Thus, there is certainly justification for the maintenance and enhancement of this distinct theoretical approach.

The theoretical base in rural nursing must move beyond simply focusing on the unique aspects of rural nursing in various settings and situations. Further work needs to clarify that which is common across all rural nursing and not situation specific. Integrating rural nursing theory with the larger body of nursing theory will also be important. The potential fit of rural nursing theory with major theories such as those of Orem (1991), Roy (1989), or Watson (1988) should be considered. Further, rural nursing theory should now be reconnected with knowledge from a variety of other health related fields. Just as rural nursing practice must be coordinated with multiple disciplines, the knowledge base should also be integrated. Rural nursing theory has developed to a point where it can contribute to interdisciplinary knowledge and practice. One clear example is the generalist orientation to health care that has been a hallmark of rural nursing and is now valued by a variety of health care provider and financing systems. Scharff (chapter 2) describes this broad, adaptable approach and focuses on the distinctiveness of rural nursing. The next step may well be the theoretical and practical translation of this knowledge so that it can become more useful to a variety of disciplines.

THEORY READY FOR TESTING

A theory is only an intellectual artifact unless hypotheses can be generated from it and then tested to determine fit with reality. Aspects of rural nursing theory appear ready for such testing. Several chapters in the text provide examples of data sets and theoretical constructs that could yield testable hypotheses. Koehler's (chapter 19) work provides a framework for understanding the variable of protecting independence which appears closely related to the previously identified rural nursing variable of self-reliance. Koehler's qualitative work describes health maintenance strategies used by rural elders to achieve the goal of independent living. Specific hypotheses could be developed to test predicted outcomes about the types of health promotion and health maintenance services that rural elders will use based on their desire to protect independence. Health status outcomes of such uses can be measured. In this way, rural nursing theory can be moved from descriptive to predictive, and applications for rural nursing practice can emerge.

The text contains several other good examples of theory that is ripe for testing. Beuhler, Malone, and Majerus (chapter 24) provide a well-organized framework for understanding how rural persons determine the severity of their symptoms and what circumstances prompt them to seek health care. Their qualitative study was limited to specific rural subgroups and, therefore, needs to be replicated with many other rural populations. In addition, however, hypotheses can be generated for the subgroups studied, namely rural Caucasian and Native American women. Specific questions about how and when these women will seek health care for themselves and their family members should now be addressed prospectively. This type of theory testing will allow for the expansion of theoretical knowledge, the examination of the validity of the original premises, and consideration of the theory's usefulness in guiding practice.

Another example of work that should be further developed is the study that focuses on factors related to the retention of nurses in rural hospitals. The theoretical links are not yet fully developed, but the authors, Derwinski-robinson, Lee, Ballantyne, and Scharff (chapter 33), introduce the idea that the insider/outsider concept may be relevant in retention of nursing and other health care professionals. Interesting theoretical questions can be derived and examined regarding the similarities and differences in the insider/outsider concept as applied to rural people in patient verses provider roles. Further, the descriptive research completed thus far can and should be expanded to examine strategies for both recruiting and retaining rural health care professionals in a variety of health care settings. The insider/outsider framework could be used to generate relatively low cost interpersonal strategies that enhance recruitment or retention, and these strategies could be applied and evaluated.

APPLICATIONS OF THEORY

While rural nursing theory is clearly still a work in progress, much of what has been learned to date can be applied, albeit with caution, in nursing practice. The text contains several good examples of work that can help nurses, and all health care providers, in understanding rural patients and in assessing their health status and health care needs. For example, the chapters on health (Running; chapter 18), independence (Koehler; chapter 19), and hardiness (Wirtz, Lee, & Running; chapter 20) provide a remarkably rich data base for understanding rural elderly clients, ranging from the "young old" (age 50 and over) to those well into their 80s and 90s. The combined studies in these three chapters clarify and reinforce several characteristics that are relevant for health care delivery. The self-reliance and hardiness of older rural dwelling adults become apparent through the studies, as does their desire to maintain privacy and a sense of control over their own lives. What is available in these chapters, and other work like them, is an important frame of reference that can guide clinicians in understanding how older rural patients are likely to express and manage both states of health and episodes of illness. A few implications for practice are addressed briefly by Running (chapter 18) and Koehler (chapter 19). However, actual applications in terms of specific interventions for individuals or unique community-based health care programs remain to be further developed.

In addition to understanding rural patients and rural populations overall, the work completed to date in rural nursing theory provides valuable information about how to organize nursing practice and deliver health care in rural areas. Scharff's (chapter 2) work is a thorough and clear discussion of the distinctiveness of rural nursing. It provides a framework that those in rural practice can use to understand the circumstances, challenges, and opportunities of their work environment, and it could be used effectively to orient those who plan to enter a rural practice setting. It can guide established and new rural nurses in analyzing work-setting constraints and developing effective approaches for addressing them.

Hovey and Doll's work (chapter 25) is a good example of how basic concepts and premises for rural nursing theory can be used to improve practice in a specific nursing role. Shreffler's (chapter 32) analysis of professional isolation has clear implications for the organization of rural nursing practice. The antecedents and consequences of professional isolation are identified, and the significance of this concept in rural practice is explicated by model cases. The need for organizing practice in ways that can lessen professional isolation is made clear.

Ballantyne's (chapter 14) analysis of health resources for rural clients is a complement to Shreffler's (chapter 32) work and shows a kind of isolation experienced by seriously ill persons and their families in rural areas. While specific implications for practice are not developed in the chapter, they can readily be derived from the work. The importance, for rural nurses and rural patients, of developing strategies and networks for accessing supportive resources is made evident. The need to develop nursing care systems that can link patients with both local and distant resources is exemplified.

A final example of theoretical work that can and should guide the organization of rural practice is found the concept work by Turnbull (chapters 15) and Grossman and McNerney (chapter 16). Lay and informal networks are analyzed, and their significance in rural health care delivery is identified. The importance of linking formal and informal health care resources is apparent, and implications can and should be derived for the ways in which rural nurses can most effectively organize and deliver care.

THEORY AND RESEARCH TO EXPAND PRACTICE

Some of the rural nursing theory work completed to date does not simply *apply* to rural practice but actually expands or stretches the understanding of that practice. Buehler, Malone and Majerus's work (chapter 24) on a symptom-action-time-line provides a new conceptualization and helps the reader understand how important self-diagnosis is in determining the health and well-being of rural dwellers. The nursing role in using this symptom-action-time-time to predict patient behavior should be further developed through specific applications and evaluations, as well as through broader studies with multiple rural subpopulations. The potential benefits for both patient health and cost-savings for the health care system are substantial.

Buehler's (chapter 26) work on containing disruption provides an insightful critique, showing the subtle ways in which nurses can become agents rather than patient advocates of a health care system. This study and its findings have relevance beyond rural practice to the socialization and resocialization of nurses in all settings. Wenger's (chapter 27) work expands the understanding of both homelessness and rurality and the implications of these circumstances for health status and health care delivery. By examining the role of students and faculty members in addressing preventive health care for rural homeless clients, Wenger's work offers new insights about concepts such as hardiness and provider distrust. Similarly, Ballantyne and Buehler's (chapter 28) descriptions of health care for HIV-infected men in rural areas dismantle old stereotypes of rural practice that might have led providers to imagine a more idyllic setting, where problems such as AIDS and drug abuse are relatively nonexistent. Instead the reader is challenged actually to see and understand the plight of HIV-infected men from their own perspective and to realize the stigma and lack of care that characterize many rural settings.

Each of these expanding works is a meaningful starting point for changes in practice that can and should be made. Rural nursing theory provided a framework for the analyses and research conducted thus far and can be a mechanism for continuing theoretical and empirical work.

LOOKING FORWARD

Rural nursing theory was born of a desire to prepare graduate level nursing students with the knowledge, skills, and abilities necessary to understand and care for people in a sparsely populated state. Its development included a truly shared process that engaged nationally prominent scholars, practicing rural nurses, rural dwellers, and students. This text is, in a sense, a tribute to these individuals and a significant milestone in the development of a knowledge base to inform health care practice in rural areas.

There are significant challenges ahead. The existing set of concepts and premises needs to be assembled into a coherent theory. Descriptive research needs to be expanded to explanatory work. Research focused on specific rural populations must be replicated across geographic settings and cultural boundaries. The *nursing* aspect of rural nursing theory needs to be both connected with the theory base of nursing in general and expanded to become a useful framework for interdisciplinary work. Most importantly, the *theory* aspect of rural nursing theory needs to be further translated, applied, and tested, with the goal being improved rural nursing practice. Fortunately the characteristics often associated with rural people in general—hardiness, self-reliance, devotion to work—are seemingly characteristics of rural nursing theorists, scientists, and clinicians, as well. This bodes well for the future of rural nursing!

REFERENCES

Elison, G. (1986). Frontier areas: Problems for the delivery of health care services. *Rural Health Care, 8* (5), 1–3.

Hewitt, M. (1992). Defining "rural" areas: Impact on health care policy and research. In W.M. Gesler & T.C. Ricketts (Eds.). *Health in Rural North America: The geography of health care services and delivery* (pp. 25–54). New Brunswick, CN: Rutgers Univ. Press.

Orem, D.E. (1991). *Nursing Concepts of Practice.* St. Louis: Mosby.

Roy, C. (1989). An explication of the philosophical assumptions of the Roy Adaptation Model. *Nursing Science Quarterly, 2* (3), pp. 26–34.

Watson, J. (1988). *Nursing: Human science and human caring.* New York: National League for Nursing.

INDEX